Dedication

This book is dedicated to my husband Jim, for his ceaseless love and support; and to our daughter Alex who makes us proud every single day.

Mary Lynn McPherson

Demystifying Opioid Conversion Calculations

A Guide for Effective Dosing

Mary Lynn McPherson, Pharm.D., BCPS, CPE
Professor and Vice Chair
Department of Pharmacy Practice and Science
University of Maryland School of Pharmacy
Adjunct Professor
University of Maryland School of Nursing
Hospice and Ambulatory Care Pharmacist
Baltimore, Maryland

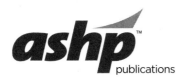

ashp™
publications

Any correspondence regarding this publication should be sent to the publisher, American Society of Health-System Pharmacists, 7272 Wisconsin Avenue, Bethesda, MD 20814, attention: Special Publishing.

The information presented herein reflects the opinions of the contributors and advisors. It should not be interpreted as an official policy of ASHP or as an endorsement of any product.

Because of ongoing research and improvements in technology, the information and its applications contained in this text are constantly evolving and are subject to the professional judgment and interpretation of the practitioner due to the uniqueness of a clinical situation. The editors, contributors, and ASHP have made reasonable efforts to ensure the accuracy and appropriateness of the information presented in this document. However, any user of this information is advised that the editors, contributors, advisors, and ASHP are not responsible for the continued currency of the information, for any errors or omissions, and/or for any consequences arising from the use of the information in the document in any and all practice settings. Any reader of this document is cautioned that ASHP makes no representation, guarantee, or warranty, express or implied, as to the accuracy and appropriateness of the information contained in this document and specifically disclaims any liability to any party for the accuracy and/or completeness of the material or for any damages arising out of the use or non-use of any of the information contained in this document.

Director, Special Publishing: Jack Bruggeman
Senior Editorial Project Manager: Dana Battaglia
Editorial Resources Manager: Bill Fogle
Design Manager: Carol A. Barrer
Cover and page design: DeVall Advertising

Library of Congress Cataloging-in-Publication Data

McPherson, Mary Lynn M.
 Demystifying opioid conversion calculations : a guide for effective dosing / Mary Lynn McPherson.
    p. ; cm.
 Includes bibliographical references and index.
 ISBN 978-1-58528-198-5
1. Opioids--Administration. 2. Pharmaceutical arithmetic. 3. Drugs--Dosage. 4. Drugs-
-Therapeutic equivalency. I. American Society of Health-System Pharmacists. II. Title.
 [DNLM: 1. Analgesics, Opioid--administration & dosage. 2. Analgesics, Opioid--thera-
peutic use. 3. Drug Dosage Calculations. QV 89 M478d 2009]
 RM328.M37 2009
 615'.7822--dc22
                                    2009027866

ASHP is a service mark of the American Society of Health-System Pharmacists, Inc.; registered in the U.S. Patent and Trademark Office.
ISBN: 978-1-58528-198-5
                                                    10 9 8 7 6 5

Foreword

"To boldly go where no man (nor woman) has gone before." With apologies to Star Trek fans everywhere, this book truly represents the definitive effort to explore the strange world of opioid conversions, to seek out new knowledge about these essential compounds, and to share this information with fellow pain clinicians. Dr. Mary Lynn McPherson takes the reader on the voyages and adventures of opioid conversions with the skill of an exceptionally brave commander.

It takes extreme courage to tackle this topic. Most of us who work in the field would enthusiastically agree to speak on any topic related to pain—with the exception of opioid conversions. This is the most complicated topic to share with others, in part because it entails equations and math. Nothing makes a trainee's eyes glaze over like numbers, particularly when the information does not seem relevant to practice.

Yet, the information provided in this outstanding text is not only relevant, it is critical to the safe and effective delivery of opioids. Every clinician who comes in contact with patients needs this information. And Dr. McPherson makes this journey uncomplicated and painless. The text is concise, practical, and grounded in the author's many years of clinical experience. The material is scholarly and well referenced, with clear tables and figures to illustrate key concepts. Practice problems with answers appear within each chapter to allow readers to test their newly acquired knowledge and skills. And yet, the tone is conversational with humor dispensed liberally throughout.

Dr. McPherson effortlessly transforms complex concepts into simple, practical solutions. Opioid conversions, routes of administration, the use of around-the-clock vs. prn dosing, and definitions regarding breakthrough pain are translated for new and experienced clinicians entering the world of pain management. Methadone, a complex but essential opioid, is described in detail, as well as delivery methods such as patient controlled analgesia, and epidural and intrathecal administration.

Very few have the credentials to undertake this mission. Mary Lynn McPherson, Pharm.D., BCPS, CPE, is a full professor at the University of Maryland School of Pharmacy and a well-known expert in the area of pain management and palliative care. She has lectured and published extensively on the topic of opioid therapy. In addition, Dr. McPherson has directed a pain management and palliative care residency for over a decade, and her remarkable teaching skills are evident throughout this text. Thanks to her knowledge and talent, opioid management is no longer an uncharted civilization. The final frontier has been conquered for all to go forth and put into practice.

Judith A. Paice, Ph.D., RN
Director, Cancer Pain Program
Division of Hematology-Oncology
Northwestern University; Feinberg School of Medicine
Past President, American Pain Society

Preface

Writing a book such as this one is like purposely walking around with a bull's eye painted on your forehead. If you ask five "experts" about a specific opioid conversion calculation, you'll probably get fifteen different answers! Even though this book deals with drug math, which usually means there is ONE correct answer, that's not always the case with conversion calculations. As a matter of fact, after spending a fair amount of time banging my head on the desk wrestling with the limited, yet frequently conflicting, information published on opioid conversion calculations, I decided there had to be a better way to consistently address these situations! So I went looking for a resource that pulled together all this information, only to find there was none! We have a handful of facts, a few more semi-solid facts, and a LOT of "that's what we've always done!" when it comes to opioid conversions.

What can we agree on? First, patients frequently need to switch from one opioid to another, from one route of administration to another, or from one dosage formulation to another. Second, the data used to generate opioid equivalency charts is often anecdotal, unidirectional, based on single dose studies, and without regard for patient variability. The last and most important thing we can agree on is the absolute need to carefully consider our calculations and interpret them with a big dose of common sense. Good pain management is a basic human right, but I believe "safety first" even supersedes that edict.

Another thing we can agree on is that this book will be an indispensable resource for a wide range of clinicians, particularly physicians, nurses, and pharmacists. This resource could easily become the new best friend of acute care practitioners (converting to various opioids and dosage formulations on admission and discharge), those caring for chronic non-cancer pain patients, and clinicians working in end of life care. Being able to accurately and safely convert among opioids is a mandatory competency for physicians and other prescribers, as well as nurses caring for patients with chronic non-cancer pain and pain from advanced illness, such as hospice and palliative care nurses. This text will also be very useful for students and residents in training. As a matter of fact, you could easily become known as a smarty-pants with this information under your belt!

In writing this book, no stone was left unturned in an attempt to find evidence-based information. Unfortunately there are still things we don't understand about the opioid conversion process, and the variability among human beings doesn't help either! After writing each chapter, it was shipped off to a highly-respected, spooky-smart cadre of practitioners to evaluate critically. Reviewers included nurses, nurse practitioners, physicians, and pharmacists. These practitioners were from practice areas ranging from acute care to home-based hospice, education, and research. Tough love is a beautiful thing, believe you me!

My vision for the book was for the reader to learn about a systematic process for these calculations that relies not only on available evidence, but also on a healthy dose of common sense. You will learn about a five-step process to perform opioid conversion calculations, first practicing on conversions between routes of administration and dosage formulations for the same opioid, then branching out to converting between various opioids and dosage formulations. You will learn how to titrate opioid dosages up and down (including magnitude of dosage change and timing), and how to calculate doses for rescue opioid therapy. Specific chapters devoted to calculations with fentanyl, methadone, high-tech parenteral infusions (including neuraxial) and oral solutions are included in this book. The text is written in an easy-to understand conversational tone, with numerous illustrated examples and practice problems. Just to keep you on your toes, you will encounter a variety of "pearls," "pitfalls," and "fast facts" as you journey through this book! I hope you find these tips useful and feel they can save you time, improve patient outcomes (safety and efficacy), and keep you from stepping into potholes others have probably encountered. Many of the reviewers read the pearls, pitfalls, and fast facts and commented "Oh, yes, I've been there before!" Here's a really important fast fact: even though this text is as evidence-based as possible, it is not a substitute for excellent clinical judgment!

Writing a book on drug math is a daunting prospect, and it couldn't be completed without the help of numerous people. Thanks to the administration and staff at the University of Maryland School of Pharmacy for encouraging me to indulge in this adventure. Special kudos to Barbara Hunter, who could find an article under a rock! Special thanks to Dana Battaglia, Rebecca Olson, and Bill Fogle at the American Society of Health-Systems Pharmacists for keeping me on track, and for their invaluable guidance and suggestions for strengthening this book.

I am eternally grateful to the aforementioned reviewers who gave of their time and talent to read and critique every chapter in the book. I am very fortunate to have had such a wide range of compassionate and gifted clinicians on board. Special thanks to Dr. D, my guardian angel! I am very appreciative of Dr. Judy Paice's very kind comments in the foreword to this book. Thanks to my family and friends for supporting me during the birthing of this book, despite their ponderings about my mental health (oh, no, not another book!).

Last, I would like to share any success this book may achieve with the clinicians I have worked with over the years, in doing a million or so opioid conversion calculations, and all the pharmacy students who have embraced this particular skill as an opportunity for pharmacists to shine. But most especially, I am humbled by the patients who have allowed me to share in their final journal, which may or may not have included the need for an opioid conversion calculation.

Mary Lynn McPherson
June, 2009

Contents

Dedication iii

Foreword v

Preface vii

Reviewers xi

2011 Update xiii

Chapter 1 1
Introduction to Opioid Conversion Calculations

Chapter 2 17
Converting Among Routes and Formulations of the Same Opioid

Chapter 3 41
Converting Among Routes and Formulations of Different Opioids

Chapter 4 57
Titrating Opioid Regimens: Around the Clock and to the Rescue!

Chapter 5 83
Transdermal and Parenteral Fentanyl Dosage Calculations
   and Conversions

Chapter 6 107
Methadone: A Complex and Challenging Analgesic, But It's Worth It!

Chapter 7 145
Patient-Controlled Analgesia and Neuraxial Opioid Therapy

Chapter 8 167
Calculating Doses from Oral Solutions and Suspensions

Glossary 183

Appendix 185

Index 191

Reviewers

Nancy A. Alvarez, Pharm.D., BCPS, FAPhA
Director, Medical Information
Medical Affairs Department
Endo Pharmaceuticals, Inc.
Chadds Ford, Pennsylvania

Kathleen Broglio, MN, ANP-BC, ACHPN, CPE
Nurse Practitioner Pain
Management
New York University School of
Medicine
Bellevue Hospital Center, Pain
Management Center
New York, New York

B. Eliot Cole, MD, MPA
Executive Director
American Society of Pain
Educators
Montclair, New Jersey

Constance Dahlin, ANP, BC, ACHPN, FPCN
Clinical Director
Palliative Care Service
Massachusetts General
Hospital
Boston, Massachusetts

Mellar P. Davis, MD, FCCP
Director, Palliative Medicine
Research
Palliative Medicine and
Supportive Oncology
Services
Division of Solid Tumor
Taussig Cancer Center
The Cleveland Clinic
Foundation
Cleveland, Ohio

Perry G. Fine, MD
Professor of Anesthesiology
Pain Research Center
School of Medicine
University of Utah
Salt Lake City, Utah

Phyllis Grauer, Pharm.D., CGP
Assistant Clinical Professor
College of Pharmacy
The Ohio State University
Columbus, Ohio

Holly M. Holmes, MD
Assistant Professor of
Medicine
The University of Texas M. D.
Anderson Cancer Center
Houston, Texas

Karen Snow Kaiser, Ph.D., RN-BC, CHPN, AOCN®
University of Maryland Medical
Center
Baltimore, Maryland

Kathleen N. Kappler BSN, CHPN
Liaison/Case Manager
Hospice of the Chesapeake
Annapolis, Maryland

Susan B. LeGrand MD, FACP
Section of Palliative Medicine
and Supportive Oncology
Solid Tumor Oncology
Taussig Cancer Institute
Cleveland Clinic
Cleveland, Ohio

Douglas Nee, Pharm.D., MS
President/Consultant
OptiMed, Inc.
San Diego, California

Annice O'Doherty, MS, BSN, CHPN
Case Manager
Hospice of the Chesapeake
Annapolis, Maryland

Patrice Roberts RN, OCN
Infusion RN
Sidney Kimmel Comprehensive
Cancer Center
Baltimore, Maryland

Laura Scarpaci, Pharm.D., BCPS
Manager, Clinical Performance
Improvement
excelleRx, Inc., an Omnicare
Company
Philadelphia, Pennsylvania

Scott A. Strassels, Pharm.D., Ph.D., BCPS
Assistant Professor, Division of
Pharmacy Practice
College of Pharmacy,
University of Texas at Austin
Adjunct Assistant Professor in
Public Health
University of Texas School
of Public Health, Austin
Regional Campus
Austin, Texas

Lynn V. Tieu, Pharm.D., BCPS, CPE
Department of Pharmacy
Union Memorial Hospital
Baltimore, Maryland

Kathryn A. Walker, Pharm.D., BCPS, CPE
Assistant Professor
University of Maryland School
of Pharmacy
Baltimore, Maryland

Douglas J. Weschules, Pharm.D., BCPS
Senior Medical Information
Scientist II
GlaxoSmithKline
Philadelphia, Pennsylvania

Suzanne B. Wortman, BS, Pharm.D., BCPS
DuBois Regional Medical
  Center
DuBois, Pennsylvania

Mark Yurkofsky, MD, CMD
Chief of Extended Care Facility
Home Visit and Palliative
  Medicine Programs
Harvard Vanguard Medical
  Associates
Medical Director, Seasons
  Hospice
Medical Director, Boston
  Center for Rehabilitative and
  Subacute Care
Instructor of Medicine, Harvard
  Medical School
Boston, Massachusetts

2011 Update to *Demystifying Opioid Conversion Calculations: A Guide for Effective Dosing*

Since the publication of this reference in August 2009, time has unsurprisingly marched on! During that time we have seen a new opioid come to market (tapentadol) as well as several new opioid formulations (refer to Table 1) that may influence our opioid conversion calculations! The purpose of this update is to provide a quick review of these developments for the reader.

New Opioid (Tapentadol)

Tapentadol (Nucynta) is a novel analgesic that is classified as having "opioidergic" and "monoaminergic" mechanisms of action. It acts as a mu-opioid receptor agonist and a norepinephrine reuptake inhibitor. It also weakly inhibits serotonin reuptake but to a clinically insufficient degree to contribute to pain relief.[1] Tapentadol is indicated for the relief of moderate to severe acute pain in patients 18 years of age or older.[2] At present, there are three immediate-release (IR) tablet formulations on the market in the United States: 50, 75, and 100 mg. While dosing should be individualized to meet specific patient needs, the appropriate dose is 50, 75, or 100 mg every 4 to 6 hours. On the first day of dosing, if the first dose does not adequately relieve the pain, a second dose may be administered as soon as one hour after the first dose. Total daily doses in excess of 700 mg the first day, or 600 mg on subsequent days have not been studied.

Unfortunately, there is no published data that can clearly guide us in converting between tapentadol and other opioids. Tapentadol is less potent than morphine; the prescribing information states it is 18 times less potent than morphine in binding to the human mu-opioid receptor and is 2–3 times less potent in producing analgesia in animal models.[2] Tapentadol has been shown to be superior to placebo, and has been compared to oxycodone in the management of both orthopedic surgical pain and musculoskeletal pain.[1] When dosed every 4 to 6 hours for orthopedic (bunionectomy) surgical pain, tapentadol 50 and 75 mg dose groups were found to be noninferior to the oxycodone 10 mg dose group. The tapentadol 100 mg dose group, but not the tapentadol 75 mg dose group, was found to be noninferior to the oxycodone 15 mg dose group. In a post-hoc exploratory analysis, the tapentadol 100 mg dose was found to be more effective than oxycodone 10 mg. In the management of moderate to severe pain associated with osteoarthritis of the knee, tapentadol 50 or 75 mg was found to be noninferior to oxycodone 10 mg in a ten-day treatment trial. In a 90-day treatment trial, tapentadol 50 or 100 mg and oxycodone 10 or 15 mg demonstrated similar analgesic effectiveness.[1]

It is important to recognize that demonstrating "noninferiority" does not constitute proof of equianalgesic dosing. A noninferiority clinical trial is somewhat one-sided by design: the purpose is to show that the new intervention (e.g., in this case, tapentadol) is "no worse" than a reference intervention (e.g., in this case, oxycodone) within a pre-specified noninferiority interval (in other words, the clinical response is

Table 1.

Opioid Formulations

Opioid	Oral Tablet or Capsule	Extended Release Tablet or Capsule	Oral Solution, Suspension or Elixir	Sublingual Tablet	Sublingual Film	Rectal Suppository	Injectable	Transdermal	Transmucosal	Intranasal
Buprenorphine				X	X		X	X		
Codeine	X		X				X			
Codeine plus non-opioid	X		X							
Fentanyl				X			X	X	X	X
Hydrocodone plus non-opioid	X		X							
Hydromorphone	X	X	X			X	X			
Methadone	X		X				X			
Morphine	X	X	X			X	X			
Oxycodone	X	X	X				X*			
Oxycodone plus non-opioid	X		X							
Oxymorphone	X	X					X			
Tramadol	X	X					X*			
Tapentadol	X	X								

*Not available in the U.S.

"close enough for government work" as the expression goes).[3] However, a noninferiority trial design is very useful when an untreated control group (such as untreated pain) is not pleasant or even ethical.

Based on these noninferiority trials, however, some healthcare systems have suggested the following therapeutic interchange when tapentadol is prescribed (and is nonformulary):

- tapentadol 50 mg po every 4–6 hours → oxycodone 5 mg po every 4–6 hours
- tapentadol 75 mg po every 4–6 hours → oxycodone 10 mg po every 4–6 hours
- tapentadol 100 mg po every 4–6 hours → oxycodone 15 mg po every 4–6 hours

Again, this guideline does not suggest equianalgesia either as shown or in reverse. Further research is necessary to determine more conclusive equianalgesia guidance with tapentadol.

An extended-release (ER) formulation of oral tapentadol (Nucynta ER) has recently been approved in the United States in several tablet strengths: 50 mg, 100 mg, 150 mg, 200 mg and 250 mg. The recommended starting dose in patients who are opioid-naïve is 50 mg every 12 hours. The conversion from immediate-release to extended-release tapentadol tablets is 1:1; the extended-release tablets are administered every 12 hours. The indication for tapentadol ER is for the management of moderate to severe chronic pain in adults when a continuous, around-the-clock opioid analgesic is needed for an extended period of time. Several clinical trials have been completed demonstrating efficacy of extended-release tapendatol in osteoarthritis, chronic low back pain, and diabetic neuropathy.[5] One clinical trial evaluated the conversion between tapentadol IR and ER for low back pain.[6] Patients were titrated to an effective level of pain control over a 3-week period using tapentadol IR. On day 22, half the group received their effective total daily dose of tapentadol as the IR formulation plus and ER placebo, and the other half received this dose of tapentadol as the ER formulation plus an IR placebo. The same exact dose was given whether the active treatment was given as tapentadol IR or ER (basically a 1:1 conversion). This continued for two weeks, and then the groups switched to the alternate strategy for an additional two weeks. Tapentadol ER was available as a 100, 150, 200, or 250 mg tablet, and dosed twice daily. Their conclusion was that approximately equivalent total daily doses of tapentadol IR and ER provided equivalent analgesia for the relief of moderate to severe chronic low back pain. Armed with this information you'll be able to convert patients from immediate-release to extended-release tapentadol with the greatest of ease!

New Opioid Delivery Systems

Transdermal Buprenorphine (Butrans)

Buprenorphine is a mu-opioid partial agonist used by the parenteral route of administration for moderate to severe acute pain and the oral route of administration to treat opioid addiction. It is now available in the United States as a new delivery system: transdermal buprenorphine (Butrans). Butrans is indicated for the management of moderate to severe chronic pain in patients requiring a continuous, around-the-clock opioid for an extended period of time.[7] Transdermal buprenorphine has been shown to be effective in treating a wide variety of moderately to severely painful conditions including chronic cancer and non-cancer pain, ischemic pain, osteoarthritis pain, and neuropathic pain.[8] Butrans is meant to be worn for 7 days, after which time a new transdermal patch should be applied to a different location (wait a minimum of 3 weeks before reapplying to the same site). Recommended application sites include the upper outer arm, upper chest, upper back or the side of the chest (eight possible application sites). This opioid delivery system is available in three strengths: 5 mcg/hour, 10 mcg/hour and 20 mcg/hour.

Butrans therapy may be initiated in opioid-naive patients with the 5 mcg/hour system. Because it takes three days to achieve steady-state serum levels of buprenorphine with the transdermal system, the dosage should not be increased for at least 72 hours, although many practitioners will wait a full week. The decision to move to the next higher Butrans strength should be based on the patient's need for supplemental short-acting opioid use and their level of pain control. The maximum dose of Butrans is 20 mcg/hour; higher doses (e.g., 40 mcg/hour) have resulted in prolongation of the QTc interval.

So what guidance do we have for switching an opioid-tolerant patient from their current opioid to Butrans? The manufacturer's guideline is as follows[7]:

- Oral morphine equivalent < 30 mg a day → Butrans 5 mcg/hour
- Oral morphine equivalent 30–80 mg a day → Butrans 10 mcg/hour

The prescribing information advises that there is a potential for buprenorphine to precipitate withdrawal in patients who are already on opioids. The manufacturer recommends tapering the patient's current around-the-clock opioid, for up to 7 days, to no more than the equivalent of 30 mg of oral morphine before switching to Butrans. It is unclear if the rationale is concern that buprenorphine theoretically has a greater affinity for mu-opioid receptors than other opioids such as morphine, or acknowledgement that the recommended conversion ratio is low. The prescribing information further recommends using caution when prescribing Butrans to opioid-tolerant patients receiving > 80 mg/day of morphine or its equivalent. The concern is that Butrans 20 mcg/hour may not provide adequate analgesia for patients receiving > 80 mg/day of oral morphine or an equivalent.

An equipotency ratio of oral morphine to transdermal buprenorphine of 1:75 has been proposed, however, in recent years some data have suggested the ratio may range from 1:70 to 1:100.[8-10] As a reminder, an equipotency ratio is defined as the ratio of the doses of two opioids required to achieve the same degree of analgesia. As discussed above, the oral morphine transdermal buprenorphine equipotent ratio that has been proposed is 1:75, explained by the following mathematical equation:

mg buprenorphine/day x 75 = mg oral morphine/day

For example, consider the Butrans 10 mcg/hour patch:

$$\frac{(\text{buprenorphine 10 mcg})}{\text{hr}} \times \frac{(24\ \text{hr})}{\text{day}} \times \frac{(1\ \text{mg})}{1000\ \text{mcg}} = 0.24\ \text{mg buprenorphine/day}$$

0.24 mg buprenorphine/day x 75 = 18 mg oral morphine/day

Sittl and colleagues calculated an equipotency ratio of oral morphine to transdermal buprenorphine by comparing "identical-cohort" groups of patients with cancer and non-cancer pain, using a drug utilization database.[10] Using this methodology, they determined an oral morphine to transdermal buprenorphine ratio of 1:110 or 1:115. However, remember that their methodology was to use retrospective data from "identical-cohort" groups, not a methodology where patients served as their own control.

Mercadente and colleagues evaluated the equianalgesic ratio between oral morphine and transdermal buprenorphine in cancer patients receiving oral morphine ranging from 120 to 240 mg a day.[9] Patients served as their own control, and were switched from oral morphine (patients had stable doses for at least 6 days) to transdermal buprenorphine using a 1:70 ratio. Pain levels were assessed on days 3 and 6 post-switch. This was a small study (four patients), but all patients maintained good control of their pain and other symptoms, and the only clinical difference in switching to transdermal buprenorphine was an improvement in constipation. Their conclusion was that the proposed conversion ratio from oral morphine to transdermal buprenorphine of 1:70 was appropriate.[9]

If we believe that the oral morphine : transdermal buprenorphine ratio is 1:70 as shown by Mercadente and colleagues, or if we accept Sittl and colleagues' conclusion that the ratio is 1:100 (or more), clearly the conversions recommended by the manufacturer of Butrans are low. Look at the following table:

Buprenorphine TD Dose (using 1:70 ratio)		Equipotent Oral Morphine Dose (mg)	Buprenorphine TD Dose (using 1:100 ratio)		Butrans Recommended Conversion (mcg/hour)
mcg/hour	mg/day		mcg/hour	mg/day	
17.9	0.43	30 mg	12.5	0.3	5
47.6	1.14	80 mg	33.3	0.8	10

For example, if a patient was receiving 30 mg/day of oral morphine, using the 1:70 ratio, it calculates to a hypothetical equivalent potency of 17.9 mcg/hour transdermal buprenorphine. Using the 1:100 ratio, it would be 12.5 mcg/hour transdermal buprenorphine. However, the manufacturer of Butrans, in this example, would recommend starting with the 5 mcg/hour transdermal system. Similarly, for total daily oral morphine doses up to 80 mg a day, the manufacturer of Butrans recommends starting with a 10 mcg/hour patch. However, the data that support a 1:70 ratio would suggest a 47.6 mcg/hour patch and the 1:100 ratio would suggest a 33.3 mcg/hour patch. The bottom line from all this is that we should follow the prescribing guidelines, but know that the recommended Butrans dosage conversion is very conservative, and an analgesic for breakthrough pain should also be prescribed simultaneously.

Mercadente also considered the conversion of patients receiving transdermal fentanyl (TDF) 50 to 100 mcg/hour to transdermal buprenorphine (TDB), using a transdermal fentanyl : transdermal buprenorphine ratio of 0.6 : 0.8.[9] Six patients receiving TDF for 6 or more days with stable pain control were switched to TDB as follows:

■ TDF 50 mcg/hour → TDB 70 mcg/hour

■ TDF 75 mcg/hour → TDB 105 mcg/hour

■ TDF 100 mcg/hour → TDB 140 mcg/hour

Pain and other symptoms were evaluated at days 3 and 6, and no significant changes were noted (except improvement in reported constipation with TDB). These findings are again considerably more aggressive that those from the manufacturer of Butrans.

The only other issue to consider is that of QTc prolongation associated with use of Butrans in excess of 20 mcg/hour. The risk associated with QTc prolongation is the development of torsades de pointes, a potentially fatal ventricular arrhythmia. According to the prescribing information, a Butrans dose of 40 mcg/hour (given as two 20 mcg/hour Butrans Transdermal Systems) prolonged the mean QTc by up to 9.2 ms across 13 assessment time points. For this reason, in the United States, Butrans is only approved for dosages up to 20 mcg/hour. However, higher concentration buprenorphine patches have been available in Europe for almost ten years (Transtec 35 mcg/hour, Transtec 52.5 mcg/hour and Transtec 70 mcg/hour).[11] According to the FDA document "Guidance for Industry: E14: Clinical evaluation of QT/QTc interval prolongation and proarrhythmic potential for non-antiarrhythmic drugs" the threshold level for regulatory concern "is around 5 ms as evidenced by an upper bound of the 95% confidence interval around the mean effect on QTc of 10 ms."[12] Prescribers should be mindful of the other risk factors for the development of torsades or prolongation of the QTc when using Butrans in their patients.

Transdermal Fentanyl (TDF) Formulations and Contemporary Issues

As discussed on page 84 of this book, TDF patches were designed to provide long-lasting opioid therapy to control stable, chronic pain of moderate to severe intensity. The majority of patients achieve pain relief for 72 hours after TDF patch application, while a small number of patients seem to require changing to a new patch(es) after 48 hours. Notwithstanding, practitioners continue to inappropriately use TDF in practice. The most common errors are use of TDF for acute pain management, or for intermittent or mild pain. Probably even more common (and inappropriate) is the use of TDF for patients who are not considered to be "opioid tolerant." This is defined as a patient who has been taking, for a week or longer, at least 60 mg of oral morphine, 30 mg of oral oxycodone, 8 mg of oral hydromorphone, or an equianalgesic dose of another opioid. It is imperative that prescribers follow these guidelines to avoid patient or prescriber harm (e.g., avoiding a lawsuit!).

As shown on page 85, the first TDF product on the market (Duragesic) was a gel-containing reservoir. There are now many generic formulations of TDF on the market, many of which use a different formulation known as the drug-in adhesive matrix layer formulation. The following is a depiction of a drug-in-matrix formulation of fentanyl[13]:

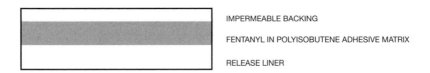

IMPERMEABLE BACKING

FENTANYL IN POLYISOBUTENE ADHESIVE MATRIX

RELEASE LINER

As you can see, the patch has three layers: a release liner, an adhesive drug formulation, and a backing film. This is the most common design for transdermal drug delivery and is often used with drugs that are relatively easy to deliver transdermally, such as fentanyl.[14]

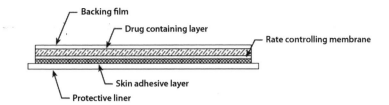

Backing film

Drug containing layer

Rate controlling membrane

Skin adhesive layer

Protective liner

Another transdermal fentanyl formulation was approved in 2011, described as a rate-controlling membrane, or a "matrix-membrane" patch. This system contains a protective liner and four function layers: a backing film, a drug containing layer, a rate-controlling membrane, and a silicone adhesive (see depiction).[15]

The reservoir and matrix transdermal fentanyl products are bioequivalent (i.e., interchangeable) and produce similar therapeutic outcomes.[16]

Rapid-Acting Fentanyl Products

In Chapter 4 of this book, you will learn about the management of breakthrough pain, which is defined as a transitory flare of pain that occurs against a background of otherwise controlled pain.[17] Breakthrough pain can further be characterized as spontaneous (no precipitating stimulus identified), volitional incident pain (an identified cause that is under the patient's control), nonvolitional incident pain (an identified cause that the patient cannot control), and end-of-dose failure from a long-acting opioid. For breakthrough pain that is fairly slow in evolution (e.g., 30 minutes from start to peak), or volitional incident pain, we can use traditional opioids as oral solution (e.g., oral morphine or oxycodone solution) or oral tablets. However, for idiopathic or quickly evolving breakthrough pain, or nonvolitional incident pain, we may need to consider a more rapid-acting opioid. In Chapter 4, we discuss two oral transmucosal fentanyl products that were available at the time of the original writing: oral transmucosal fentanyl citrate lozenge (OTFC, ACTIQ, generic) and fentanyl buccal tablet (Fentora). Since the original writing, three new rapid-acting fentanyl products have been approved by the FDA: Onsolis (fentanyl buccal soluble film), Abstral (fentanyl sublingual tablet), and Lazanda (fentanyl nasal spray). Just like the OTFC and buccal tablet, all three of the newer products are ONLY approved to treat breakthrough pain in patients with cancer who are 18 years and older and who are opioid tolerant. Opioid tolerance for all three products is defined as a patient taking at least one of the following for a week or longer:

- 60 mg of oral morphine per day
- 25 mcg/hr of TDF
- 30 mg of oral oxycodone per day
- 8 mg of oral hydromorphone per day
- 25 mg of oral oxymorphone per day
- or an equianalgesic dose of another opioid

These three products (like the previously approved other two) are not approved for acute or postoperative pain. Also, similar to the first two products, there is no approved dosing strategy for converting to these three new products from other opioids; practitioners must start with the lowest dose and follow the approved titration schedule. Let's take a closer look at the particulars for these three delivery systems.

Fentanyl Buccal Soluble Film (Onsolis)[18]

Initial dose and titration instructions	■ For opioid-tolerant patients ONLY (patients taking at least 60 mg of oral morphine/day, 25 mcg/hr of TDF, 30 mg of oral oxycodone daily, 8 mg of oral hydromorphone daily, 25 mg oral oxymorphone per day, or an equianalgesic dose of another opioid for a week or longer).
	■ Initial dose of Onsolis is 200 mcg in all patients (even when switching from a different transmucosal fentanyl product).
	■ Use the tongue to wet the inside of the cheek or rinse the mouth with water. Using a dry finger with the pink side facing up, place the pink side of the Onsolis film against the inside of the cheek, press and hold in place for 5 seconds.
	■ Single doses should be separated by at least two hours; Onsolis can only be used *once per episode of breakthrough cancer pain*. Onsolis cannot be re-dosed within an episode of breakthrough pain.
Initial dose and titration instructions	■ If adequate pain relief is not achieved after one 200 mcg Onsolis film, titrate using multiples of the 200 mcg Onsolis film (for doses of 400, 600, or 800 mcg) in subsequent breakthrough pain episodes.
	■ When multiple 200 mcg films are used, do not place them on top of each other; they may be placed on both sides of the mouth.
	■ If adequate pain relief is not achieved after 800 mcg Onsolis (four of the 200 mcg Onsolis films simultaneously), treat the next episode of breakthrough pain with one 1200 mcg Onsolis film. Doses above 1200 mcg have not been evaluated.
	■ Once adequate pain relief is achieved with a dose between 200 and 800 mcg Onsolis, the patient should receive the appropriate dose using ONE Onsolis film (e.g., 200, 400, 600, 800, or 1200 mcg Onsolis film: one per episode).
Maintenance dosing	■ Once a successful dose of Onsolis has been identified, each episode of breakthrough pain should be treated with a single film.
	■ During any episode of breakthrough pain, if adequate pain relief is not achieved within 30 minutes, the patient may use a different rescue medication as directed (e.g., a different short-acting opioid).
	■ Onsolis should be limited to four or fewer doses per day; if this is insufficient then consider increasing the around-the-clock opioid prescribed.

Fentanyl Sublingual Tablet (Abstral)[19]

Initial dose and titration instructions	■ For opioid-tolerant patients ONLY (patients taking at least 60 mg of oral morphine/day, 25 mcg/hr of TDF, 30 mg of oral oxycodone daily, 8 mg of oral hydromorphone daily, 25 mg oral oxymorphone per day, or an equianalgesic dose of another opioid for a week or longer).
	■ Initial dose of Abstral is 100 mcg in all patients (even when switching from a different transmucosal fentanyl product).
	■ Place the Abstral tablet on the floor of the mouth directly under the tongue immediately after removal from the blister unit. Allow the tablet to completely dissolve in the sublingual cavity. Do not drink or eat anything until the tablet is dissolved.

Fentanyl Sublingual Tablet (Abstral)[19] (contd.)

Initial dose and titration instructions	■ If breakthrough pain is not relieved within 30 minutes of the first dose, one additional 100 mcg ABSRAL tablet may be administered.
	■ No more than two doses of Abstral may be used to treat an episode of breakthrough pain.
	■ Patients must wait at least 2 hours before treating another episode of breakthrough pain with Abstral.
	■ If the 100 mcg dose was insufficient to treat the episode of breakthrough pain, increase the dose by 100 mcg multiples up to 400 mcg as needed. If adequate analgesia is not achieved with a 400 mcg dose, the next titration step is 600 mcg, then 800 mcg. Doses above 800 mcg have not been evaluated.
Maintenance dosing	■ Once an appropriate dose for treating an episode of breakthrough pain has been established, instruct patients to use only one Abstral tablet of the appropriate strength.
	■ No more than two doses of Abstral may be used to treat an episode of breakthrough pain.
	■ If more than four episodes of breakthrough pain are experienced per day then consider increasing the around-the-clock opioid prescribed.
	■ Limit the use of Abstral to treat four or fewer episodes of breakthrough pain per day.

Fentanyl Nasal Spray (Lazanda)[20]

Initial dose and titration instructions	■ For opioid-tolerant patients ONLY (patients taking at least 60 mg of oral morphine/day, 25 mcg/hr of TDF, 30 mg of oral oxycodone daily, 8 mg of oral hydromorphone daily, 25 mg oral oxymorphone per day, or an equianalgesic dose of another opioid for a week or longer).
	■ Initial dose of Lazanda is a 100 mcg spray in all patients (even when switching from a different transmucosal fentanyl product). This refers to one spray in one nostril.
	■ Instruct the patient to prime the device before use by spraying into the included carbon-lined pouch (4 sprays in total). Patients should insert the nozzle of the Lazanda bottle a short distance (1/2-1 cm) into the nose and point towards the bridge of the nose, tilting the bottle slightly. They then press down firmly on the finger grips until patient hears a "click" and the number in the counting window advances by one.
	■ Single doses should be separated by at least two hours; Lazanda can only be used *once per episode of breakthrough cancer pain*. Lazanda cannot be re-dosed within an episode of breakthrough pain.

Fentanyl Nasal Spray (Lazanda)[19] (contd.)

Initial dose and titration instructions	■ If adequate analgesia is not achieved with the first 100 mcg dose, dose escalate in a step-wise manner over consecutive episodes of breakthrough pain until adequate analgesia is achieved as follows: • Lazanda 100 mcg (1 x 100 mcg spray) • Lazanda 200 mcg (2 x 100 mcg sprays; 1 in each nostril) • Lazanda 400 mg (1 x 400 mcg spray) • Lazanda 800 mcg (2 x 400 mcg sprays; 1 in each nostril) • Doses higher than 800 mcg have not been evaluated.
Maintenance dosing	■ Once an appropriate dose for treating an episode of breakthrough pain has been established, instruct patients to use that dose for subsequent breakthrough cancer pain episodes.
Maintenance dosing	■ During any episode of breakthrough pain, if adequate pain relief is not achieved within 30 minutes following Lazanda dosing or if a separate episode of breakthrough cancer pain occurs before the next dose of Lazanda is permitted (e.g., within 2 hours), the patient may use a different rescue medication as directed (e.g., a different short-acting opioid). ■ Limit the use of Lazanda to treat four or fewer episodes of breakthrough pain per day. ■ If more than four episodes of breakthrough pain are experienced per day, re-evaluate the dose of the long-acting opioid used for persistent underlying cancer pain.

Extended-Release (ER) Hydromorphone (Exalgo)

Exalgo is a once-daily, ER oral tablet available as 8, 12, or 16 mg. It is indicated for the management of moderate to severe pain in opioid tolerant patients who require continuous, around-the clock analgesia for an extended time period.[21] A similar definition of "opioid tolerance" is described in the prescribing information for Exalgo: a patient taking 60 mg oral morphine/day, 25 mcg/hr TDF, 30 mg oral oxycodone/day, 8 mg oral hydromorphone/day, 25 mg oral oxymorphone/day, or an equianalgesic dose of another opioid, for a week or longer. This opioid formulation has been shown to be efficacious in a variety of cancer and non-cancer pain states, including osteoarthritis and low back pain, and comparable to ER oxycodone in treating osteoarthritis pain.[22] Exalgo is not approved for the management of acute or postoperative pain, intermittent pain, or for "as needed" use (i.e., breakthrough pain).

When converting from unmodified IR hydromorphone to Exalgo, determine the total daily dose of the IR hydromorphone and switch to an equivalent total daily dose of Exalgo (as described in Chapter 2). The absolute bioavailability of IR hydromorphone and Exalgo (compared to IV hydromorphone) is 19% ± 5%, and 24% ± 6%, respectively.[22] With single doses of Exalgo, the median Tmax ranges from 12 to 16 hours and the mean half-life is approximately 11 hours (range from 8 to 15 hours).[21] Steady-state plasma concentrations are reached after 3 to 4 days of once-daily dosing with Exalgo. Therefore, when switching to Exalgo, the dose should not be adjusted before 3 days of continuous therapy. It would be reasonable to provide IR hydromorphone for breakthrough pain, dosed as 10% to 15% of the total daily long-acting hydromorphone (Exalgo).

Converting from other opioids to Exalgo is just as described in Chapter 3. Data evaluating the conversion of patients from oral morphine to Exalgo confirm the conversion ratio shown in the Equianalgesic Opioid Dosing table provided with this book (and shown below in Table 2). In a study by Wallace et al., 336 patients were enrolled in a conversion trial, using an oral morphine:hydromorphone (Exalgo) ratio of 5:1.[23] Two hundred twenty two patients completed the trial, and the investigators did not reduce the calculated dose of hydromorphone to allow for cross tolerance. Dosage adjustments (titrating up to achieve maximal pain relief) were allowed, and 87% of patients required two or fewer dosage increases. The conclusion was the 5:1 ratio was safe and effective when converting from morphine to Exalgo. This is further consistent with the footnote of the Equianalgesic Opioid Dosing table in this book that states the morphine:hydromorphone conversion is not bidirectional; when switching from morphine to hydromorphone the ratio is 5:1 (M:HM), whereas the conversion from hydromorphone to morphine is 3.7:1 (HM:M). Wallace et al. did not evaluate converting patients back from Exalgo to oral morphine.[23]

Wallace et al. also evaluated patients being switched from TDF to Exalgo.[23] They used a ratio of TDF 25 mcg/hr to Exalgo 8 mg orally daily. This is consistent with our discussion of converting to/from TDF in Chapter 5, where we see "every 2 mg oral morphine per day is approximately 1 mcg/hr TDF" (e.g., 50 mg per day oral morphine is approximately 25 mcg/hr TDF). We can use this approximation in the other direction as well, so TDF 25 mcg/hr is roughly equivalent to 50 mg oral morphine/day. Using the M:HM ratio of 5:1, this would be approximately 10 mg oral hydromorphone/day. It would be entirely reasonable to reduce the hydromorphone dose to 8 mg per day (and Exalgo is available as an 8 mg tablet). Patients in this group fared equally as well. The manufacturer's guidelines recommend starting Exalgo 18 hours after removal of the TDF.[21] This makes sense because 17 hours after removal of TDF, 50% of the fentanyl is eliminated from the body. If you begin Exalgo at that time, it takes about 12 hours to the maximum hydromorphone serum concentration, at which point 75% of the fentanyl has been eliminated from the body (see page 96). When switching from Exalgo to TDF, it would make sense to apply the TDF approximately 18–24 hours after the last dose of Exalgo If it takes 3–4 days to reach steady-state with Exalgo, the terminal half-life once at steady state is likely between 14–19 hours. Let's work through this: assume at time zero the patient takes one last dose of Exalgo. At hour 18, about 50% of the hydromorphone has been eliminated, and the transdermal fentanyl patch is applied. Over the next 12–16 hours the transdermal fentanyl patch is beginning to deliver therapeutic fentanyl serum concentrations. Eighteen hours after applying the transdermal fentanyl patch (36 hours after the last dose of Exalgo), the hydromorphone serum level has declined to about 25% of the steady state serum concentration. Of course it would be prudent to supply an IR opioid for breakthrough pain.

Abuse-Deterrent Opioid Formulations

In the United States, the abuse and misuse of opioids is as critical an issue as unresolved pain. One new tool to help limit the former while fighting the latter is the development of abuse-deterrent opioid formulations. Of course, it is impossible to guarantee that a tablet or capsule is "abuse proof," but even small steps in the right direction

Table 2.

Equianalgesic Opioid Dosing

Drug	Equianalgesic Doses (mg)		Formulation Comments
	Parenteral	Oral	
Morphine[a]	10	30	Available as short-acting tablets and capsules, and oral solution (including oral concentrate Roxanol, 100 mg/5 mL).
			Available as oral long-tablet tablets and capsules (MS Contin, Oramorph SR, Kadian, Embeda, Avinza, generic).
			Available as rectal suppositories (equivalent dosing to oral).
Buprenorphine[b]	0.3	0.4 (sl)	Available as sublingual (sl) tablets and injection.
			Transdermal 4- and 7-day patches available in Europe. Butrans 7-day patch available in the United States.
Codeine	100	200	Codeine is a prodrug, metabolized to morphine by the liver.
			Available as injectable, tablets and oral solution; most commonly administered in combination with acetaminophen (e.g., Tylenol #3).
Fentanyl[c]	0.1	NA	Available as injection, transmucosal, intranasal and transdermal. Refer to chapters 4 and 5 for further discussion of transmucosal/intranasal and transdermal dosing of fentanyl, respectively.
Hydrocodone[d]	NA	30	Only available as a combination product (e.g., hydrocodone plus acetaminophen or ibuprofen). Oral solution (Hycodan) contains hydrocodone and homatropine.
			Most commonly given in combination with acetaminophen (Lorcet, Lortab, Vicodin, others).
Hydromorphone[e]	1.5	7.5	Available as oral tablets, long-acting tablet (Exalgo), solution, injection and rectal suppository.
Meperidine	100	300	Available as tablets, syrup, oral solution and injection.
			Not recommended for routine clinical use.
Methadone[f]	See methadone chapter		Available as oral tablets and oral solution (including oral concentrate, 20 mg/1 mL).
			Dispersible tablet (40 mg) not used for chronic pain management (only for opioid treatment programs).

Table 2. (contd.)
Equianalgesic Opioid Dosing

Drug	Equianalgesic Doses (mg)		Formulation Comments
	Parenteral	**Oral**	
Oxymorphone[h]	1	10	Available as a short-acting tablet, oral long-acting tablet, and parenteral formulation.
Tramadol[i]	100	120	Available as a short-acting tablet, extended-release oral tablet, and injectable.
			Parenteral formulation is not available in the United States.

Note: Equianalgesic data presented in this table is that which is most commonly used by health care practitioners, but it is *approximate*. The clinician is urged to read the following caveats, along with the text, and use good clinical judgment at all times.

Data adapted from:

Carr DB, Jacox AK, Chapman CR, et al. Acute Pain Management: Operative or Medical Procedures and Trauma. Clinical Practice Guideline No. 1. AHCPR Pub. No. 92-0032. Rockville, MD: Agency for Health Care Policy and Research, Public Health Service, U.S. Department of Health and Human Services. Feb. 1992.

Jacox A, Carr DB, Payne R, et al. Management of Cancer Pain. Clinical Practice Guideline No. 9. AHCPR Publication No. 94-0592. Rockville, MD. Agency for Health Care Policy and Research, U.S. Department of Health and Human Services, Public Health Service, March 1994.

[a]With chronic morphine dosing, the average relative potency of intravenous (IV) or subcutaneous (SC) morphine to oral morphine is between 1:2 and 1:3 (e.g., 20-30 mg of morphine orally or sublingually is equianalgesic to 10 mg IV or SC). *(Kalso E, Vainio A. Morphine and oxycodone hydrochloride in the management of cancer pain. Clin Pharmacol Ther. 1990;47:639-646.)*

Oral:rectal bioavailability is considered to be approximately equivalent. *(Westerling D, et al. Absorption and bioavailability of rectally administered morphine in women. Eur J Clin Pharm. 1982;23(1):59-64. Brook-Williams P. Morphine suppositories for intractable pain. CMA J. 1982;126:14.)*

[b]Sublingual buprenorphine 0.4 mg has been shown to be equivalent to 0.3 mg buprenorphine given parenterally. *(Bullingham RES, et al. Sublingual buprenorphine used postoperatively: clinical observations and preliminary pharmacokinetic analysis. Br J Clin Pharma. 1981;12:117-122.)*

Buprenorphine 0.3 mg given intramuscularly (IM) has been shown to be equivalent to morphine 10 mg IM. *(Kjaer M, et al. A comparative study of intramuscular buprenorphine and morphine in the treatment of chronic pain of malignant origin. Br J Clin Pharmacol. 1982;13:487-492.)* Similar findings have been seen with IV doses of both opioids. *(Zacny J, et al. Comparing the subjective, psychomotor and physiological effects of intravenous buprenorphine and morphine in healthy volunteers. J Pharm and Exper Ther. 1997;282:1187-1197.)*

Buprenorphine is available as a 4- and 7-day transdermal patch in Europe. Butrans (a 7-day patch) is available in the United States. Both brands (Butrans and Transtec) recommend starting with the lowest strength patch (e.g., 5 mcg/hr in the United States) when switching to transdermal buprenorphine. In the reference *Palliative Drugs*, a conversion of 100:1 (morphine:buprenorphine) is suggested. Example: multiply 24-hour oral morphine dose in mg by 10 to obtain 24-hour buprenorphine dose in micrograms; divide answer by 24 to obtain mcg/hr patch strength; round down to closest patch strength. *(Palliative Drugs; www.palliativedrugs.com/opioid-dose-conversion-ratios.html, Accessed January 9, 2009).* The U.S. manufacturer of Butrans has a more conservative recommendation when switching to transdermal buprenorphine (see text).

[c]Although parenteral MS:fentanyl is shown as 10:0.1 mg (which is a 100:1 ratio) based on a mg-to-mg ratio, in clinical practice the ratio is described as 15-112.5:1; many clinicians use an equivalency of 4 mg/hr IV morphine equivalent to 100 mcg/hr parenteral or transdermal fentanyl. *(Indelicato RA, Portenoy RK. Opioid rotation in the management of refractory cancer pain. JCO 2003;21:87s-91s. Patanwala AE, Duby J, Waters D et al. Opioid conversions in acute care. Ann Pharmacother. 2007;41:255-67. Lawlor P, Pereira J, Bruera E. Dose ratios among different opioids: underlying issues and an update on the use of equianalgesic table. In: Bruera E, Portenoy RK, eds. Topics in Palliative Care, Volume 5. Oxford University Press, 2001. New York.)*

Transdermal fentanyl (TDF) patch (used for chronic pain) dosed in mcg, is roughly equivalent to 50% of the total daily dose of oral morphine in mg (e.g., TDF 25 mcg/hr patch is roughly equal to 50 oral morphine/day). Refer to Chapter 5 for additional information on dosing transdermal fentanyl. *(Breitbart W, Chandler S, Eagel B, et al. An alternative algorithm for dosing transdermal fentanyl for cancer-related pain. Oncology. 2000;14:695-705.)*

[d]Equivalence to oral morphine not clearly defined; generally thought to be equal to or less potent than oxycodone. *(Hallenbeck JL. Palliative Care Perspectives. New York: Oxford University Press; 2003:71).*

[e]Oral bioavailability may be as high as 60%, particularly with chronic dosing; ranges from 29% to 95%. *(Vallner JJ, et al. Pharmacokinetics and bioavailability of hydromorphone following intravenous and oral administration to human subjects. J Clin Pharmcol. 1981;21:152-156. Ritschel WA, et al. Absolute bioavailability of hydromorphone after peroral and rectal admin-*

Table 2. (contd.)
Equianalgesic Opioid Dosing

istration in humans: saliva/plasma ratio and clinical effects. J Clin Pharmacol 1987;27:647-653. Parab PV, et al. Pharmacokinetics of hydromorphone after intravenous, peroral and rectal administration to human subjects. Biopharm Drug Dispos. 1988;9:187-199).

Research has shown a lower dose ratio and a directional influence seen when converting between morphine and hydromorphone. It is suggested that when switching from morphine (M) to hydromorphone (HM) (using the same route of administration; e.g., SC to SC or oral to oral), a conversion ratio of 5:1 (M:HM) for morphine to hydromorphone and a dose ratio of 3.7:1 (M:HM) when switching from morphine to hydromorphone (again, using the same route of administration). *(Lawlor P, et al. Dose ratio between morphine and hydromorphone in patients with cancer pain: a retrospective study. Pain 1997;72:79-85. Anderson R, et al. Accuracy in equianalgesic dosing: conversion dilemmas. J Pain Symptom Manage 2001;21:397-406).*

Oral:rectal bioavailability approximately equal; the FDA-approved dosing interval for rectal hydromorphone is every 6 hours.

[f]Methadone dosing is highly variable, and conversion to/from other opioids is NOT linear. Refer to Chapter 6 for additional information on methadone dosing.

[g]Because of the variations in bioavailability between morphine (15% to 64%) and oxycodone (60% or more), the equianalgesic ratio for oral morphine:oxycodone ranges from 1:1 to 2:1, partially dependent on the patient's ability to absorb the opioid. A ratio of 1:1.5 is used clinically as a compromise. *(Anderson R, et al. Accuracy in equianalgesic dosing: conversion dilemmas. J Pain Symptom Manage. 2001;21:397-406).*

Parenteral oxycodone is not available in the United States. According to manufacturer's information (Mundipharma New Zealand Limited, Distributed by Pharmaco (N.Z.) Ltd,) 2 mg of oral oxycodone is approximately equivalent to 1 mg parenteral oxycodone. *(Medsafe: Information for Health Professionals, Oxynorm Injection. Available at: http://www.medsafe.govt.nz/profs/Datasheet/o/OxyNorminj.htm). Accessed January 8, 2009.* This ratio may be somewhat conservative because the oral bioavailability of oxycodone has been shown to be 60% or greater. *(Poyhia R, et al. The pharmacokinetics and metabolism of oxycodone after intramuscular and oral administration to healthy subjects. Br J Clin Pharmacol. 1992;33:617-621.).*

[h]Conversion from oral morphine or oral oxycodone to oxymorphone is shown as 30:10 and 20:10, respectively per package labeling. Some data suggests the conversion ratio when switching to oxymorphone is closer to 18:10 for morphine, and 12:10 for oxycodone, especially once at steady state. *(Sloan P, et al. Effectiveness and safety or oral extended-release oxymorphone for the treatment of cancer pain: a pilot study. Support Care Cancer. 2005;13:57-65.).*

[i]Parenteral tramadol has been shown to be approximately equipotent to parenteral morphine in a 10:1 (tramadol:morphine) ratio. *(Wilder-Smith C, et al. Effects of morphine and tramadol on somatic and visceral sensory function and gastrointestinal motility after abdominal surgery. Anesthesiology 1999;91:639-647).* With chronic dosing, oral tramadol achieves between 90% and 100% bioavailability. *(Grond S, et al. Clinical pharmacology of tramadol. Clin Pharmacokinet 2004;31:879-923.)* Despite bioavailability data, equipotent use of oral morphine and oral tramadol ranges from 1:4 to 1:10 (morphine:tramadol). Therefore, using an equivalence of 120 mg oral tramadol may be very conservative. *(Grond S, et al. High-dose tramadol in comparison to low-dose morphine for cancer pain relief. J Pain Symptom Manage 1999;18:174-179).*

are welcomed. There are several examples of opioids that have been reformulated or newly formulated for this purpose. By and large, these pharmaceutical changes do not influence our opioid conversion calculations. A few examples are as follows:

- OxyContin (ER oxycodone tablet) has been reformulated with the intent to prevent the tablets being cut, broken, chewed, crushed or dissolved in an attempt to release the opioid all at one time (as opposed to the intended 8-12 hour release time).[24]

- The long-acting capsule of Kadian (ER beads containing morphine in a capsule) have been reformulated as Embeda. With Embeda, the core of each bead contains naltrexone, an opioid antagonist. If the capsule or the beads are swallowed whole, the naltrexone has no pharmacologic effect. However, if the capsules or beads are crushed, cut or chewed, the naltrexone negates the effect of the morphine, both euphoric and analgesic. There are six strengths of this combination (20 mg/0.8 mg, 30 mg/1.2 mg, 50 mg/2 mg, 60 mg/2.4 mg, 80 mg/3.2 mg, and 100 mg/4 mg, morphine sulfate/naltrexone hydrochloride); however, as of this writing, EMBEDA is not available in the United States. It is anticipated that this is a temporary situation and it will be back on the market.[25]

- The FDA recently approved an IR oxycodone tablet (Oxecta), which is indicated for the management of acute and chronic pain of moderate to severe intensity.

Oxecta uses technology designed to discourage common methods of medication tampering. An added ingredient causes the oxycodone to gel, thus preventing injection, or to irritate the nasal passages to discourage inhalation.[26]

- Several other abuse-deterrent opioid formulations are in various stages of development and approval.

Lagniappe (A Small Gift or Unexpected Benefit)[27]

I frequently get calls from hospice and palliative care providers about patients with very difficult-to-control pain problems. In these cases, we occasionally use ketamine parenterally (either intravenous [IV] or subcutaneous [SC]), or the parenteral formulation of ketamine mixed in orange juice and given orally) to reduce hyperalgesia or opioid-induced neurotoxicity, usually with very good effect. Benitez-Rosario and colleagues evaluated a 1:1 conversion from to oral ketamine in cancer patients.[27] In a cohort of 29 cancer pain patients, after establishing good pain control with a continuous SC infusion of ketamine, the investigators calculated the total dose of ketamine administered subcutaneously. This total daily dose was divided into thirds and administered orally every 8 hours, using the parenteral formula mixed with fruit juice. The first oral ketamine dose was given 4 to 8 hours after the SC infusion was discontinued. After switching to oral ketamine, 27 of the 29 patients maintained good pain control; 2 patients required a dose increase (to a ratio of 1:1.3 and 1:1.5) to maintain analgesia. There were no additional adverse effects and, in fact fewer adverse effects were experienced when the patients were switched to oral ketamine.

While it is exciting that we are beginning to see data accumulate on the effective use of ketamine for difficult pain cases, it is still early days. Ketamine should not be used by the uninitiated or the faint of heart due to the need for close attention to detail in dosing, and monitoring. It is important to also point out that ketamine would likely only be initiated in an inpatient facility. But this piece of research is a welcomed addition, as we continue to explore the analgesic properties of ketamine.

Conclusion

Given the magnitude of the pain problem in the United States and worldwide, and the competing problem of opioid misuse and abuse, it is not unexpected that new analgesics and dosage formulations will continue to be introduced to the market. Well-designed clinical trials that help practitioners calculate safe and effective opioid doses when converting between drugs, routes of administration, and formulations are always welcomed.

References

1. Frampton JE. Tapentadol immediate release: A review of its use in the treatment of moderate to severe acute pain. *Drugs*. 2010;70(13):1719-1743.

2. Nucynta Prescribing Information. Available at: http://www.nucynta.com/sites/default/files/pdf/Nucynta-PI.pdf. June 30, 2011.

3. Gotzsche PC. Lessons from and cautions about noninferiority and equivalence randomized trials. *JAMA*. 2006;295(10):1172-1174.

4. EPG Online. Available at: http://www.epgonline.org/viewdrug.cfm/drugId/DR004554/search_text/tapentadol/search/drug/CurrentPage/1/language/LG0001/drugName/Palexia®-SR-100-mg-prolonged-release-tablets. Accessed June 30, 2011.

5. Johnson & Johnson. Available at: http://prod-web02.jnj.cl.datapipe.net/connect/NewsArchive/product-news-archive/20100204_090000. Accessed June 30, 2011.

6. Etropolski MS, Okamoto A, Shapiro DY, Rauschkolb C. Dose conversion between tapentadol immediate and extended release for low back pain. *Pain Physician.* 2010;13:61-70.

7. Butrans Prescribing Information. Available at: http://www.purduepharma.com/pi/prescription/ButransPI.pdf. Accessed July 1, 2011.

8. Hans G, Robert D. Transdermal buprenorphine: a critical appraisal of its role in pain management. *J Pain Res.* 2009;2:117-134.

9. Mercadente S, Casuccio A, Tirelli W, Ciarrantano A. Equipotent doses to switch from high doses of opioids to transdermal buprenorphine. *Support Care Cancer.* 2009;17:715-718.

10. Sittl R, Likar R, Nautrup BP. Equipotent doses of transdermal fentanyl and transdermal buprenorphine in patients with cancer and noncancer pain: results of a retrospective cohort study. *Clin Ther.* 2005;27:225-237.

11. Transtec transdermal patch. Drugs.com. Available at: http://www.drugs.com/uk/transtec-transdermal-patch-1358.html. Accessed July 4, 2011.

12. U.S. Department of Health and Human Services, Food and Drug Administration, Center for Drug Evaluation and Research (CDER), Center for Biologics Evaluation and Research (CBER), October 2005. Guidance for Industry: E14 Clinical Evaluation of QT/QTc Interval Prolongation and Proarrhythmic Potential for Non-Antiarrhythmic Drugs. Available at: http://www.fda.gov/downloads/RegulatoryInformation/Guidances/ucm129357.pdf. Accessed July 4, 2011.

13. U.S. National Library of Medicine, DailyMed. Fentanyl patch, extended release (TEVA Pharmaceuticals USA Inc.). Available at: http://dailymed.nlm.nih.gov/dailymed/drugInfo.cfm?id=12150. Accessed July 4, 2011.

14. Gordon RD. Backing films for transdermal and topical patches: more than pieces of plastic. *TransDermal.* 2010;2(2):13-23.

15. Fentanyl Transdermal System Prescribing Information. Available at: http://pharmaceuticals.covidien.com/imageServer.aspx/doc201802.pdf?contentID=18643&contenttype=application/pdf. Accessed July 24, 2011.

16. Freynhagen R, von Giesen JH, Busche P, Sabatowski R, Konrad C, Grond S. Switching from reservoir to matrix systems for the transdermal delivery of fentanyl: a prospective, multicenter pilot study in outpatients with chronic pain. *J Pain Symptom Manage.* 2005;30(3):286-297.

17. Portenoy RK, Hagen NA. Breakthrough pain: definition, prevalence and characteristics. *Pain.* 1990;41:273-281.

18. Onsolis (fentanyl buccal soluble film) Prescribing information. Available at: http://www.Onsolis.com/assets/downloads/Onsolis_pi.pdf. July 4, 2011.

19. Abstral (sublingual fentanyl tablets) Prescribing information. Available at: http://www.Abstral.com/pdfs/Abstral-PI-MedGuide.pdf. Accessed July 4, 2011.

20. Lazanda (fentanyl nasal spray) Prescribing information. Available at: http://www.lazanda.com/Lazanda_PI.pdf. Accessed July 4, 2011.

21. Exalgo (Hydromorphone HCl) Extended-Release Tablets Prescribing Information. Available at: http://www.exalgo.com/media/pdf/Exalgo_FullPrescribingInformation.pdf. Accessed July 4, 2011.

22. Guay DRP. Oral hydromorphone extended-release. *Consult Pharm.* 2010;25(12):816-828.

23. Wallace M, Rauck RL, Moulin D, Thipphawong J, Khanna S, Tudor IC. Once-daily OROS hydromorphone for the management of chronic nonmalignant pain: a dose-conversion and titration study. *Int J Clin Pract.* 2007;61(10):1671-1676.

24. FDA U.S. Food and Drug Administration. FDA approved new formulation for OxyContin. Available at: http://www.fda.gov/NewsEvents/Newsroom/PressAnnouncements/2010/ucm207480.htm. Accessed July 4, 2011.

25. EMBEDA Prescribing Information. Available at: http://www.kingpharm.com/products/product_document.cfm?brand_name=Embeda&product_specific_name=CII&document_type_code=PI. Accessed July 4, 2011.

26. Medscape. FDA approves tamper-resistant oxycodone. Available at: http://www.medscape.com/viewarticle/744935. Accessed July 4, 2011.

27. Benitez-Rosario MA, Salinas-Martin A, Gonzalez-Guillermo T, Feria M. A strategy for conversion from subcutaneous to oral ketamine in cancer pain patients: effect of a 1:1 ratio. *J Pain Symptom Manage.* 2011;41:1098-1105.

Introduction to Opioid Conversion Calculations

OBJECTIVES

After reading this chapter, the participant will be able to:

1. Identify common clinical scenarios that are appropriate for opioid conversion.

2. Compare and contrast the concepts of potency and equianalgesia.

3. Explain the principles used to develop an Equianalgesic Opioid Dosing Table, and describe the limitations of this tool.

4. Use a five-step process to switch a patient from one opioid to a different opioid.

INTRODUCTION

Consider these scenarios:

■ MJ is a 72 year old woman with breast cancer who has grown too weak to swallow her MS Contin tablets. How do you convert her to oral morphine solution? How often is it administered? What happens when she can't swallow the oral morphine solution?

■ WE is a 54 year old man with an end-stage malignancy referred to hospice with an implanted intrathecal pump, which is delivering 1 mg of morphine per day. The hospice nurse calls you and wants to know what would be an appropriate dose of oral morphine to give the patient for breakthrough pain?

■ SA is a 94 year old woman with end-stage dementia and severe osteoarthritis. She has been maintained on a transdermal fentanyl patch for the past year, but she now weighs 72 pounds and doesn't seem to be receiving the expected continued benefit. How do you convert her to oral oxycodone solution? When do you start the oral oxycodone solution relative to removing the transdermal fentanyl patch?

■ JR is a 68 year old man with prostate cancer with significant metastatic disease. He is referred to your outpatient palliative care clinic for a pain consult. He is receiving MS Contin 100 mg po q12h, hydromorphone 4 mg po q4h prn (using about 5 doses per day), a transdermal fentanyl patch 100 mcg every 3 days, and a morphine subcutaneous infusion at 1 mg/hour with 0.5 mg bolus (using about 12 per day). His physician asks your advice on converting all this to a simpler regimen, specifically using methadone. Where do you start?

Ah…drug math. Those two little words can make a strong health care professional clench their bowel and want their Mommy. But this doesn't have to be the case! Armed with an understanding of conversion calculations, some semi-solid facts about equivalencies, and a healthy sense of "does that LOOK right?" you'll be just fine! Just like much of health care, there is both science and art involved in performing opioid conversion calculations. This book is designed to teach you how to do opioid conversion calculations safely AND effectively. Jump in, the water's fine!

Opioids are the mainstay of pain management in patients with moderate to severe pain. Morphine is practically mother's milk to practitioners who work with patients with advanced illness due to its familiarity, availability of multiple dosage formulations, low cost, and proven effectiveness. However, morphine is not always the answer. For example, we know that up to 30% of cancer patients show poor responsiveness to a given opioid such as morphine during routine administration.[1] This is only one reason why health care practitioners must be able to transition patients from one opioid to another, which may require changing the route of administration and/or dosage formulation. A large recent multicenter study conducted with palliative care patients showed that 12% of patients required a change to a different opioid (not counting a change in route of administration) for reasons including lack of pain control (64%), development of adverse effects (51%), and medication application problems (22%).[2] Let's take a closer look at the clinical situations that result in the need to switch a patient from one opioid to another.

Reasons for Changing Opioids

Lack of Therapeutic Response

If the patient's pain is not responding adequately to the opioid, and a repeat assessment indicates that opioid therapy continues to remain appropriate, a dose increase would be the most likely intervention. The increase in pain may be due to disease progression, or the development of opioid analgesic tolerance. If the patient cannot tolerate an increase in dose due to the development of adverse effects, or an increase in dose does not produce a reduction in pain, switching to a different opioid may be beneficial.

Occasionally a patient is receiving a combination analgesic (e.g., Percocet, which contains oxycodone and acetaminophen), and an increase would exceed the maximum recommended daily dose of acetaminophen (4 grams). In this case, switching to a tablet or capsule containing just oxycodone would be appropriate, with subsequent dosage titration.

Development of Adverse Effects

If the patient develops an adverse effect to an opioid, the health care professional must consider plan B. Opioid-induced adverse effects are well-recognized and include:

- Gastrointestinal effects (nausea, vomiting, constipation)

- Autonomic (xerostomia, urinary retention, postural hypotension)

- Cutaneous (pruritus, sweating)
- Central nervous system (sedation, confusion, dizziness, hallucinations, delirium, myoclonus, hyperalgesia, seizures, and respiratory depression)
- Rarely, opioid allergy (rash, hives, difficulty breathing)

Faced with an opioid-induced adverse effect, management options include the following:

- Reduction of opioid dose if pain adequately controlled (monitor patient response carefully)
- Aggressive management of the opioid-induced toxicity
- Addition of a non-pharmacologic intervention or co-analgesic to allow reduction of the opioid dose
- Switch to a different route of administration to minimize adverse effect
- Switch to a different opioid which will hopefully be as or more effective and better tolerated

Change in Patient Status

As patients with advanced illness decline, they may not be able to tolerate their current opioid formulation or route of administration. For example, a patient may develop difficulty swallowing (dysphagia) or pain with swallowing (odynophagia). Although somewhat controversial, patients who are very cachectic or who have poor peripheral circulation may not receive the full expected benefit of a transdermally-delivered opioid. On the other hand, a transdermal patch may be more convenient for, and acceptable to the patient or family, and switching would enhance quality of life.

A patient may require a very high dose of an oral, rectal or transdermal opioid, necessitating a change to parenteral therapy. Conversely, a patient being discharged home who is able to swallow would likely prefer oral opioid therapy over parenteral.

Other Considerations

Availability of the opioid and/or particular formulation at the patient's pharmacy, and cost and formulary issues may influence prescribing. Also, patients, families and caregivers may hold health care beliefs about certain opioids that affect prescribing such as a previous bad experience with a particular opioid (e.g., severe nausea or vomiting), or a stigma associated with a particular opioid (e.g., "Isn't morphine just for dying patients?" or "Isn't methadone only used by drug addicts?").

Opioid Switching vs. Rotation

Historically, moving a patient from one opioid to a different opioid has been referred to as "**opioid rotation**." Other terms include "**opioid switching**" or "**opioid substitution**."[3] These terms are used interchangeably, although some practitioners use the term "opioid rotation" to describe one or sequential trials of opioid therapy to maximize analgesia while minimizing adverse effects. Regardless of the term that is used, getting the job done will require a calculation, hence the name of this book—**Opioid Conversion Calculations!**

Regardless of what we call it, the big question is, **DOES IT WORK?** A Cochrane review concluded "the effectiveness of opioid switching to manage pain relief inadequacies and intolerable side effects could not be assessed because of a lack of randomized controlled trials."[4] However, the case reports, retrospective studies and audits and prospective controlled trials considered in the Cochrane review generally showed positive results, with improvement in pain and adverse effects with opioid switching. A prospective trial published since the Cochrane review evaluated the benefits of switching from morphine to another opioid in 186 palliative care patients.[3] Forty-seven of the 186 patients were switched to a different opioid after experiencing inadequate pain relief or unacceptable morphine-related adverse effects. Of these, 37 (79%) achieved a good clinical outcome when switched to oxycodone.[3] Therefore, we can conclude that switching from one opioid to another is a valuable clinical exercise.

Equianalgesic Opioid Dosing

OK, so we want to switch from one opioid to another. How do we get from point A to point B? To understand that, we must first explore several definitions. **Opioid responsiveness** has been defined as "the degree of analgesia achieved as the dose is titrated to an endpoint defined either by intolerable side effects or the occurrence of acceptable analgesia."[5] Obviously, we want a high degree of opioid responsiveness so the patient can achieve pain relief. Can opioid responsiveness be determined solely by opioid potency? What the heck is potency?

Potency refers to the intensity of analgesic effect for a given dose, and is dependent on access to the opioid receptor and binding affinity (or "fit") at the receptor site.[6] Several **physicochemical** and **pharmacokinetic** properties affect the access of the opioid to the receptor, which accounts for differing potency among opioid agonists. **Physicochemistry** describes the physical and chemical processes of a drug binding to a receptor. The term **"pharmacokinetics"** describes what the human body "does" to the drug: how we absorb, distribute, metabolize and excrete a drug.

Different opioid doses can be made **equipotent** (having equivalent potency), resulting in an **"equianalgesic"** effect (the two opioids provide the same degree of pain relief). Equipotent doses of opioids can be determined by correcting for these physicochemical and pharmacokinetic differences through dosage corrections and different routes of administration.[6] Therefore, the potency of an opioid does not solely define opioid responsiveness or efficacy. For opioids that are less "potent" we can simply increase the dose of the drug to get similar efficacy to a more potent opioid. For example, oral oxycodone is generally considered to be more "potent" than oral morphine. One commonly used conversion ratio is that 30 mg of oral morphine will achieve approximately the same degree of pain relief as 20 mg of oral oxycodone. By knowing this we can switch from oxycodone to morphine (or vice-versa) and achieve a similar clinical outcome by adjusting the dose to allow for this difference.

Doses of two different opioids (or two different routes of administration of the same opioid) are considered to be **equianalgesic** if they provide approximately the same degree of pain relief. Table 1-1 is an Equianalgesic Opioid Dosing chart, that lists opioid doses that provide approximately the same analgesic response based on potency and bioavailability. The term **bioavailability** refers to the percentage of drug that is detected in the systemic circulation after its administration and is available to provide pain relief. For a drug administered intravenously, the bioavailability is 100%. Drugs administered by other routes of administration, such as the oral route, may have reduced bioavailability because the drug must be absorbed through the gut and circulate through the liver where it may be subject to metabolism, prior to entering the systemic circulation.

Table 1-1

Equianalgesic Opioid Dosing

Drug	Equianalgesic Doses (mg)		Formulation Comments
	Parenteral	Oral	
Morphine[a]	10	30	■ Available as short-acting tablets and capsules, and oral solution (including oral concentrate Roxanol).
			■ Available as oral long-tablet tablets and capsules (MS Contin, Oramorph SR, Kadian, Avinza).
			■ Available as rectal suppositories (equivalent dosing to oral).
Buprenorphine[b]	0.3	0.4 (SL)	■ Available as sublingual (SL) tablets and injection.
			■ Transdermal 4- and 7-day patches available (not in the United States).
Codeine	100	200	■ Codeine is a prodrug, metabolized to morphine by the liver.
			■ Available as injectable, tablets, and oral solution; most commonly administered in combination with acetaminophen (e.g., Tylenol #3).
Fentanyl[c]	0.1	NA	■ Available as injection, transmucosal and transdermal. Refer to Chapters 4 and 5 for further discussion of transmucosal and transdermal dosing of fentanyl, respectively.
Hydrocodone[d]	NA	30	■ Only available as a combination product (e.g., hydrocodone plus acetaminophen or ibuprofen). Oral solution (Hycodan) contains hydrocodone and homatropine.
			■ Most commonly given in combination with acetaminophen (Lorcet, Lortab, Vicodin, others).
Hydromorphone[e]	1.5	7.5	■ Available as oral tablets, solution, injection and rectal suppository.
Meperidine	100	300	■ Available as tablets, syrup, oral solution and injection.
			■ Not recommended for routine clinical use.

Table 1-1 (contd.)
Equianalgesic Opioid Dosing

| Drug | Equianalgesic Doses (mg) | | Formulation Comments |
	Parenteral	Oral	
Methadone[f]	See Chapter 6		■ Available as oral tablets and oral solution (including oral concentrate). ■ Dispersible tablet not used for chronic pain management (only for opioid treatment programs).
Oxycodone[g]	10	20	■ Available as short-acting oral tablets, capsules, oral solution (including oral concentrate OxyFast, Roxicodone). ■ Available as a long-acting oral tablet (OxyContin). ■ Frequently given in combination with acetaminophen (e.g., Percocet). ■ Parenteral formulation is not available in the United States.
Oxymorphone[h]	1	10	■ Available as a short-acting tablet, oral long-acting tablet, and parenteral formulation.
Tramadol[i]	100	120	■ Available as a short-acting tablet, extended-release oral tablet, and injectable. ■ Parenteral formulation is not available in the United States.

Equianalgesic data presented in this table is that which is most commonly used by health care practitioners, but it is *approximate*. The clinician is urged to read the following caveats, along with the text, and use good clinical judgment at all times.

[a]With chronic morphine dosing, the average relative potency of intravenous or subcutaneous morphine to oral morphine is between 1:2 and 1:3 (e.g., 20–30 mg of morphine by mouth is equianalgesic to 10 mg IV or SQ). (Kalso E, Vainio A. Morphine and oxycodone hydrochloride in the management of cancer pain. *Clin Pharmacol Ther.* 1990;47:639–646.)

Oral:rectal bioavailability is considered to be approximately equivalent. (Westerling D Lindahl S, Andersson KE, Andersson A. Absorption and bioavailability of rectally administered morphine in women. *European J Clin Pharmacol.* 1982;23(1):59–64.) (Brook-Williams P. Morphine suppositories for intractable pain. *CMA J.* 1982;126:14.)

[b]Sublingual buprenorphine 0.4 mg has been shown to be equivalent to 0.3 mg buprenorphine given parenterally. (Bullingham RE, McQuay HJ, Porter EJ, Allen MC, Moore RA. Sublingual buprenorphine used postoperatively: clinical observations and preliminary pharmacokinetic analysis. *Br J Clin Pharmacol.* 1981;12:117–122.)

Buprenorphine 0.3 mg given IM has been shown to be equivalent to morphine 10 mg IM. (Kjaer M, Henriksen H, Knudsen J. A comparative study of intramuscular buprenorphine and morphine in the treatment of chronic pain of malignant origin. *Br J Clin Pharmacol.* 1982;13:487–492.) Similar findings have been seen with IV doses of both opioids. (Zacny J, Conley K, Galinkin J. Comparing the subjective, psychomotor and physiological effects of intravenous buprenorphine and morphine in healthy volunteers. *J Pharm Exp Ther.* 1997;282:1187–1197.)

Buprenorphine is available as a 4- and 7-day transdermal patch in Europe. Both brands (BuTrans and Transtec) recommend starting with the lowest strength patch when switching to transdermal buprenorphine. In the reference *Palliative Drugs*, a conversion of 100:1 (morphine:buprenorphine) is suggested. Example: multiply 24 hour oral morphine dose in mg by 10 to obtain 24 hour buprenorphine dose in micrograms; divide answer by 24 to obtain microgram/hour patch strength; round down to closest patch strength. (Palliative Drugs; www.palliativedrugs.com/opioid-dose-conversion-ratios.html, Accessed January 9, 2009).

[c]Although parenteral MS:fentanyl is shown as 10:0.1 mg (which is a 100:1 ratio) based on a mg-to-mg ratio, in clinical practice the ratio is described as 15-112.5:1; many clinicians use an equivalency of 4 mg/hour IV morphine equivalent to

Table 1-1 (contd.)
Equianalgesic Opioid Dosing

100 mcg/hour parenteral or transdermal fentanyl. (Indelicato RA, Portenoy RK. Opioid rotation in the management of refractory cancer pain. *JCO.* 2003;21:87s–91s.) (Patanwala AE, Duby J, Waters D, et al. Opioid conversions in acute care. *Ann Pharmacother.* 2007;41:255–267.) (Lawlor P, Pereira J, Bruera E. Dose ratios among different opioids: underlying issues and an update on the use of equianalgesic table. In: Bruera E, Portenoy RK, ed. *Topics in Palliative Care.* Volume 5. New York: Oxford University Press, 2001.)

Transdermal fentanyl (TDF) patch (used for chronic pain) dosed in mcg, is roughly equivalent to 50% of the total daily dose of oral morphine in mg (e.g., TDF 25 mcg patch is roughly equal to 50 oral morphine per day). Refer to Chapter 5 for additional information on dosing transdermal fentanyl. (Breitbart W, Chandler S, Eagel B, et al. An alternative algorithm for dosing transdermal fentanyl for cancer-related pain. *Oncology.* 2000;14:695–705.)

[d]Equivalence to oral morphine not clearly defined; generally thought to be equal to or less potent than oxycodone. (Hallenbeck JL. *Palliative Care Perspectives.* New York: Oxford University Press; 2003:71.)

[e]Oral bioavailability may be as high as 60%, particularly with chronic dosing; ranges from 29–95%. (Vallner JJ, et al. Pharmacokinetics and bioavailability of hydromorphone following intravenous and oral administration to human subjects. *J Clin Pharmcol.* 1981;21:152–156.) (Ritschel WA, Parab PV, Denson DD, Coyle DE, Gregg RV. Absolute bioavailability of hydromorphone after peroral and rectal administration in humans: saliva/plasma ratio and clinical effects. *J Clin Pharmacol.* 1987;27:647–653.)(Parab PV, Ritschel WA, Coyle DE, Gregg RV, Denson DD. Pharmacokinetics of hydromorphone after intravenous, peroral and rectal administration to human subjects. *Biopharm Drug Dispos.* 1988;9:187–199.)

Research has shown a lower dose ratio and a directional influence seen when converting between morphine and hydromorphone. It is suggested that when switching from morphine (M) to hydromorphone (HM) (using the same route of administration; e.g., SQ to SQ or oral to oral), a conversion ratio of 5:1 (M:HM) when switching from morphine to hydromorphone and a dose ratio of 3.7:1 (M:HM) when switching from hydromorphone to morphine (again, using the same route of administration). (Lawlor P, Turner K, Hanson J, Bruera E. Dose ratio between morphine and hydromorphone in patients with cancer pain: a retrospective study. *Pain.* 1997;72:79–85. Anderson R, Saiers JH, Abram S, Schlicht C. Accuracy in equianalgesic dosing: conversion dilemmas. *J Pain Symptom Manage.* 2001;21:397–406).

Oral:rectal bioavailability approximately equal; the FDA-approved dosing interval for rectal hydromorphone is every 6 hours.

[f]Methadone dosing is highly variable, and conversion to/from other opioids is NOT linear; refer to Chapter 6 for additional information on methadone dosing.

[g]Because of the variations in bioavailability between morphine (15–64%) and oxycodone (60% or more), the equianalgesic ratio for oral morphine:oxycodone ranges from 1:1 to 2:1, partially dependent on the patient's ability to absorb the opioid. A ratio of 1.5:1 is used clinically as a compromise. (Anderson R, Saiers JH, Abram S, Schlicht C. Accuracy in equianalgesic dosing: conversion dilemmas. *J Pain Symptom Manage.* 2001;21:397–406.)

Parenteral oxycodone is not available in the United States. According to manufacturers information (Mundipharma New Zealand Limited, Distributed by Pharmaco (N.Z.) Ltd,) 2 mg of oral oxycodone is approximately equivalent to 1 mg parenteral oxycodone. (Medsafe: Information for Health Professionals. Oxynorm Injection. Accessed online January 8, 2009, at http://www.medsafe.govt.nz/profs/Datasheet/o/OxyNorminj.htm.) This ratio may be somewhat conservative because the oral bioavailability of oxycodone has been shown to be 60% or greater. (Pöyhiä R, Seppälä T, Olkkola KT, Kalso E. The pharmacokinetics and metabolism of oxycodone after intramuscular and oral administration to healthy subjects. *Br J Clin Pharmacol.* 1992;33:617–621.)

[h]Conversion from oral morphine or oral oxycodone to oxymorphone is shown as 30:10 and 20:10, respectively per package labeling. Some data suggests the conversion ratio when switching to oxymorphone is closer to 18:10 for morphine, and 12:10 for oxycodone, especially once at steady state. (Sloan P, Slatkin N, Ahdieh H. Effectiveness and safety or oral extended-release oxymorphone for the treatment of cancer pain: a pilot study. *Support Care Cancer.* 2005;13:57–65).

[i]Parenteral tramadol has been shown to be approximately equipotent to parenteral morphine in a 10:1 (tramadol:morphine) ratio. (Wilder-Smith CH, Hill L, Wilkins J, Denny L. Effects of morphine and tramadol on somatic and visceral sensory function and gastrointestinal motility after abdominal surgery. *Anesthesiology.* 1999;91:639–647.) With chronic dosing, oral tramadol achieves between 90 and 100% bioavailability. (Grond S, Sablotzki A. Clinical pharmacology of tramadol. *Clin Pharmacokinet.* 2004;31:879–923.) Despite bioavailability data, equipotent use of oral morphine and oral tramadol ranges from 1:4 to 1:10 (morphine:tramadol). Therefore, using an equivalence of 120 mg oral tramadol may be very conservative. (Grond S, Radbruch L, Meuser T, Loick G, Sabatowski R, Lehmann KA. High-dose tramadol in comparison to low-dose morphine for cancer pain relief. *J Pain Symptom Manage.* 1999;18:174–179).

Source: Data adapted from (1) Carr DB, Jacox AK, Chapman CR, et al. "Acute Pain Management: Operative or Medical Procedures and Trauma. Clinical Practice Guideline No. 1." AHCPR Pub. No. 92-0032. Rockville, MD: Agency for Health Care Policy and Research, Public Health Service, U.S. Department of Health and Human Services. Feb. 1992; and (2) Jacox A, Carr DB, Payne R, et al. Management of Cancer Pain. Clinical Practice Guideline No. 9. AHCPR Publication No. 94-0592. Rockville, MD. Agency for Health Care Policy and Research, U.S. Department of Health and Human Services, Public Health Service, March 1994.

Therefore, looking at this chart, doses listed *across* a row for a given opioid show equipotent doses (e.g., 30 mg oral morphine is approximately equivalent to 10 mg parenteral morphine). Doses for different opioids in a *column* are also equipotent (e.g., 10 mg parenteral morphine is approximately equivalent to 1.5 mg parenteral hydromorphone). We can even use this chart to look at equivalent doses between opioids AND routes of administration (e.g., 10 mg parenteral morphine is approximately equivalent to 20 mg oral oxycodone). You will learn more about actually using this table in subsequent chapters. Even though we have just spoken in terms of equivalent "doses" we're really referring to equivalencies or ratios; the values in this table are not patient-specific doses. For example, even though "10 mg" is shown in the "parenteral morphine" box in the table below, this does *not* mean it is necessarily the appropriate *dose* for a given patient.

For completeness sake, it is important to remember that a patient's response to an opioid (the **"pharmacodynamic effect"**: what the drug does to the body), despite our very best estimate of equianalgesic dosing, may be different than expected. We are created as unique individuals; how we react to drugs varies from person to person based on our genetics and other factors.

The Problem with "Those Charts"

All the left-brain thinkers are no doubt, delighted with the Equianalgesic Opioid Dosing Table shown above. It makes so much sense, doesn't it? Someone figured out the potency differences, put it in this chart, we do the math, and we're home free with our opioid conversion calculations! Well, it's not quite that simple! Unfortunately, there are some caveats to "those charts" such as the one above. Let's explore the issues.

Source of Equianalgesic Data

Much of the data in this chart was obtained from single-dose cross-over studies in opioid-naïve patients with acute pain. An example would be a clinical trial where a healthy volunteer or patient received one dose of Opioid A and their clinical response was observed. Then they received one dose of Opioid B and their clinical response was observed and compared to the dose of Opioid A. Obviously these individuals had limited opioid exposure (both duration and dose). Very few studies have evaluated equianalgesia in chronic pain patients, and we know that accumulation of opioids and/or their metabolites may contribute to the overall effectiveness of the opioid. For example, with repeated dosing, the active metabolite of morphine (morphine-6-glucuronide) also has analgesic properties.

Patient-specific Variables

Patient-related variables such as age, sex, pharmacogenomics (polymorphism of opioid receptors), organ function (liver and kidney), level and stability of pain control, duration and extent of opioid exposure, interacting medications, and co-morbid conditions have not been considered in putting together a chart such as the one shown above. No consideration has been given as to why the patient is no longer responding to the original opioid, or the influence of existential pain (e.g., suffering) in patients with advanced illness. All of these factors can influence the pharmacokinetics (absorption, distribution, metabolism and excretion) and pharmacodynamics (pharmacologic effect) of the opioid, and they are largely unaccounted for in the Equianalgesic Opioid Dosing Table.

Unidirectional vs. Bidirectional Equivalencies

In looking at the Equianalgesic Opioid Dosing Table we assume that the data is bidirectional. For example, we see that the oral morphine:hydromorphone ratio is approximately 4:1 (30 mg oral morphine is about equal to 7.5 mg oral hydromorphone) and we assume that ratio holds whether we are converting from morphine to hydromorphone or from hydromorphone to morphine. However, well-crafted cross-over trials have shown the oral morphine:hydromorphone ratio is actual 5-8:1, while the oral hydromorphone:morphine ratio is 1:3-4.[7] I'm sure you're holding your head in your hands right now, thinking "WHAT do I do about this?" We'll discuss this later in the chapter, but basically you do the best you can, and you **MONITOR** your patient closely!

 PITFALL •••
Be Careful Which Rule You Slide On

Many pharmaceutical manufacturers of opioid products will provide a "conversion calculator" for ease of converting to *their* product. Generally speaking, the guidelines they provide are fairly conservative for switching from other opioids to *their* product. Therefore it is imperative that practitioners *not* use these conversion calculators to convert *from* the manufacturer's opioid to other opioids, or between other opioids. Obviously if the conversion calculator is *conservative* going to the manufacturers opioid, when used erroneously it would be too *aggressive* when converting from their opioid.

Introduction to the Process of Opioid Conversion Calculations

We will discuss opioid conversion calculations (OCC) at length in subsequent chapters, but it is important to recognize that there is a *process* to doing these calculations. This discussion includes the <u>art</u> as well as the <u>science</u> in OCC. Gammaitoni et al. recommended a five-step approach to OCC, which is shown in Table 1-2.[8] This five step process illustrates the importance of calculating not only an effective dose, but even MORE importantly, a safe dose. As shown in Figure 1-1, your best option would be to calculate a safe AND effective dose (top right quadrant). Barring that, a less effective, but safer dose is your next best goal. Importantly, when calculating a new opioid regimen, it is perfectly acceptable to be conservative with the scheduled, or long-acting opioid dose. However, if you are being conservative (which is a good thing), the patient must have adequate rescue rapid- or short-acting analgesics available for breakthrough pain.

	Less Effective	More Effective
Safer	Most safe dose, but not as effective as it could be. **This is an acceptable quadrant.** Have a rescue plan in place (e.g., rapid or short-acting opioid).	Most effective and most safe dose. **This is the preferred quadrant.**
Less Safe	Dose not safe or effective; clearly a place you do NOT want to be! **This is your LEAST acceptable quadrant!**	Most effective dose, but not as safe as it could be. **This is not an acceptable quadrant.**

Figure 1-1. Opioid conversion calculations should be as safe AND effective as possible.

Table 1-2

Five-Step Approach to Opioid Conversion

1. Step 1—Globally assess the patient (i.e., PQRSTU) to determine if the uncontrolled pain is secondary to worsening of existing pain or development of a new type of pain.

2. Step 2—Determine the total daily usage of the current opioid. This should include all long-acting and breakthrough opioid doses.

3. Step 3—Decide which opioid analgesic will be used for the new agent and consult the established conversion tables to arrive at the proper dose of the new opioid, recognizing the limitations of the data.

4. Step 4—Individualize the dosage based on assessment information gathered in Step 1 and ensure adequate access to breakthrough medication.

5. Step 5—Patient follow-up and continual reassessment, especially during the first 7–14 days, to fine-tune the total daily dose (long-acting + short-acting) and increase or decrease the around the clock long-acting dosage accordingly.

Source: Reprinted with permission from: Gammaitoni AR, Fine P, Alvarez N, et al. Clinical application of opioid equianalgesic data. *Clin J Pain.* 2003;19:286–297.

Let's look at the five-step approach to opioid conversions.

Step 1

Lack of effectiveness is probably one of the most common reasons we switch to a new opioid. Before jumping in with your calculator however, it is important to assess the pain. This will help the health care practitioner determine if continuing opioid therapy (including possibly switching to a new opioid) is the best course of action, vs. adding a co-analgesic.

There are many proposed methods to assess a report of pain, but one of the most common is the "PQRSTU" method. The letters represent elements of symptom analysis that help the patient characterize the pain, and include:

- P—*precipitating and palliating*—what brings on or worsens the pain? What relieves the pain (non-pharmacologic and pharmacologic)? If pharmacologic, ask what the patient has taken (including breakthrough analgesics), what the response was, and if any side effects developed. What medications have been tried to treat the pain?

- Q—*quality*—can you describe the pain in your own words? You're looking for words such as stabbing, shooting, throbbing, aching, gnawing, etc.

- R—*region and radiation*—where is the pain? Does the pain move anywhere else? Is the pain deep inside, or more superficial?

- S—*severity*—there are many severity rating scales. For example, if 0 is no pain, and 10 is the worst pain you can imagine, how would you rate your pain right now? What is the BEST the pain is over the course of a day? The worst? The average? One hour after taking your rapid- or short-acting pain medication? You may need to consider non-verbal indicators of pain for patients who cannot describe it for you.

- T—*temporal*—is the pain constant, or does it come and go? If it comes and goes, how many times per day does it occur? How long does it last? Is it increasing in frequency or duration over the past few days/weeks?

- U—you—*how is the pain affecting your life*? How has the pain affected your ability to sleep, your appetite, your ability to ambulate, your mood, etc.?

This information, along with physical inspection of the painful areas will help you determine if this is the same pain the patient originally complained of, or if this is a new pain.

Step 2

Part of effective medication reconciliation is to get a complete and accurate list of all medications the patient is taking. You know what analgesics were <u>prescribed</u> for the patient, but this does not guarantee that's the way the patient has been taking these medications. Be sure to include both the long-acting and rapid- or short-acting analgesics the patient has been taking when determining the total daily dose of opioid. Of course you will also ask about nonprescription, complementary and alternative product use.

FAST FACT Do You Know What I Know (About Your Medications)?

Unsurprisingly, patients frequently lack basic knowledge about their analgesics; this can frequently be a barrier to good pain management. When performing medication reconciliation, you can use this time to assess the patient's knowledge of their medications as well as ask how they are actually taking the medication (which may or may not reflect what is typed on the medication label). Taking it one medication at a time, show the patient the medication and say "Tell me how and when you take this medication." You can also ask if the patient knows the purpose, administration precautions, and potential adverse effects of the medications. This information will help you make clinical decisions (the "art") about the calculation.

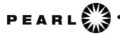

PEARL •••

I Spy With My Little Eye... Patients tend to forget to tell you about medications taken by the non-oral route of administration. This includes inhaled medications (e.g., metered dose inhalers or nebulized medications), injected medications (e.g., insulin), and topical products (e.g., ointments, creams, and transdermal medications). Detection of any transdermal opioids is critical when performing OCC. It is not uncommon for a patient to be admitted to the hospital, or to hospice care and not tell the admitting nurse s/he has a transdermal fentanyl patch on. If the nurse does not physically inspect the patient, s/he may miss this important piece of information. The health care team is often left scratching their heads wondering why the patient's pain control deteriorates one or two days later.

 PITFALL ••••••••••••••••••••••••••••••••••••

The Whole Truth and Nothing But the Truth

It is critically important to ask the patient about ALL doses of rapid- or short-acting analgesic they are taking. Frequently patients want to impress the health care provider with how severe the pain has been, so when asked, they claim "Doc, I've been taking that liquid medicine every two hours, just like it says on the label." This is a red flag—is the patient really, truly, taking the rapid- or short-acting opioid EVERY two hours around the clock? Literally 12 doses on average over a 24-hour period? Patients are generally referring to the hours they are awake. If you take the "every two hours around the clock" report at face value and base your OCC calculation on that, you may be calculating too aggressive a dose and put the patient at risk for toxicity. Encourage use of a pain diary so the patient or caregiver records all doses of rapid- or short-acting opioid taken for breakthrough pain. Then you can average their use over 24 hours.

•••

Step 3

Using your knowledge of drug therapy selection, decide which opioid to switch to. This decision may be influenced by the patient's ability to swallow medications or apply a transdermal system, their renal function (drugs with pharmacologically-active metabolites, such as morphine, are not the best choice in patients with end-stage renal disease), or the nature of the pain (perhaps you want to choose methadone because there is anecdotal evidence suggesting it is more effective for neuropathic or mixed nociceptive-neuropathic pain than other opioids). The decision may be driven by the availability of dosage formulations that are best suited to your patients needs (e.g., oral concentrated solution, parenteral infusion). The potential for drug interactions (e.g., methadone can interact with many medications) and the patient's previous history of response to various opioids should also be considered. Last, the decision may be influenced by formulary or financial limitations, or safety concerns (e.g., children in home, risk of drug abuse and diversion).

Once you have decided which opioid you are switching to, consult the Equianalgesic Opioid Dosing Table, and calculate the equianalgesic dose of the new opioid (this will be discussed at length in subsequent chapters). As stated earlier, using the Equianalgesic Opioid Dosing Table is a ballpark estimate of the opioid dose you are switching to. Let's take the ballpark analogy and run with it. Buying a ticket to the ballgame held in a stadium that seats 70,000 people is equivalent to consulting the Equianalgesic Opioid Dosing Table and doing your calculation. Now you have your new opioid dose – but what do you do with it? It's like arriving at the ballpark with your ticket in hand. Now what? You have to consult your ticket to see what section you're in, which row, which seat. How quickly you get to your seat depends on how quickly the game is going to start. You may have to get to your seat immediately, maybe even run and increase your risk of falling if you want to catch the early action. On the other hand, if you're early, you can probably score a hotdog and popcorn as you meander to your seat. Similarly, if the patient is in pain crisis, you will want to act immediately, be a bit more aggressive, and monitor them extremely closely. If you are switching to a new opioid for a less urgent reason, you can be more conservative and methodical. Integrating the art and science of OCC will help you hit this one out of the ballpark!

Step 4

Once you do your calculation, you will need to individualize the dose for the patient. Using the information you gathered in step 1, you basically have three choices. You can use the dose you calculated, you can increase it, or decrease it. When converting from one opioid to another because of unacceptable adverse effects (where pain control was not an issue), it would be advisable to reduce the newly calculated dose by 25–50%. Patients likely develop some degree of **tolerance** to the therapeutic effects of an opioid, but when they convert to a new opioid, they will not show the same degree of tolerance. Tolerance is defined as a phenomenon where continued exposure to a drug reduces its effectiveness, occasionally necessitating a dosage increase. The increased opioid sensitivity seen with switching is known as "**incomplete cross-tolerance.**" Therefore, if you calculate an equivalent dose, but don't reduce it, the patient may experience an enhanced and possibly toxic effect from the new opioid. Another reason for reducing the dose of the new opioid has to do with the "ballpark" nature of the equivalency values in the Equianalgesic Opioid Dosing Table discussed above.

If you are switching the patient because their pain was not controlled on the original opioid, you can consider using the calculated dose of the new opioid. The patient will experience a greater sensitivity to the new opioid, but this is a welcome effect, since their pain was not controlled. In the case of severe pain at the time of the switch, you may occasionally even decide to increase the dose over what you calculated.

So which of the three roads do you take: run with the newly calculated dose, cut it back, or increase it? Here's where the art comes in (as in "art and science!"). We know that one size really *doesn't* fit all, therefore you must consider your patient and his or her specific situation. Are they at home? In the hospital? In a long term care facility or assisted living? Is there a competent caregiver present or adequate nursing staff to assess for opioid-related adverse effects? How acute is the need to make this switch? How severe is the pain? Is the patient a 42 year old man or a 94 year old woman? Trust your gut!

Once you've decided on the optimal total daily dose of the new opioid, you need to divide the 24 hour dose as appropriate for the new dosing interval. For example, if you're switching to an hourly infusion, you would calculate the dose to be delivered per hour by dividing the total daily dose by 24. If you will be advising the patient to take their opioid every 4 hours, you need to divide the total daily dose by 6. The individual dosage amount you calculate will then need to be rounded up or down to be a reasonable number: it must be "doable" with commercially available tablets, capsules, oral solution, or whatever dosage formulation you are going to be using. You can be Albert Einstein and do complicated conversion calculations all day long, but there's no way in the world you can accurately give 12.75 mg of oxycodone every 4 hours with a tablet or capsule! The last step in individualization (and a very important step) is to account for residual drug in the patient's system (if any) during the conversion process. This is especially important when converting FROM long-acting oral opioids or transdermal patches. Starting the new drug, particularly a regularly scheduled, long-acting opioid basal (known as the "**basal**" dose), should be delayed if significant residual drug is in the body. In the meantime, the patient can use their rapid- or short-acting opioid should the pain recur. This will become clearer as you work through the problems included in this book.

Step 5

OK, you've done the deed! You've assessed the patient, picked the best opioid, sharpened your pencil, calculated a dose, adjusted it if necessary, and implemented your plan. But your work is NOT done! This is where the real skill comes in: monitoring the patient for several days to two weeks after a medication change (duration of vigilant monitoring depends on time to achieve steady-state serum drug levels). Because the Equianalgesic Opioid Dosing Table is not set in concrete you may have been a bit over- or under-aggressive with your dosing. You need to monitor the subjective and objective monitoring parameters for both therapeutic effectiveness (pain control) and potential toxicity from the opioid. Every patient's situation is different. Figure 1-2 is an example of a monitoring plan.

Armed with this information, you can fine-tune the opioid regimen over the ensuing hours/days. You may also make adjustments to both the long- and short-acting

	Subjective Parameters	Objective Parameters
Monitoring for therapeutic effectiveness	■ Pain rating ■ Patient subjectively states s/he is better able to perform ADLs (e.g., personal care), sleep, ambulate, etc.	■ Patient objectively reports s/he sleeps longer and does not awaken in pain ■ Patient can objectively ambulate further without pain ■ Limited use of rescue opioid
Monitoring for potential toxicity from an opioid	■ Complaints of constipation, nausea, sedation, dizziness, confusion, itching, hallucinations, vomiting, dry mouth, urinary retention, sweating, rash or hives	■ Level of arousal/sedation ■ Respiratory rate ■ Pinpoint pupils ■ Bowel movement frequency ■ Episodes of emesis ■ Mini-mental state exam ■ Hours spent sleeping ■ Signs of excoriation

Figure 1-2. Example of a patient monitoring plan.

opioid in the regimen as you monitor the patient's response. It is important to share your monitoring and titration plan with the patient/family/caregiver; you are more likely to experience success if you explain the transition from one opioid to another, the importance of the rescue medications, and so forth.

Conclusion

In this chapter we have introduced the idea of opioid conversion calculations. There are many clinical situations where OCC is an appropriate intervention. It is important to use a systematic process when switching a patient from one opioid to another, and strongly consider patient variables when instituting a new regimen. Follow-up is critical to patient success. We will discuss numerous specific examples of opioid conversions in upcoming chapters.

REFERENCES

1. Indelicato RA, Portenoy RK. Opioid rotation in the management of refractory cancer pain. *J Clin Oncol.* 2002;20:348–352.
2. Muller-Busch HC, Lindena G, Tietze K, Woskanjan J. Opioid switch in palliative care, opioid choice by clinical need and opioid availability. *Eur J Pain.* 2005;9:571–579.
3. Riley J, Ross JR, Rutter D, et al. No pain relief from morphine? Individual variation in sensitivity to morphine and the need to switch to an alternative opioid in cancer patients. *Support Care Cancer.* 2006;14:56–64.
4. Quigley C. Opioid switching to improve pain relief and drug tolerability. Cochrane Database of Systematic Reviews 2004, Issue 3. Art. No.:CD004847. DOI: 10.1002/14651858.CD004847.
5. Mercadante S, Portenoy RK. Opioid poorly-responsive cancer pain. Part 1: Clinical considerations. *J Pain Symptom Manage.* 2001;21:144–150.
6. Ferrante FM. Principles of opioid pharmacotherapy: practical implications of basic mechanisms. *J Pain Symptom Manage.* 1996;11:265–273.
7. Patanwala AE, Duby J, Waters D, Erstad BL. Opioid conversions in acute care. *Ann Pharmacother.* 2007;41:255–267.
8. Gammaitoni AR, Fine P, Alvarez N, et al. Clinical application of opioid equianalgesic data. *Clin J Pain.* 2003;19:286–297.

ADDITIONAL RECOMMENDED READING

Berdine HJ, Nesbit SA. Equianalgesic dosing of opioids. *J Pain Palliative Care Pharmacother.* 2006;20:79–84.

Gordon DB, Stevenson KK, Griffie J, et al. Opioid equianalgesic calculations. *J Palliative Med.* 1999;2:209–218.

Mercadante S, Bruera E. Opioid switching: a systemic and critical review. *Cancer Treat Rev.* 2006;32:304–315.

Pereira J, Lawlor P, Vigano A, et al. Equianalgesic dose ratios for opioids: a critical review and proposals for long-term dosing. *J Pain Symptom Manage.* 2001;22:672–687.

CHAPTER 2

Converting Among Routes and Formulations of the Same Opioid

OBJECTIVES

After reading this chapter and completing all practice problems, the participant will be able to:

1. List the advantages and disadvantages of potential routes of administration for opioid analgesics.

2. Define bioavailability and explain factors that influence medication bioavailability such as the first pass effect, solubility, gastrointestinal influences, and drug formulation considerations.

3. Given an actual or simulated patient with a complaint of pain, convert between dosage formulations and routes of administration for the same opioid (e.g., morphine, hydromorphone, oxycodone and oxymorphone).

INTRODUCTION

In Chapter 1 we discussed the reasons why a patient may need to be switched from one opioid to another. Frequently, a patient's pain is controlled on his/her current opioid, but he/she requires, or would benefit from, a different dosage formulation or route of administration. For example, approximately 70% of patients with advanced illness will require a non-oral route of administration prior to death due to difficulty swallowing.[1] Conversely, patients who receive parenteral opioid therapy post-procedure or to control a pain crisis would likely prefer the convenience of oral opioid therapy as soon as possible. The purpose of this chapter is to learn how to switch a patient between routes of administration or dosage formulations, using the same opioid.

Routes of Administration

As you can see from Table 2-1, most opioids are commercially available in a variety of dosage formulations, giving us flexibility in opioid administration. Morphine, for example, can be given by the oral route (short-acting tablets, capsules and oral solution, and long-acting tablets and capsules), rectal route (rectal suppositories and rectal insertion of long-acting tablets [not an FDA-approved route of administration]), parenterally (intramuscular, subcutaneous, or intravenous), or via the neuroaxis (epidural or intrathecal routes; to be discussed in Chapter 7). Let's consider route of administration and formulation-specific issues that guide dosing equivalency considerations.

Table 2-1

Opioid Formulations

Opioid	Oral Tablet or Capsule	Extended Release Tablet or Capsule	Oral Solution, Suspension or Elixir	Sublingual Tablet	Rectal Suppository	Injectable	Transdermal	Transmucosal
Buprenorphine				X		X	X*	
Codeine	X		X			X		
Codeine plus non-opioid	X		X					
Fentanyl						X	X	X
Hydrocodone plus non-opioid	X		X					
Hydromorphone	X		X		X	X		
Methadone	X		X			X		
Morphine	X	X	X		X	X		
Oxycodone	X	X	X			X*		
Oxycodone plus non-opioid	X		X					
Oxymorphone	X	X				X		
Tramadol	X	X				X*		

*Not available in the U.S.

Oral

Oral dosage formulations are preferred when feasible and effective, particularly for the management of chronic pain. Oral medications are usually cost effective, convenient, portable, flexible, reliable, result in relatively steady blood levels, and are less associated with the sick role.

Most opioids are short-acting, requiring frequent dosing (e.g., every 4 hours). Some practitioners may purposely choose to use a short-acting opioid to titrate to adequate pain relief, and then switch the patient to a long-acting oral opioid formulation. At present, morphine, oxycodone, oxymorphone, and tramadol are available in a variety of long-acting, modified-release oral formulations. Methadone is inherently a long-lasting opioid (e.g., 8–12 hours) and will be discussed in Chapter 6.

For patients who have difficulty swallowing tablets or capsules, they can be switched to a liquid opioid formulation. Alternately, long-acting morphine capsules such as Kadian or Avinza may be opened, and the contents sprinkled on soft food such as applesauce. Kadian is also approved for administration through a 16 French gastrostomy tube (flush tube with water to ensure it is wet; sprinkle Kadian pellets into 10 mL of water; swirl to pour pellets and water into gastrostomy tube through a funnel; rinse beaker and pour into funnel until no pellets remain in beaker). Importantly, neither long-acting tablets or the long-acting particles inside Kadian or Avinza should ever be crushed, chewed, or allowed to dissolve. Doing so would render a dose of opioid intended to be delivered over 12–24 hours to be immediately available. The patient would likely be REALLY comfortable, but this will probably cause adverse effects which may be fatal (patients hate that side effect!).

:::::::::::::: **FAST FACT** Timing of Long-Acting Opioid Administration

Researchers have long recognized that pain exhibits a diurnal variation, or circadian rhythm, although it is likely variable among patients and disease states. One recent study evaluated the impact of administering a once-daily oral morphine first thing in the morning vs. at bedtime to patients with opioid-responsive advanced cancer pain. Their results showed no difference in overall pain control, pain during the day, pain disturbing sleep or use of breakthrough medications. The researchers concluded that any differences between AM and PM administration of this once-daily oral morphine product to advanced cancer patients were small, and unlikely to be clinically significant for most people. This data allows us to dose once-daily oral morphine products when it is most convenient for the patient/family.[11]

The primary disadvantage to oral dosage formulations, particularly opioids, is reduced **bioavailability** (see sidebar "Bioavailability"). **Bioavailability** is defined as "the rate and extent to which the active ingredient or active **moiety** [the active part of the drug molecule] is absorbed from a drug product and becomes available at the site of action."[2] In simpler terms, the bioavailability of a drug refers to the percentage of drug that eventually ends up in the systemic circulation. Intravenous injection of a drug (where you PUT the drug in the systemic circulation) is considered to have 100% bioavailability. The bioavailability of other dosage formulations is determined by administering the same dose in a different formulation and determining how much of the dose ends up in the systemic circulation. The average bioavailability of oral morphine is approximately 30–40% but may be quite variable (e.g., 16–68%).[2] Oral hydromorphone has approximately 50% bioavailability (range 29–95%), while oral oxycodone is about 80% and oral oxymorphone is about 10%.[3-4] This means that you must give considerably more opioid by the oral route than by intravenous injection to get the same amount into the systemic circulation, and a similar therapeutic effect. As shown on our Equianalgesic Opioid Dosing Table (Table 1-1), the dose equivalency ratio between parenteral and oral morphine is 10:30 – we must give three times as much morphine by tablet or capsule as we do by intravenous injection to achieve an equivalent blood level, and by inference, a similar level of analgesia. Things get a bit more complicated when we consider the role of morphine metabolites with chronic dosing however. In single dose studies, the ratio of IV to oral morphine is closer to 10:60. Accumulation of morphine-6-glucuronide (M6G) with repeated morphine dosing (especially oral) contributes to the analgesic activity of morphine, therefore a true comparison of oral and IV morphine includes consideration of M6G. For patients with normal kidney function, and consequently adequate clearance of M6G, the 10:30 IV:oral ratio holds up under conditions of repeated dosing. In patients with compromised renal function, a more correct conversion would be 10:20 when going from intravenous to oral morphine, and conversely 20:10 when going from oral to intravenous morphine.[6]

There are many variables that affect the extent of drug absorption. One major influence on oral medication administration is the **"first pass"** effect. When a medication is given by the oral route of administration, after being absorbed from the gastrointestinal tract it first goes through the liver (see Figure 2-1). During transit through

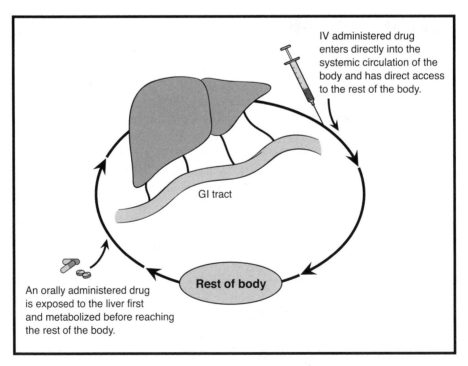

Figure 2-1. Medications administered by the oral route of administration may be subject to "first pass" metabolism by hepatic enzymes, reducing the amount of administered drug that reaches the systemic circulation

the gastrointestinal tract, and the "first pass" through the liver, a considerable portion of the administered dose can be metabolized to pharmacologically inactive metabolites by the gastrointestinal enzymes and microsomal (P450) or glucuronide enzymes in the liver. Other factors that affect bioavailability are discussed in the sidebar.

BIOAVAILABILITY

As discussed in the text, **bioavailability** is defined as "the rate and extent to which the active ingredient or active moiety [the active part of the drug molecule] is absorbed from a drug product and becomes available at the site of action."[2] Put more simply, **bioavailability** is expressed as a percent and represents the fraction of administered drug that eventually reaches the systemic circulation. For example, if 30 mg of oral morphine were administered by mouth, and 10 mg of the drug was absorbed unchanged, the bioavailability would be 1/3, or 33%.

You learned how the **"first pass effect"** can dramatically affect bioavailability, as is the case with drugs such as fentanyl (metabolized to inactive metabolites by the P450 system), morphine (metabolized to active and potentially toxic metabolites via glucuronidation), lidocaine and nitroglycerin. We can minimize this effect by giving nitroglycerin by the sublingual route, bypassing the liver prior to absorption, or administering lidocaine topically (LidoDerm transdermal patch) or intravenously.

Another factor that influences the bioavailability of drug is its **solubility**. Medications that are either extremely water-soluble (hydrophilic) or extremely lipid-soluble (hydrophobic or lipophilic) are poorly absorbed either because they cannot cross the lipid-rich cell membranes or they cannot dissolve into solution. For optimal drug absorption it must be primarily lipophilic, but be sufficiently soluble in aqueous solutions.

Some medications are unstable in the pH of gastric contents, such as penicillin G. Other medications, such as insulin, are <u>degraded</u> by enzymes in the gastrointestinal tract.

Last, the nature of the **drug formulation** (e.g., tablet or capsule) can influence the bioavailability. This includes factors such as drug particle size, salt form, crystal polymorphism and the presence of various excipients. **Excipient** is a fancy word for "all the stuff aside from the drug itself in the tablet or capsule." Examples include the following:

- Lubricants
- Granulating agent
- Filler (to bulk up tablet or capsule so it's not too small)
- Wetting agent (to assist with penetration of water into the tablet)
- Disintegration agent (helps the tablet break apart)

Excipients can enhance tablet or capsule dissolution, and therefore alter the rate and extent of absorption.

Buccal or Sublingual

Occasionally we need to administer opioids in the buccal or sublingual cavity. Fentanyl is now available as a transmucosal tablet and lozenge on a stick intended for buccal administration. Highly concentrated oral opioid solutions are frequently instilled in the buccal or sublingual cavity. Only a small portion of the oral solution is actually absorbed transmucosally, but the portion that does get absorbed through the mucosal members in the mouth bypasses the liver, therefore is not subject to a first pass effect. Transmucosally absorbed opioids have a rapid onset of action due to the good blood supply to the area of absorption. The rest of the medication is swallowed and absorbed subject to the first pass effect. Disadvantages to buccal/sublingual opioid administration include the inconvenience of holding the dosage formulation in the mouth, and the relatively poor transmucosal absorption of morphine and oxycodone. Rapid-acting fentanyl products will be discussed in greater detail in Chapter 4, and they have a much higher degree of transmucosal absorption than morphine or oxycodone solution.

Rectal

Medications administered by the rectal route are commonly suppositories or enemas. Morphine and hydromorphone are commercially available as rectal suppositories. Opioid suppositories inserted just past the rectal sphincter avoid first-pass hepatic metabolism, although suppositories inserted higher into the rectal vault are absorbed into the superior rectal vein that empties into the hepatic circulation, resulting in first-pass metabolism. Morphine rectal suppositories are approximately bioequivalent to oral morphine (1:1 dosing conversion), and are usually dosed every 4 hours.[7] There is less data on the bioequivalence of rectal hydromorphone, however most practitioners would consider hydromorphone suppositories bioequivalent to oral hydromorphone due to similar pharmacokinetics as morphine. Rectal hydromorphone seems to have a longer duration of action possibly due to reduced first-pass metabolism or slower absorption, so the FDA approved dosing interval is every 6 hours. Although rectal methadone is not commercially available, evidence shows it is approximately bioequivalent to oral methadone.

Although not approved by the FDA, controlled-release oral morphine tablets have been administered rectally to cancer patients (every 12 hours) and provided as good or better absorption than when administered orally. Generally practitioners use a 1:1 ratio for oral:controlled-release morphine tablets administered rectally, although the rectal dose may require dosage reduction due to increased sedation from better absorption.[8-9] Controlled-release oxycodone tablets have also been administered by rectum, and show a significantly higher "area under the curve" (39% increase) and a higher maximum concentration (9%) due to enhanced drug absorption.[10]

The rectal route of administration is not appropriate for all patients. First, patients tend not to LIKE this route, and it makes for uncomfortable family dynamics when a 60 year old man has to administer a rectal suppository to his 85 year old mother. In addition to emotional discomfort, rectal products can be physically uncomfortable for patients with advanced illnesses. Patients who are dehydrated may have insufficient fluid in the rectal vault to absorb medications delivered by this route. Rectal drug products should not be administered into surgically created openings, and are less helpful in patients with diarrhea, colostomy, hemorrhoids, anal fissures or in neutropenic patients.[8]

Last, it is important to recognize that there is a high degree of inter-individual absorption variability in rectally-administered medications. Even though the rectal administration of oral controlled-release morphine and oxycodone is possible, it is important to remember that this is not an FDA-approved route of administration, and is probably not a good long-term drug administration strategy. Rectal doses can be expelled before they are fully absorbed and if the lower rectum is filled with stool, absorption will also be limited. This can only be proven by performing a rectal examination, and for obvious reasons, this creates an additional burden for the patient and caregiver.

Parenteral

When we speak of parenteral drug administration we are generally referring to intravenous (IV), subcutaneous (SQ) and intramuscular (IM) administration, which are injected into the vein, subcutaneous tissue or a muscle respectively (Figure 2-2). As discussed previously, medications administered by the IV route are 100% bioavailable. Drugs can be injected into a peripheral vein over several minutes, or administered by an intermittent or continuous infusion. The IV route allows the fastest onset of drug action. Disadvantages to the IV route of administration include the need to find a suitable vein, which in turn requires trained personnel and more expensive equipment to administer the drug. Patients are also frequently fearful of more invasive or painful medications given by injection.

Subcutaneous administration of a medication involves much less equipment and may be administered by the patient or a family member. While absorption is slower than an IV injection, it is usually complete. Opioids may be administered by intermittent SQ injections, or continuous SQ infusion. Disadvantages to this route of administration include potential discomfort, local tissue irritation, and probably most importantly, the need to limit the volume injected (because the subcutaneous tissue has a limited capacity to absorb fluid). Some references site a maximum of 2 mL per injection, or 1–2 mL/hour of continuous SQ infusion.

What do plastic silverwear, jumbo shrimp, and an intramuscular opioid all have in common? They are all oxymorons! An IM injection is painful, which is kind of a kick in the pants when we're administering an analgesic! The American Pain Society

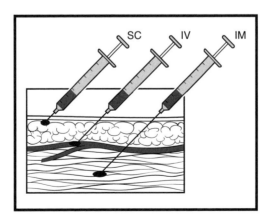

Figure 2-2. Commonly used parenteral injections include subcutaneous (SC), intravenous (IV), and intramuscular (IM).

recommends that the IM route of administration be abandoned for this reason, as well as wide fluctuations in absorption from the site of injection, a 30- to 60-minute lag time to peak analgesic effect, and rapid falloff of action when compared to oral administration. Chronic use of IM injections can also lead to nerve injury with persistent neuropathic pain, sterile abscess formation and muscle/soft tissue fibrosis.[11]

As you can see in the Equianalgesic Opioid Dosing Table, there is no differentiation between IV, SQ and IM dosing in the "parenteral" column. Therefore, this implies a 1:1:1 ratio in dosing. If only life were that straightforward! Since we have already voted IM opioids off the island, let's focus on IV and SQ comparisons. Pharmacokinetic studies comparing SQ vs. IV continuous infusions of identical doses of both morphine and hydromorphone have shown comparable plasma concentrations. Further, the SQ and IV route provided equivalent analgesia and adverse effects.[12-13] The subcutaneous route is preferred for the reasons described above, particularly for a patient at home without established IV access. With high doses however, absorption may be more variable with SQ injections/infusion, and may require dosage adjustment. Some literature suggests that the relative potency ratio of SQ to oral morphine is between 1:2 and 1:3 with doses in excess of 10 mg/hour (our table states it is 1:3 regardless of the parenteral route of administration, but this data bears consideration), while IV to oral morphine is predictably closer to the 1:3 ratio.[7]

Well, I'm sure that discussion left you holding your head in your hands! Let's jump into some calculations to clear the water! You can start by wearing your life vest and you'll be swimming with the sharks by the end of the chapter!

Remember the steps outlined in Chapter 1 Table 1-2 that summarize the five steps in opioid conversion calculations. Table 2-2 shows FOUR possible conversion calculation methods; what a deal! You can do a simple ratio in your head (not recommended) or on paper (A), a mathematical proportion using cross-multiplication (B and C), or a mathematical proportion using ratios (D). We'll use methods B and D primarily, but method A is a good way to check yourself!

 CASE 2.1

. . . .

Same Opioid, Same Route of Administration (Oral), Different Formulation

HW is an 84 year old man in a long term care facility with general debility. He has moderate pain from spinal stenosis, and other general aches and pains. HW has been having transient ischemic attacks (TIAs) and he has had increasing difficulty swallowing solid food and medications. Up to this point, his pain was well controlled on Percocet (5 mg oxycodone/325 mg acetaminophen per tablet), six tablets daily. To accommodate his difficulty swallowing, HW just had a feeding tube placed, and his physician asked that you convert HW to a liquid formulation to provide an equivalent degree of pain relief. HW tells you that the six Percocet tablets per day did a good job controlling his pain. You decide to switch HW to the Roxicet oral solution, which contains 5 mg oxycodone and 325 mg acetaminophen per 5 mL. What would be the correct regimen to recommend to HW's physician? Let's look at our five-step opioid conversion calculation process.

Step 1—HW's pain is well controlled on six Percocet tablets per day. When he was able to take the tablets he was able to do his limited activities of daily living, and he reported

Table 2-2
Calculating the New Opioid Dose

Just as there are several ways to pluck a chicken, so are there several ways you can use the Equianalgesic Opioid Dosing Table data to calculate the dose of the opioid you are switching to. Several examples are as follows:

- **Simple ratio (Method A)**

  - Oral morphine to oral morphine is a 1:1 conversion (or 30 mg:30 mg conversion). There is no dividing or multiplying to be done; oral morphine is oral morphine!

  - Oral morphine to parenteral morphine is a 3:1 conversion (or 30 mg:10 mg conversion)

  - You can apply the simple ratio practically in your head (not recommended) by dividing or multiplying by three.

  - Even when switching from one opioid to another you can do a simple ratio. For example, oral hydromorphone to oral morphine is a 1:4 ratio (or 7.5 mg:30 mg conversion). If the patient is getting 8 mg of oral hydromorphone per day, this would be approximately 32 mg of oral morphine per day

- **Mathematical proportion using cross multiplication (Methods B and C)**

  - Set up a simple mathematical proportion using ratios. This can be done several ways, but the important thing is that the ratios on both sides of the equation are parallel. Here are two examples (reminder: TDD = total daily dose):

  - Method B:

    Actual Drug Doses: Equianalgesic Data from Chart:
    $$\frac{\text{``X'' mg TDD new opioid}}{\text{mg TDD current opioid}} = \frac{\text{equianalgesic factor of new opioid}}{\text{equianalgesic factor of current opioid}}$$

  - Method C

    New Opioid   Current Opioid
    $$\frac{\text{``X'' mg TDD new opioid}}{\text{equianalgesic factor of new opioid}} = \frac{\text{mg TDD current opioid}}{\text{equianalgesic factors of current opioid}}$$

- **Mathematical proportion using ratio (Method D)**

  - Instead of cross-multiplying, you can directly apply the ratio to the current total daily dose, and end up with the new opioid total daily dose as follows:

    $$\text{TDD current opioid} \times \frac{\text{equianalgesic factor of new opioid}}{\text{equianalgesic factor of current opioid}} = \text{TDD new opioid}$$

Wow! So many possible equations, so little time! I suggest you stick with method B or D, and keep method A as your "does that LOOK right?" method. Or, use method B, and use method D to check yourself! Whatever you pick, be consistent!!

he was comfortable. There appears to be no reason to suspect he should be switched to a different opioid, or have any co-analgesics added.

Step 2—HW has been consistently taking six Percocet tablets (5 mg oxycodone/325 mg acetaminophen per tablet) per day, giving a total daily dose (TDD) of oxycodone of 30 mg. The acetaminophen dose is less important, but should always be less than 4 grams per day (and lower in some patients).

Step 3—We have already chosen our new formulation (Roxicet Oral Solution, 5 mg oxycodone/325 mg acetaminophen per 5 mL). This conversion is very straight forward! Oral oxycodone is oral oxycodone, and the amount of oxycodone (5 mg) in one tablet HW was taking happens to be the same as the amount of oxycodone (5 mg) in a teaspoon of the solution. This makes your life a bit easier, but don't get used to it—things won't always be this easy! The bioavailability of oxycodone from the tablet formulation is very similar to that of the oral solution, therefore the dose is the same: 30 mg TDD oxycodone.

Step 4—In this step we individualize the dose for the patient. There is no need to increase the dose because HW's pain was well controlled on 30 mg oxycodone per day, and there is no need to decrease the dose due to increased sensitivity to the new opioid (because we're not SWITCHING opioids—we're going from oxycodone to oxycodone—same drug!). Therefore HW's new regimen is the same TDD (30 mg oxycodone), given as Roxicet Oral Solution, 5 mg oxycodone/325 mg acetaminophen (5 mL) every 4 hours by feeding tube. The last piece of business in individualizing the dose for HW is determining when to begin therapy with the new formulation. Since Percocet tablets only last approximately 4 hours, HW can begin the Roxicet Oral Solution anytime four or more hours after his last Percocet tablet.

Step 5—HW begins therapy with the Roxicet Oral Solution. The nursing staff in the long term care facility monitor HW closely. He has no complaints of sedation, confusion, nausea, or any other adverse effects. It has been 24 hours since his last Percocet tablet was administered (he received a very small dose of SQ morphine when the feeding tube was placed), but by the time HW had been receiving the Roxicet Oral Solution for 24 hours, he said he pain control was acceptable. You would continue to monitor HW and adjust his regimen as clinically indicated. Of course, if he continued to require more oxycodone you would have to be cautious of the acetaminophen dose, and perhaps switch to a single ingredient oxycodone oral solution product.

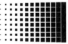 **CASE 2.2**
•••
Same Opioid, Same Route of Administration (Oral), Different Formulation

RS is a 62 year old man with a history of renal cancer, no metastatic disease noted. He has been experiencing visceral pain for the past several months, and his physician prescribed Opana IR (immediate-release oxymorphone hydrochloride 5 mg), 1–2 tablets every 4–6 hours as needed for pain. He has been taking six or seven tablets daily with fairly good pain control. He rates his pain as a daily best of 3 (on a scale of 0 = no pain, 10 = worst imaginable pain), a daily worst pain of 7, and an average of 4 or 5. He states that this level of pain control allows him to perform most of his activities of daily living, but he feels that the pain management could be improved. He does complain about having to either get up during the night to take another dose of Opana IR, or of awakening in pain. What should be done?

Step 1—You have carefully assessed RS's pain and have determined that he continues to experience nociceptive pain that is unlikely to be metastatic bone pain. You do not suspect neuropathic pain because the patient does not use any descriptors suggestive of neuropathic pain (stabbing, shooting, burning pain), and he has a normal neurologic exam. The pain has responded fairly well to six or seven Opana IR tablets, but there is room for improvement.

Step 2—We can calculate the total daily dose (TDD) of oxymorphone RS is receiving as follows: six or seven tablets of oxymorphone, 5 mg per tablet for a TDD of 30–35 mg. He is taking no other analgesic medications.

Step 3—Oxymorphone is available as a sustained-release tablet (Opana ER), which is dosed every 12 hours. This would allow RS to sleep through the night without having to redose, and hopefully to not awaken in pain. Oral oxymorphone has approximately 10% bioavailability, and the immediate-release and extended-release tablets are equivalent. Therefore, the equivalent TDD of extended-release oxymorphone would be 30–35 mg.

Step 4—Because RS's pain is likely visceral, he shown good response to oxymorphone, and his pain is not quite controlled, a dosage increase would seem reasonable. Opana ER is available as 5-, 10-, 20- and 40-mg tablets. An increase in the TDD to 40 mg seems reasonable, which could be accomplished with a regimen of Opana ER 20 mg po q12h. RS could keep the Opana IR 5 mg tablets for additional or unanticipated pain. The Opana ER could be started approximately 4 hours after the last Opana IR tablet.

Step 5—RS should be monitored clinically, and he should be encouraged to use a pain diary to record his pain ratings, and his use of Opana IR tablets. This will assist his health care team in titrating his long-acting oral opioid regimen.

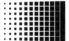

CASE 2.3

· ·

Same Opioid, Same Route of Administration (Oral), Different Formulation

PL is an 82 year old woman living in an assisted living facility with lung cancer, with widespread metastatic disease, including bone involvement. PL also has end-stage Alzheimer's disease. As her Alzheimer's disease has worsened her health care team has assessed her pain by observing her behavior, particularly during personal care. PL's pain was being managed with morphine sulfate immediate-release tablets, 15 mg po q4h until she began "pocketing" the tablets (between the cheek and the gum), which she later spit out. Her physician switched her to morphine sulfate oral solution at the same dose and dosing interval, but PL found it amusing to shoot the morphine solution out between her clenched teeth. PL's physician asks your help in treating this patient's pain.

Step 1—On close observation you determine that PL grimaces and moans loudly when receiving personal care. She seems to be guarding her right side, and is particularly disinclined to roll over on that side. Her physician agrees that it is likely that this behavior is due to painful metastatic bone disease. In response to this, you recommended adding a nonsteroidal anti-inflammatory drug such as naproxen, which PL takes with no commotion. She continues to spit out the morphine solution, and you aren't even sure how much she has been getting per day thanks to these antics. The naproxen has reduced but not eliminated behaviors that are thought to be related to pain, therefore the decision has been made to continue PL on morphine, provided an acceptable regimen can be identified.

Step 2 — Had PL been taking all the morphine prescribed for her, this would be a TDD of 90 mg (15 mg po q4h = 15 x 6 times per day = 90 mg). The aides caring for PL estimate that she has been actually swallowing about 60% of her prescribed morphine per day since she started "acting out."

Step 3 — You decide to try Kadian, a once or twice a day long-acting morphine capsule that can be swallowed whole, or opened and the contents administered by a gastrostomy tube or sprinkled on soft food such as applesauce. Since PL adores applesauce, you decide to go with this option. Based on an estimated TDD of 54 mg of morphine from the morphine solution PL was taking (60% of 90 mg TDD), it would be the same TDD of Kadian.

Step 4 — So should you keep the TDD of 54 mg, increase it, or decrease it? Since you don't know for SURE how much morphine PL was getting, it would be prudent to go with a lower TDD of Kadian. You have also decided to go with a q12h regimen so you can closely monitor PL's progress. Kadian is available as 10-, 20-, 30-, 50-, 60-, 80-, 100-, and 200-mg capsules. You decide to begin with Kadian 20 mg po q12h sprinkled on applesauce. The morphine oral solution is still available for additional breakthrough pain as needed (e.g., every 4 hours). Kadian therapy can begin at any time 4 hours after PL's last dose of oral morphine solution.

Step 5 — After instituting this plan, PL responded very well. Her pain seemed to be well controlled as evidenced by significantly less difficulty providing personal care. PL was happy to eat her applesauce twice daily (without crunching the morphine particles), with 20 mg of Kadian sprinkled on top. PL probably thought they were sprinkles — otherwise she probably would have pulled some other hijinks!

▣▣▣▣ FAST FACT ▶ Using Long-Acting Morphine Capsules

When opening a Kadian or Avinza capsule, and sprinkling the contents on applesauce there are several important things to remember.

- Do not use a large quantity of applesauce — this is not a meal, merely a drug delivery vehicle. A tablespoon or two should be sufficient.

- Never use a large quantity of applesauce with a higher strength capsule and attempt to give only a portion of the mixture. Use exactly the capsule strength prescribed ONLY.

- Make sure the patient is able to swallow the morphine/applesauce mixture without crunching or chewing the beads, which are extended-release. Have the patient rinse his/her mouth and swallow when done the morphine/applesauce mixture to avoid having a little sustained-release snack hiding behind a molar.

- Do NOT heat the applesauce! Do not sprinkle cinnamon on the applesauce! Do not get out your Easy Bake Oven and whip up a batch of Apple Cinnamon Morphine Muffins! There is no data on the stability of the morphine should you heat this mixture, and other foodstuffs should not be added to the mixture!

CASE 2.4

•••

Same Opioid, Different Formulation and Route of Administration (Oral to Rectal)

KT is a 72 year old woman with advanced stage pancreatic cancer. She had recently been in the hospital receiving a low-dose morphine IV infusion for pain control, and was converted to oral morphine solution for discharge home when she decided not to pursue any additional chemotherapy. KT's pain was well controlled on morphine 10 mg oral solution, but she started throwing up after most doses, and her pain has returned. KT's physician has prescribed haloperidol for the nausea and vomiting, but it has had little impact. KT is likely to die within the next 48 hours. What do you recommend?

Step 1—KT is very weak but she states that the pain is exactly the type and intensity she had in the hospital, which responded very well to the morphine infusion. She tells you the oral morphine solution worked well also when she was able to keep it down. She does not have complaints or physical findings that are suggestive of metastatic bone pain or neuropathy, therefore it seems appropriate to continue the morphine.

Step 2—KT achieved good pain relief with a TDD of 60 mg oral morphine when she was able to take the oral morphine solution.

Step 3—Since morphine worked well for KT, she is close to death, and she has a strong family support system and caregivers in place, you decide to switch her to rectal morphine suppositories. As you know, oral:rectal morphine is 1:1 and the dosing interval is the same for immediate-release oral morphine and rectal morphine suppositories (q4h). You can obviously figure this out in your head (morphine 10 per rectum every 4 hours), or you can set up a mathematical proportion by ratio (Method D) as follows:

$$\text{TDD current opioid} \times \frac{\text{equianalgesic factor of new opioid}}{\text{equianalgesic factor of current opioid}} = \text{TDD new opioid}$$

$$\text{TDD 60 mg oral morphine} \times \frac{30 \text{ mg rectal morphine}}{30 \text{ mg oral morphine}} = \text{TDD mg pr morphine}$$

Cancel out like units as shown below:

$$\text{TDD 60 } \cancel{\text{mg oral morphine}} \times \frac{30 \text{ mg rectal morphine}}{30 \text{ } \cancel{\text{mg oral morphine}}} = \text{TDD mg pr morphine}$$

Solve for TDD mg pr morphine: 60 × 30/30 = 60

The TDD rectal morphine is 60 mg.

Step 4—We have no reason to increase the TDD morphine dose because her pain was well controlled on this regimen previously. We have no reason to reduce the TDD because we are not switching opioids (going from morphine to morphine), so the only thing left to consider is can we DO morphine by rectal suppository 10 mg every 4 hours? By golly we can—morphine rectal suppositories are available as 5-, 10-, 20-, and 30-mg suppositories. You definitely don't want to get into the business of carving up commercially available suppositories to create new strengths. If you really feel the need for a different strength rectal suppository, talk to a pharmacist who can compound (these people are angels of mercy) and they can whip you up a batch. Fortunately, we can rock and roll with an order for "morphine 10 mg by rectal suppository every 4 hours." Since the patient threw up her last dose of MSIR, you can start the rectal morphine suppositories as soon as they are delivered.

Step 5—You would monitor KT's response as she uses the morphine suppositories for both therapeutic effect (pain relief) and potential toxicity, particularly nausea. An important point to mention is that as KT declines, she may lose consciousness. Sometimes family members, caregivers, and even other health care providers question the continued need for the opioid once a patient becomes obtunded. If the patient is free from physical signs of opioid overdose (e.g., reduced respirations, pinpoint pupils), there is no reason to suspect the pain magically went away, so you should continue the opioid throughout the duration of the patient's life. However, if the patient becomes oliguric, leading you to suspect reduced renal clearance, the dosing may be extended. Each cased must be assessed independently, since physiologic functions, especially at life's end, are variable among patients.

P E A R L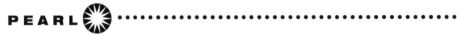

In the case of KT (Case 2.4), if she had been receiving MS Contin 30 mg po q12h and experienced nausea and vomiting, what could you have done? Certainly you could have calculated her TDD of oral morphine to be 60 mg, and again gone with the morphine 10 mg rectal suppository every 4 hours. Alternately, if KT lived far from the pharmacy, or was even closer to death, you could insert an MS Contin tablet rectally, 30 mg pr q12h. As discussed in the text, the tablet would have fairly equivalent bioavailability, and should keep KT comfortable. I generally do not order a large quantity (e.g., a month's worth) of long-acting morphine tablets with the idea of giving them rectally for as long as needed, but for a patient who is very close to death, or in a situation where you are unable to get the dosage formulation you'd prefer, this is an acceptable option. Remember, this is not an FDA-approved route of administration for these tablets.

 C A S E 2 . 5

Same Opioid, Different Formulation and Route of Administration (Oral to Parenteral)

WP is a 62 year old man with multiple myeloma and diffuse bony metastasis admitted to hospice several weeks ago. His analgesic regimen has been increased since admission to his current regimen of extended-release morphine 30 mg po q12h, plus morphine oral solution 10 mg every 2 hours as needed for breakthrough pain. WP is also receiving dexamethasone 4 mg po twice daily for bone pain, senna-S tablets twice daily to prevent constipation, temazepam 15 mg po at bedtime, and lorazepam 1 mg po q4h as needed for anxiety. Over the past few days WP's wife tells you the patient has been taking the immediate-release morphine approximately six times during a 24-hour period. When you visit the patient you review the pain diary and confirm that WP really has been taking five to six doses of the immediate-release morphine over a 24-hour period for the previous three days. Despite this, WP is complaining of pain that he rates as 5–7 (on a 0 = no pain, 10 = worst imaginable pain scale). WP has also been taking the lorazepam around the clock due to extreme agitation and worry about the pain, and he claims the bedtime temazepam is marginally effective. WP accepts your offer of in-patient admission to switch to parenteral morphine for more rapid titration.

Step 1—WP and his wife are obviously distressed over WP's pain situation. He is very fearful of the meaning of the pain (disease progression, approaching death, etc.). WP is especially terrified that the pain will never get under control and that he will die a particularly undignified death. WP's physician feels that increasing the dexamethasone is unlikely to provide significantly more relief, and that IV morphine is the best way to go. WP does not describe the pain such that the physician suspects neuropathic pain, nor are there physical findings to suggest such.

Step 2—As described in the case above, WP was receiving extended-release morphine tablets, 30 mg po q12h plus five to six daily doses of immediate-release morphine 10 mg oral solution. WP's TDD of morphine is calculated as follows: 30 mg po q12h = 30 × 2 = 60 mg, PLUS 10 mg po q2h prn × 5 doses a day = 10 × 5 = 50 mg, for a GRAND TDD of 110 mg oral morphine.

Step 3—WP's physician has asked that you calculate an appropriate starting dose of IV morphine for the patient. An IV line was started, and the plan is to dose WP every 4 hours with morphine and increase the dose as clinically indicated. The first step is to determine how much IV morphine would replace a TDD of 110 mg oral morphine. We can calculate this using the mathematical proportion by ratio (Method D) as follows:

$$\text{TDD current opioid} \times \frac{\text{equianalgesic factor of new opioid}}{\text{equianalgesic factor of current opioid}} = \text{TDD new opioid}$$

$$\text{TDD 110 mg oral morphine} \times \frac{10 \text{ mg IV morphine}}{30 \text{ mg oral morphine}} = \text{TDD mg IV morphine}$$

Cancel out like units as shown below:

$$\text{TDD 110 } \cancel{\text{mg oral morphine}} \times \frac{10 \text{ mg IV morphine}}{30 \cancel{\text{mg oral morphine}}} = \text{TDD mg IV morphine}$$

Solve for TDD mg IV morphine: 110 × 10/30 = 36.7

The TDD IV morphine is 36.7 mg.

Step 4—At this point we need to decide whether to go with the 36.7 mg TDD IV morphine, to increase the dose, or decrease the dose. First the easy one—we would NOT decrease the dose due to incomplete cross-tolerance because we are not switching opioids (we're going from morphine to morphine). We could go with the 36.7 mg, divide by 6 to get our every 4 hour dose, and increase from there, but we already KNOW the patient is in pain. We also know the pain is opioid-responsive, we just need to give MORE morphine. Therefore, it would clinically appropriate to increase the TDD of morphine at this time.

You will learn more about opioid titration in Chapter 4, but for now accept that a 25–50% increase would be appropriate. Twenty-five percent of 36.7 mg is 45.9 mg; an order for morphine 7.5 mg IV every 4 hours would be a 25% increase from his previous morphine regimen.

When should he start this new regimen? The last dose of extended-release morphine was administered about 7 hours ago, with two doses of the immediate-release morphine given since with the last one given 3 hours ago. WP is complaining of considerable pain now, thanks to the ambulance ride and all the transfer maneuvers. It would be appropriate to give WP his first IV injection of 7.5 mg morphine NOW.

Step 5—After giving an IV injection of morphine, WP's pain level should be assessed within 20-60 minutes. The onset of action of IV morphine is 2–4 minutes, with approximate time to peak of 15–20 minutes. It will take 12–24 hours to achieve steady state with this dosage increase, but WP should be getting more pain relief from this increased dose, starting with the very first dose. If he does NOT achieve pain relief with the first injection, it would be appropriate to consider a modest increase in the next injection (about 25–50%), such as 10 mg morphine IV. Continued use of the original or this higher dose requires continuous monitoring for sedation and other potential toxicities of morphine.

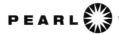 **P E A R L** ●

Monitoring for Oversedation
One method used frequently to monitor the "sleepiness" index from opioid therapy is referred to as the "Modified Ramsay Scale" for rating sedation. Originally published in 1974, Figure 2-3 is an adapted version.

Indication	Score
Patient is anxious, agitated, restless	1
Patient is awake, cooperative, oriented, tranquil	2
Patient is semi-asleep, responds to commands only	3
Patient asleep but responds briskly to glabellar tap, loud auditory stimulus, or gentle shaking	4
Patient asleep with sluggish or decreased response to glabellar tap, loud auditory stimulus, or other noxious stimuli	5
Patient does not respond to firm nailbed pressure or other noxious stimuli	6

Figure 2-3. Modified Ramsay Scale. *Source:* Adapted from references 15 and 16.

The goal would be a level of arousal rated as a 2; 3 or 4 is acceptable but warrants close monitoring, 5 is not a good look, and 6 is really bad news. If the patient is over-sedated, you would need to hold the next dose of opioid, and perhaps lower the dose and/or extend the dosing interval. Rarely do you need to resort to using an opioid antagonist such as naloxone.

CASE 2.6

•••

Same Opioid, Different Formulation and Route of Administration (Parenteral to Oral)

Let's look at the reverse of the previous case. CR is a 62 year old man recently diagnosed with colon cancer, who was admitted for surgical resection of the lesion. Post-operatively he was given hydromorphone 2 mg SQ every 4 hours as needed for pain control. On day 1 he used 12 mg of SQ hydromorphone, day 2 he used 10 mg, day 3 he used 8 mg. This is the morning of day 4 and he is preparing for discharge. CR has a past history of itching when taking oxycodone, therefore the physician does not want to transition the patient to Percocet as is her usual habit. Instead, she wants to discharge the patient with oral hydromorphone and asks your advice on dosing. What do you recommend?

Step 1—On reviewing CR's chart, you see that he has used less and less hydromorphone each day, and he reports good pain control. His last dose of hydromorphone was 3 hours ago, and he is rating his pain as a 2 or 3 (on a 0 = no pain, 10 = worst imaginable pain scale). His pain is entirely consistent with a normal post-operative course, and there does not seem to be any reason to consider adding a co-analgesic at this time.

Step 2—Over the 24-hour period of day 3, CR used 8 mg of SQ hydromorphone (TDD).

Step 3—The physician has already stated that she would like to transition CR to oral hydromorphone since hydromorphone has worked very well for this patient, and it is less likely to cause itching (which is a "pseudoallergic" reaction to opioids, probably related to histamine release).

Consulting our Equianalgesic Opioid Dosing Table, we see that 1.5 mg parenteral hydromorphone is approximately equivalent to 7.5 mg oral hydromorphone. If we use a simple ratio, this is a 5-fold difference. Therefore, we can do a simple ratio and determine that this would be 5 times the 8 mg TDD SQ hydromorphone, or 40 mg TDD oral hydromorphone. Alternately, we could use the mathematical proportion using cross multiplication method:

Actual Drug Doses: **Equianalgesic Data from Chart:**

$$\frac{\text{``X'' mg TDD new opioid}}{\text{mg TDD current opioid}} = \frac{\text{equianalgesic factor of new opioid}}{\text{equianalgesic factor of current opioid}}$$

Filling in the numbers we find:

$$\frac{\text{``X'' mg TDD new opioid}}{\text{8 mg TDD SQ hydromorphone}} = \frac{\text{7.5 mg oral hydromorphone}}{\text{1.5 mg parenteral hydromorphone}}$$

We cross multiply:

$$(8) \times (7.5) = (X) \times (1.5)$$
$$60 = X \times 1.5$$
$$X = 40$$

This method also shows the TDD oral hydromorphone would be 40 mg.

Let's do the calculation using the mathematical proportion by ratio (Method D) just for grins, as follows:

$$\text{TDD current opioid} \times \frac{\text{equianalgesic factor of new opioid}}{\text{equianalgesic factor of current opioid}} = \text{TDD new opioid}$$

$$\text{TDD 8 mg SQ hydromorphone} \times \frac{\text{7.5 mg oral hydromorphone}}{\text{1.5 mg SQ hydromorphone}} = \text{TDD mg oral hydromorphone}$$

Cancel out like units as shown below:

$$\text{TDD 8} \; \cancel{\text{mg SQ hydromorphone}} \times \frac{\text{7.5 mg oral hydromorphone}}{\text{1.5} \; \cancel{\text{mg SQ hydromorphone}}} = \text{TDD mg oral hydromorphone}$$

Doing the math shows us: $8 \times 7.5/1.5 = 8 \times 5 = 40$ mg.

Confirming for the THIRD time the TDD of oral hydromorphone is 40 mg. Eureka! I'm convinced!

 P I T F A L L •

So What IS the Bioavailability of Oral Hydromorphone?

As you learned in Chapter 1, there is wide reported range for hydromorphone bioavailability (29–95%; average 50%). In fact, many practitioners use a 1:2 (parenteral:oral) conversion, rather than the 1:5 (parenteral:oral) shown in the Equianalgesic Opioid Dosing Table. The 1:5 ratio is shown in the Equianalgesic Opioid Dosing Table because this is what *most* practitioners use, but the evidence suggests it's closer to 1:2. Just keep that in mind as we continue working through this problem!

• •

Step 4—Working from an equivalent TDD of oral hydromorphone is 40 mg, we must decide if we should increase the dose, decrease the dose, or run with the 40 mg. Since CR's pain is well controlled at this time, so there's no need to increase the dose. Further, CR has been using less and less SQ hydromorphone every day since surgery—his pain is getting better on its own. Therefore, it would be reasonable to expect he would continue to improve, and we can reduce this dose for discharge.

If we look at the oral equivalent of CR's use of hydromorphone since surgery it would be 60 mg, 50 mg, and then 40 mg. As we think ahead to discharge, hydromorphone is available as 2-, 4-, and 8- mg tablets. CR is able to swallow tablets, therefore this makes the most sense. We generally dose hydromorphone every 4 hours. If we recommend 6 mg every 4 hours that's a potential TDD of 36 mg oral hydromorphone. If we recommend 4 mg every 4 hours that's a potential TDD of 24 mg oral hydromorphone. A TDD of 36 mg seems a bit excessive given how quickly his pain is improving. Remember, however, that many practitioner follow the 1:2 (parenteral:oral hydromorphone) conversion, which would tell us that an 8 mg TDD of parenteral hydromorphine is equivalent to as little as 16 mg TDD oral hydromorphone. Therefore, we will recommend to CR's physician that she prescribe no more than hydromorphone 4 mg by mouth every 4 hours as needed for pain. We will also encourage CR to maintain a pain diary over the next few days. We could even anticipate his opioid requirements declining further over the next few days (especially if his bioavailability of hydromorphone is on the higher end), and recommend the physician prescribe the 2-mg tablet, allowing the patient to self-taper off opioids (e.g., use (one or) two 2-mg tablets every 4 hours initially for a day or two, then reduce to one 2-mg tablet every 4 hours for a day or two, then halve the tablets or discontinue therapy).

Step 5 – As discussed above, we will ask CR to maintain a pain diary, recording his pain ratings and use of hydromorphone. We will also do a phone follow-up to ask about his ability to perform activities of daily living, and his ability to sleep and ambulate. We will ask CR's wife to monitor his level of arousal/sedation to make sure he doesn't become too sedated, and we will encourage CR to use a bowel regimen if necessary and ask about constipation.

Wow! We've talked about several situations where we need to switch from one formulation or route of administration to another using the same opioid. You have learned about several methods to calculate the dose you are switching to, and have seen how all roads really do lead to Rome! It's a good idea to use one method for your calculation, and another method to check yourself. Also, ALWAYS use common sense. When you are switching from a parenteral to a non-parenteral route, the dose will ALWAYS be higher. When you are switching from a non-parenteral to a parenteral route, the TDD will ALWAYS be lower! On to the practice problems—your ears aren't ringing enough yet!

PRACTICE PROBLEMS

P2.1. Same Opioid, Same Route of Administration (Oral to Oral/Buccal), Different Formulation

IR is an 86 year old woman with dementia and uterine cancer. She is very confused and has difficulty swallowing tablets, so her prescriber put her on Avinza (once-daily extended-release morphine capsule), and titrated her to 60 mg once daily, sprinkled on applesauce. She is close to death at this point, and eating applesauce is not an option. Because IR is in a long term care facility, the prescriber would like to avoid starting parenteral morphine. You suggested switching IR to a morphine oral concentrated solution, and instilling it in the buccal cavity. The prescriber thinks that's a fabulous idea and asks you to determine an equivalent dosage regimen to Avinza 60 mg po qd.

P2.2. Same Opioid, Different Formulation and Route of Administration (Oral to Rectal)

HZ is a 92 year old man who lives at home, diagnosed with lung cancer. His pain has been well controlled on hydromorphone 2 mg, 1–2 tablets every 4 hours as needed. His average TDD over the past few days is 14–16 mg. At this time he is unable to swallow either hydromorphone tablets or oral solution, and you decide to switch him to hydromorphone rectal suppositories. What dose and regimen do you recommend and when should it start?

P2.3. Same Opioid, Same Route of Administration (Oral), Different Formulation

LK is a 42 year old man who injured his back several years ago while unloading a truck. He has had three back surgeries since his initial injury and is no longer a surgical candidate. At present LK complains of pain in his sacral area, which he rates as a best of 2 and a worst of 4 on average per day (on a 0 = no pain, 10 = worst imaginable pain) while taking his pain medications. At present LK is taking the following analgesic regimen:

- Percocet (10 mg oxycodone/650 mg acetaminophen per tablet), 2 tablets every 6 hours
- Gabapentin 900 mg po q8h
- Desipramine 75 mg po qhs

LK states he is content with his level of pain control and that it allows him to perform his desired activities of daily living. He enjoys the little "kick" he gets when he takes his two Percocet tablets every 6 hours.

As his prescriber, however, you are not as amused by the Percocet "kick." You are also concerned about the amount of acetaminophen LK is getting per day (650 mg × 8 tablets = 5.2 grams per day), especially since LK enjoys an alcoholic beverage or three on the weekends (alcohol use increases risk of acetaminophen toxicity). You decide to switch his Percocet to OxyContin. What dosage regimen do you come up with? When can it be initiated? What educational tips should you give LK about his analgesics?

P2.4: Same Opioid, Different Formulation and Route of Administration (Parenteral to Oral)

BC is a 48 year old woman who injured her back in a motor vehicle accident recently, for which she required immediate surgical repair. Post-operatively she was started on intermittent SQ injections of Opana Injection 1 mg/mL every 4 hours. It has been five days since surgery and BC has been stabilized on a TDD of 5 mg Opana Injection. BC is ready for transfer to a rehabilitation facility and it is anticipated that she will require chronic opioid therapy for the foreseeable future. What dosage regimen of Opana ER would you recommend and why? What dose of Opana should be made available to the patient for breakthrough or incident pain?

P2.5: Same Opioid, Different Formulation and Route of Administration (Oral to Parenteral)

MV is a 62 year old woman with end-stage breast cancer. She is likely within days of death and she is emphatic that she does NOT want to die at home. She is also having significant difficulty swallowing her hydromorphone tablets. Her current regimen is hydromorphone 16 mg po every 4 hours, which gives her acceptable pain control. MV is admitted to an inpatient hospice facility and will begin intermittent injections of hydromorphone. The physician at the hospice house wants to know what dose you recommend and whether the hydromorphone can be given by intermittent SQ injections, or does it have to be intermittent IV injections? What do you recommend?

REFERENCES

1. Mercadente S. Opioid rotation for cancer pain: rationale and clinical aspects. *Cancer.* 1999;86:1856–1866.

2. Food and Drug Administration, Department of Health and Human Services, Food and Drugs Chapter 1, pages 185–199. In: Code of Federal Regulations, Title 21, Volume 5, Parts 300 to 499. Accessed online November 11, 2007 at http:/www1.va.gov/oro/apps/compendium/Files/21CFR320.htm.

3. Lugo RA, Kern SE. Clinical pharmacokinetics of morphine. *J Pain Palliat Care Pharmacother.* 2002;16(4):5–18

4. Amabile CM, Bowman CJ. Overview of oral modified-release opioid products for the management of chronic pain. *Ann Pharmacother.* 2006;40:1327–1335.

5. Prommer E. Oxymorphone: a review. *Support Care Cancer.* 2006;14:109–115.

6. Patanwala AE, Duby J, Waters D, et al. Opioid conversions in acute care. *Ann Pharmacother.* 2007;41:255–267.

7. Hanks GW, DeConno F, Ripamonti C, et al. Expert Working Group of the European Association for Palliative Care. Morphine in cancer pain: modes of administration. *Br Med J.* 1996;312:823–826.

8. Mercadante SG. When oral morphine fails in cancer pain: the role of the alternative route. *Am J Hosp Palliat Care.* 1998;15:333–342.

9. Walsh D, Tropiano P. Long-term rectal administration of high-dose sustained release morphine tablets. Support Care Cancer; 2002:10:653–655.

10. About.com Drug Finder. Oxycodone. Accessed online November 20, 2007 at: http://gsm.about.com/compact/showmono.asp?cpnum=457&r=6078&monotype=full.

11. American Pain Society. *Principles of Analgesic Use in the Treatment of Acute Pain and Cancer Pain.* 5th ed. Glenview, IL: American Pain Society; 2003.

12. Moulin DE, Kfreedt JH, Murray-Parsons N, et al. Comparison of continuous subcutaneous hydromorphone infusions for management of cancer pain. *Lancet.* 1991;337:465–468.

13. Waldman CS, Eason JR, Rambohul E, et al. Serum morphine levels: a comparison between continuous subcutaneous infusion and continuous intravenous infusion in post-operative patients. *Anesthesia.* 1984;39:768–771.

14. Currow DC, Plummer JL, Cooney NJ, et al. A randomized, double-blind, multi-site, crossover, placebo-controlled equivalence study of morning versus evening once-daily sustained-release morphine sulfate in people with pain from advanced cancer. *J Pain Sympt Manage.* 2007;34:17–23.

15. Ramsay MA, Savege TM, Simpson BR, et al. Controlled sedation with alphaxalone-alphadolone. *Br Med J.* 1974;2(920):656–659.

16. Blanchard AR. Sedation and analgesia in intensive care. *Postgrad Med.* 2002;111(2):59–74.

SOLUTIONS TO PRACTICE PROBLEMS

P2.1

Step 1—Per the prescriber, IR's pain is well controlled.

Step 2—IR is receiving Avinza 60 mg once daily, so her TDD of oral morphine is 60 mg

Step 3—The prescriber has already accepted the idea of switching IR to an oral morphine concentrated solution. Because we're switching from oral morphine to oral morphine, the TDD remains the same, 60 mg oral morphine.

Step 4—The patient's pain was controlled, therefore an increase in dose is not necessary. We're not switching opioids, so a decrease is not necessary. Oral morphine concentrated solution is dosed every four hours, or six doses per day. This gives us a regimen of oral morphine solution 20 mg/mL, 10 mg (0.5 mL) every 4 hours, instilled in the buccal cavity.

Step 5—IR's upper body should be propped up 30 degrees before instilling the morphine in her buccal cavity and monitored to assure she does not aspirate the morphine solution. She should also be monitored for pain control and any potential toxicities.

P2.2

Step 1—HZ's pain is well controlled and he is doing well on his current regimen (aside from the inability to swallow).

Step 2—HZ's TDD of oral hydromorphone is between 14 and 16 mg

Step 3—We have already decided to switch HZ to rectal hydromorphone suppositories. The data on the bioequivalence of rectal hydromorphone suppositories is not as strong as it is for oral:rectal morphine, but most practitioners consider the ratio to be 1:1 for hydromorphone as well.

Step 4—Some data suggests that hydromorphone may be a bit more potent when given as a rectal suppository, and it seems to last 6 hours, as opposed to 4 hours with oral hydromorphone. For this reason, it would be prudent to switch to hydromorphone 3 mg by rectum every 6 hours, which is a TDD of 12 mg (slight less than the oral regimen).

Step 5—Monitor HZ for adverse effects to the hydromorphone, including rectal irritation, and pain control.

P2.3

Step 1—You have assessed LK's complaint of pain, and believe you have maximized his analgesic regimen at this point. More importantly, LK is feels his current analgesic regimen has met his goals for pain management.

Step 2—Focusing just on the Percocet, LK's TDD of oral oxycodone is 80 mg (two Percocet tablets every 6 hours = 20 mg oxycodone × 4 = 80 mg).

Step 3—LK admits to enjoying one or more alcoholic beverages on the weekend. Based on the tendency for individuals to underreport the amount of alcohol they consume and FDA recommendations, you have already decided to switch LK to Oxy-Contin, and to not replace the acetaminophen. Oxycodone is equally bioavailable in Percocet and OxyContin, therefore the TDD of OxyContin would be 80 mg before any TDD dose change considerations.

Step 4—As stated earlier, LK is content with his current level of pain control. Therefore, a TDD of 80 mg OxyContin should give equivalent pain relief, while only requiring twice-daily dosing. A regimen of OxyContin 40 mg po q12h would be appropriate. There is no need to increase the total daily dose, nor to decrease it. The OxyContin should be started probably at a convenient time in the evening or morning, at least 4 hours after his last dose of Percocet. Should the patient's pain not be controlled on this new regimen, it may be due to eliminating the acetaminophen. If this is the case, you can either add acetaminophen back to the regimen separately (of he is agreeable to discontinue drinking alcohol), adjust his co-analgesic regimen, or increase the opioid dose a bit.

Step 5—LK should be monitored for therapeutic effectiveness including pain rating and performance of activities of daily living (ADLs), and parameters that would indicate toxicity.

Educational points for LK include the following:

- We would rather you not appreciate the "kick" from your opioid. The opioid is to control your pain and to allow you to perform your ADLs, not for your entertainment pleasure. To show that we're not entirely hard-hearted, however, you should know that approximately 40% of the dose of an OxyContin tablet is an "immediate-release" phase, so it will disintegrate and begin to work in a time course similar to your Percocet. As the blood level of oxycodone begins to decline from this initial "bolus" of oxycodone, the second phase is being released and will continue to control your pain for 12 hours.

- It is very important to tell LK that he should take his OxyContin tablets every TWELVE hours—don't say "take twice a day." To many patients "take twice a day" means take with breakfast and dinner!

- You should advise LK to discontinue drinking alcohol. He is taking a potent medication, along with two co-analgesics, and alcohol doesn't play well in the sandbox with the others. He should avoid taking acetaminophen on top of this regimen, especially if he does not give up alcohol.

P2.4:

<u>Step 1</u>—BC's pain is stable on her current Opana Injection (oxymorphone hydrochloride) regimen, and does not require the addition of any co-analgesics at this time.

<u>Step 2</u>—BC's TDD of parenteral oxymorphone is 5 mg.

<u>Step 3</u>—The prescriber has already requested that BC be converted to oral oxymorphone, using extended-release tablets for her baseline analgesia, and to have an immediate-release oxymorphone tablet available for breakthrough or incident pain.

In comparison to IV oxymorphone, oral oxymorphone is approximately 10% bioavailable. A simple ratio tells us that we must multiply the parenteral TDD of oxymorphone by 10 to determine the TDD of oral oxymorphone, or in this case, 50 mg. Or, we you can directly apply the ratio to the current total daily dose and end up with the new opioid total daily dose as follows:

$$5 \text{ mg TDD } \cancel{\text{parenteral oxymorphone}} \times \frac{10 \text{ mg oral oxymorphone}}{1 \text{ mg } \cancel{\text{parenteral oxymorphone}}} = 50 \text{ mg TDD oral oxymorphone}$$

<u>Step 4</u>—There is no reason to increase the amount of oxymorphone the patient is receiving per day since her pain is controlled. We do not need to reduce her TDD due to incomplete cross-tolerance since we are converting from oxymorphone to oxymorphone. We will work with the TDD of 50 mg oral oxymorphone to determine her exact regimen.

Since Opana ER is dosed every 12 hours, we need to divide the TDD by 2. Unfortunately this gives us 25 mg po q12h, which is "doable" with the tablet strengths of Opana ER (5-, 10-, 20-, 40-mg tablets) but more than one tablet strength will be involved. It might be easier for the patient to recommend Opana ER 20 mg po q12h, and Opana IR 5 mg q6h prn breakthrough pain. Also, the Opana 5-mg dose can be given 1 hour before events known to produce pain (e.g., physical therapy in the rehabilitation center). BC's pain should continue to resolve as days and weeks go on.

<u>Step 5</u>—We should monitor the Medication Administration Record from the rehabilitation facility to determine how many doses of Opana the patient requires per day on top of her scheduled Opana ER. If she is consistently requiring four additional Opana tablets, we could consider increasing her Opana ER to 25 or 30 mg po q12h. Importantly, we will also monitor BC's ability to participate in physical therapy, and for any potential signs of opioid toxicity.

P2.5:

Step 1—MV states she has acceptable pain control on her current regimen, therefore it is unlikely we would need to add a co-analgesic at this time.

Step 2—MV's TDD of oral hydromorphone is 96 mg (16 mg every 4 hours $= 16 \times 6 = 96$ mg)

Step 3—We already know we want to switch MV to an intermittent injection of hydromorphone since this opioid has been beneficial for her. We are not sure of the route at this time (IV vs. SQ).

Consulting our Equianalgesic Opioid Dosing Table (Table 2-2) we see that 1.5 mg parenteral hydromorphone is approximately equivalent to 7.5 mg oral hydromorphone (a factor of 5). Using a mathematical proportion and cross-multiplying we can determine the new TDD of parenteral hydromorphone as follows:

Actual Drug Doses: **Equianalgesic Data from Chart:**

$$\frac{\text{``X'' mg TDD parenteral hydromorphone}}{\text{96 mg TDD oral hydromorphone}} = \frac{\text{1.5 mg parenteral hydromorphone}}{\text{7.5 mg oral hydromorphone}}$$

Cross-multiply and solve for "X" as follows:

$$(X)(7.5) = (96)(1.5)$$

$$X = 19.2 \text{ mg TDD parenteral hydromorphone}$$

Step 4—we have no reason to increase the hydromorphone at this time because MV's pain is controlled. Looking at the dosing interval (q4h), we need to give the TDD in six even doses. Since 19.2 mg does not divide evenly, it would be prudent to round DOWN since there is always a bit of speculation about the absolute conversion from oral to parenteral hydromorphone and vice versa. Therefore we can recommend 3 mg parenteral hydromorphone every 4 hours, for a TDD of 18 mg. Remember, the bioavailability of oral hydromorphone may be considerably higher than 20% (the assumption when using a 1:5 parenteral:oral hydromorphone conversion). If this is the case, the calculated TDD of 18 mg parenteral hydromorphone may be too LOW a TDD. The dosage may need to be increased considerably.

The physician wanted to know if the SQ route is reasonable, or if we think IV is preferred. The most important consideration in this decision is whether or not the dose can be given, and limit the volume to 1–2 mL with a SQ injection. Injectable hydromorphone is available as a 1-, 2-, 4-, and 10-mg/mL concentration. Therefore, we could use the 4 mg/mL, and 0.75 mL could be administered SQ every 4 hours. Consequently, it is possible to give MV her hydromorphone 4 mg/mL, 3 mg (0.75 mL) every 4 hours by SQ injection. MV can begin this therapy 3 or 4 hours after her last dose of oral hydromorphone.

Step 5—MV would be closely monitored for signs of over- or underdosage with this regimen.

CHAPTER 3

Converting Among Routes and Formulations of the Different Opioids

OBJECTIVES

After reading this chapter and completing all practice problems, the participant will be able to:

1. List reasons why a health care professional may need to switch a patient from one opioid to a different opioid.

2. Given an actual or simulated case of a patient in pain, calculate an equivalent regimen of a different opioid, both by the same route of administration, as well as alternate routes of administration.

INTRODUCTION

You learned all about why we switch opioids in Chapter 1, and how to switch from one route of administration or dosage formulation to a different one using the same opioid in Chapter 2. Sometimes in clinical practice we need to switch from one opioid to an entirely different opioid. Consider the case of PJ, a 22 year old man who had all four impacted wisdom teeth extracted during one procedure. The dentist realized this would cause PJ moderate pain postoperatively, and she prescribed Percocet (5 mg oxycodone/325 mg acetaminophen per tablet), 1–2 tablets every 4 hours as needed. When PJ recovered from anesthesia at home, he felt dreadful and took two Percocet tablets. Within one hour PJ was itching and scratching all over like nobody's business. The dentist realized that the pruritus PJ was experiencing was due to the oxycodone (probably due to histamine release, not a true allergy), and switched him to Vicodin (5 mg hydrocodone/325 mg acetaminophen per tablet). PJ took the Vicodin with good success and his pain resolved over the next few days. Conversion calculations weren't really necessary in this case because PJ was opioid-naïve, and received a starting dose for both the Percocet and Vicodin prescriptions.

As discussed in Chapter 1, the development of adverse effects is only one reason why we might switch opioids. Additional reasons include lack of therapeutic response, change in the patient's clinical condition (e.g., inability to use original dosage formulation), and a myriad of other reasons such as opioid product availability, formulary restriction, and patient/caregiver/prescriber health beliefs. In Chapter 2 we discussed how to switch between routes of administration and formulations of the *same* opioid; in this chapter we will make the leap *between* opioids (potentially changing the route of administration and formulation as well!). We will hold our discussions of switching to and from methadone and fentanyl until later in the book—they have very specific dosing considerations and deserve devoted discussion. We will also hold discussions of conversions to and from continuous intravenous or subcutaneous opioid infusions for a later chapter.

As you may recall, the concepts of **potency** (the intensity of analgesic effect for a given dose), **equianalgesia** (doses of two different opioids that provide the same degree of pain relief), and **bioavailability** (the percentage of drug that is detected in the systemic circulation after its administration) were discussed in Chapter 1. These concepts were considered, along with the limited primary literature we have available, to craft an "Equianalgesic Opioid Dosing Table" (see Chapter 1, Table 1-1). Remember the doses shown in Table 1-1 are *equivalent* doses, not actual doses.

Again referring to Chapter 1, charts such as Table 1-1 constitute rough estimates of dose equivalencies—most of the data used to determine these equivalencies are from single-dose cross-over studies, usually in acute pain patients, do not take into consideration patient specific variables (e.g., age, BMI, frailty, comorbidities, duration of exposure to opioids, concurrent use of other medications, etc.), and may be unidirectional. This is why we include a step in the opioid conversion calculation process where we carefully consider whether we should reduce the calculated dose (which is usually the case), use the calculated dose, or (rarely) increase the dose from that calculated. As a reminder, the five steps we use in opioid conversion calculations are shown in Chapter 1, Table 1-2. Enough talking already, let's jump into some calculations—you scream, I scream, we all scream for morphine (calculations!).

CASE 3.1
• •
Switching from Oral Acetaminophen/Oxycodone to Oral Extended-Release Morphine

PA is a 44 year old man with chronic low back pain, a consequence of a work-related injury in construction. He has undergone surgery several times, and his health care team doesn't believe his pain will improve with further surgical interventions. He has completed numerous physical therapy sessions, and is adherent to his exercise plan. PA's current analgesic regimen consists of Percocet (10 mg oxycodone/650 mg acetaminophen per tablet), 1–2 tablets every 6 hours as needed, and pregabalin (Lyrica) 100 mg three times a day. PA tells you, his community pharmacist, that taking the Percocet every 6 hours means he always awakens in pain, and he would really prefer to take medications less often. He's tried cutting back, but that causes his pain to get much worse.

<u>Step 1</u>—When you ask PA about the pain he tells you that it is an achy, occasionally "grabbing" pain localized in the lumbosacral area (he points to the small of his back, down into his buttocks). Lifting anything greater than 15 or 20 pounds increases the pain and he can only stand about 30 minutes before his back starts to hurt, and his left leg tingles, and eventually becomes numb. Rest, the analgesics, and the application of heat

relieve the pain. When he tries to go without the Percocet, or when he awakens 4–6 hours after taking a dose he rates the pain as a 7 or 8 (on a 0–10 scale; 0 = no pain, 10 = worst imaginable pain). When he takes eight Percocet tablets per day his average pain rating is a 3 or 4 (on a 0–10 scale), which he finds to be acceptable. He also tells you that the Lyrica has reduced the tingling and numbness in his leg, and it is tolerable at this point. This analgesic regimen allows him to perform the majority of his activities of daily living, and sleep fairly well (aside from awakening in pain). He denies incontinence of bowel or bladder, fever, weight loss, or other constitutional symptoms.

Step 2—PA is consistently taking eight Percocet tablets a day, along with pregabalin (Lyrica) 100 mg three times daily. You are very concerned about the amount of acetaminophen PA is receiving (5200 mg per day; patient denies taking acetaminophen from any other source). You also want PA to be able to sleep through the night without awakening in pain.

Step 3—You check PA's prescription drug coverage and discover that extended-release oxycodone is not on the formulary, however extended-release morphine is. PA has no history of morphine intolerance, and his renal function is normal for his age. You consult with the prescriber who agrees with your plan to switch PA's Percocet to extended-release morphine, and she asks you to calculate an equivalent dose. Yikes—what do we do first?

Clearly what you must do now is calculate the total daily dose (TDD) of oxycodone PA is receiving. He tells you he's taking 2 tablets every 6 hours around the clock. Therefore, we determine the TDD as follows:

2 tablets every 6 hours means PA is taking 2 tablets four times daily, which is a total daily dose of oxycodone.

$$\frac{8 \text{ tablets}}{\text{day}} \times \frac{10 \text{ mg oxycodone}}{\text{tablet}} = \frac{8 \text{ \sout{tablets}}}{\text{day}} \times \frac{10 \text{ mg oxycodone}}{\text{\sout{tablet}}} = \frac{80 \text{ mg oxycodone}}{\text{day}}$$

Therefore, PA's TDD of oxycodone = 80 mg. Please note that we are ignoring the acetaminophen component at this point. If necessary, the patient can take acetaminophen separately (e.g., an 8-hour formulation, 1300 mg every 8 hours). The contribution of acetaminophen to the patient's overall analgesia should not be underestimated or forgotten.

Now we need to magically convert the 80 mg TDD oxycodone to a TDD of morphine.

Let's use the mathematical proportion method using cross multiplication (Method B) as follows:

$$\frac{\text{"X" mg TDD new opioid}}{\text{mg TDD current opioid}} = \frac{\text{equianalgesic factor of new opioid}}{\text{equianalgesic factor of current opioid}}$$

As you recall from Chapter 1 and consulting our Equianalgesic Opioid Dosing Table (Table 1-1), the doses listed **across** a row for a given opioid show equipotent doses. Also, doses for different opioids in a **column** are also equipotent. We can also use this chart to look at equivalent doses between opioid and routes of administration. Therefore, looking at the table we can fill in the appropriate data as follows:

$$\frac{\text{"X" mg TDD new opioid (morphine)}}{80 \text{ mg TDD oral oxycodone}} = \frac{30 \text{ mg oral morphine}}{20 \text{ mg oral oxycodone}}$$

Cross-multiplication gives us:

(80) × (30) = (X) × 20

2400 = 20X

X = 120

Using this method we see a TDD of 120 mg oral morphine is approximately equipotent to 80 mg TDD of oxycodone.

Before we move on to Step 4, let's consider the answer we calculated. Does it LOOK right? Fire up those synapses and think it through. If 20 mg oral oxycodone is approximately equivalent to 30 mg oral morphine, then 80 mg oral oxycodone (which is 4 times 20) must be about equivalent to 120 mg morphine (which is 4 times 30). Yep—checks out using common sense. It takes about one and a half as many milligrams of oral morphine as it does oral oxycodone to get the same job done (20 mg oral oxycodone ~ 30 mg oral morphine; therefore 80 mg oral oxycodone ~ 120 mg oral morphine). Excellent, let's press on.

Step 4—As you read in Chapter 1, once you do your mathematical computation, you will need to individualize the dose for the patient. We can either go with a TDD of 120 mg oral morphine per day, reduce the morphine TDD dose, or rarely increase the TDD. Because there are discrete differences in the way different opioid binds and/or activates receptors, there is not complete "cross-tolerance" among opioids. In other words, PA will be more sensitive to the pharmacologic effects of morphine, therefore giving him 120 mg per day of morphine would cause a greater pharmacologic effect than the 80 mg of oral oxycodone per day despite the fact that they are approximately equipotent. This would be a good plan (e.g., no dose adjustment) if we were switching because his pain was not controlled on the oxycodone, but that's not the case. Therefore, it would be prudent to reduce his TDD oral morphine by 25–50%. For argument's sake, let's choose a 33% reduction (one third). Reducing a 120 mg TDD oral morphine by one third leaves us with about 80 mg TDD oral morphine.

We already discussed that we want to recommend an extended-release morphine tablet or capsule. Our options include:

- 12-hour formulations of morphine sulfate controlled or extended-release tablets (MS Contin, Oramorph SR, generic products); 45 mg by mouth, every 12 hours
  - In this case, since we only have 15-, 30-, 60-, 100-, and 200-mg tablets available, we have to either round up or down. Rounding up to 90 mg TDD oral morphine seems reasonable.
- 24-hour formulation of morphine sulfate extended-release pellets in capsule; Avinza 90 mg po once daily
  - Same discussion as above; Avinza is available as 30-, 60-, 90-, and 120-mg capsules
- 12–24 hour formulation of morphine sulfate extended-release pellets in capsule; Kadian 40 mg po every 12 hours, OR Kadian 80 mg po once daily

- Kadian is available as 10-, 20-, 30-, 50-, 60-, 80-, 100-, and 200-mg capsules, and can be dosed once or twice daily, with no need to round up or down

Step 5—Once the prescriber agrees with the recommendation, the pharmacist can counsel the patient about how to transition from Percocet to the extended-release morphine product. Percocet is a short-acting product, and modified-release morphine products take several hours to reach therapeutic levels after the first dose. Therefore the extended-release morphine could be started the very next morning, and at *most* one additional dose of Percocet could be taken within the first 4 hours after starting morphine, if pain is not sufficiently controlled and there is no appreciable sedation, nausea, or other untoward CNS effects from the morphine. The patient should maintain a pain diary, and make a note of pain intensity, relationship to activity, and any adverse effects experienced, if any. The pharmacist will follow-up with a phone call to ask if the patient is able to sleep through the night without awakening in pain, and assess his continued ability to perform activities of daily living. The pharmacist will also ask about adverse effects (e.g., constipation, sedation, confusion, pruritus, etc.).

 PITFALL ••
Double-Check Those Dosing Intervals!

Always stop yourself and make SURE you are CLEAR on how many doses the patient is actually taking per day. A common mistake is to hear "every 6 hours" and think "SIX" doses—or "every 4 hours" and think "FOUR" doses per day. Remember to divide the hourly dosing interval into 24 (hours per day)—obviously "every 6 hours" means four doses per day (24 hours divided by 6-hour intervals) and "every 4 hours" means six doses per day (24 hours divided by four hour intervals). This is a **common** mathematical error that could result in overdosage or undertreatment of pain.

••

 CASE 3.2
••
Switching from Oral Oxymorphone to Oral Oxycodone

ZH is a 68 year old woman who is being discharged from a rehabilitation center after left total knee replacement. She has received extensive physical therapy, which caused some discomfort. Her physiatrist wants the patient to continue opioid therapy at home, but finds that the Opana IR (immediate-release oxymorphone hydrochloride) and Opana ER (extended-release oxymorphone hydrochloride) she has been receiving in the facility are not on formulary with the patient's pharmacy plan. Extended-release and immediate release oxycodone are on formulary, however, so the physiatrist finds himself needing to switch from the patient's current regimen of oxymorphone to oxycodone instead.

Step 1—ZH describes her pain as being well-localized to her left knee. She says the physical therapy exacerbates the pain, and rest, ice, and the opioid regimen relieve the pain. She describes the pain as achy, and sometimes throbbing immediately after physical therapy. On her current analgesic regimen she rates the pain as 1–2 (on a 0–10 scale) at rest, 4 with normal movement, and 6-7 toward the end of a physical therapy session; she finds this level of pain control acceptable. She states the opioid regimen is necessary to allow her to continue physical therapy, which she will continue on an outpatient basis. ZH denies any burning, tingling, or numbness. The pain does not prevent her from sleeping, although her limited mobility at this time prevents her from several activities of daily living (e.g., housecleaning, grocery shopping) and hobbies (gardening, walking for exercise).

Step 2—ZH is currently receiving Opana ER 10 mg po every 12 hours, and Opana IR 5 mg every 4 hours as needed for breakthrough pain. She usually takes two of the 5 mg short-acting tablets per day, for a TDD of oral oxymorphone of 30 mg.

Step 3—When we consult the Equianalgesic Opioid Dosing Table (Table 1-1), we see the following data (abstracted from table):

Drug	Equianalgesic Doses (mg)	
	Parenteral	Oral
Morphine	10	30
Oxycodone	10*	20
Oxymorphone	1	10

*Not available in the United States.

We are switching from oxymorphone to oxycodone—can we do this in one jump, or do we need to switch from oxymorphone to morphine, then from morphine to oxycodone? Some practitioners feel that it should be a two step process (the latter scenario), but whether you do it in one step or two, you end up with the same answer. This being the case, it seems much easier just to make the leap. But for all you Doubting Thomases out there, let's do it both ways, so we can put this to bed!

Let's use method B and go from oxymorphone to morphine, then morphine to oxycodone.

$$\frac{\text{“X” mg TDD oral morphine}}{30 \text{ mg TDD oral oxymorphone}} = \frac{30 \text{ mg equianalgesic factor of oral morphine}}{10 \text{ mg equianalgesic factor of oral oxymorphone}}$$

Cross multiply:

(X)(10) = (30)(30)

10X = 900

X = 90

This calculation shows a TDD of oral morphine 90 mg is approximately equivalent to 30 mg TDD oral oxymorphone.

OK, now let's take this morphine dose and convert to oxycodone.

$$\frac{\text{“X” mg TDD oral oxycodone}}{90 \text{ mg TDD oral morphine}} = \frac{20 \text{ mg equianalgesic factor of oral oxycodone}}{30 \text{ mg equianalgesic factor of oral morphine}}$$

Cross multiply:

(X)(30) = (20)(90)

30X = 1800

X = 60

This calculation shows a TDD of **60 mg oral oxycodone** is approximately equivalent to 90 mg TDD oral morphine.

So doing the two-step (via morphine) takes us from:

Oral oxymorphone 30 mg TDD → oral morphine 90 mg TDD → oral oxycodone 60 mg TDD

Gee, I wonder how this would work if we just switched right from oral oxymorphone to oral oxycodone? I can't stand the suspense, how about you? Let's do it by golly!

$$\frac{\text{"X" mg TDD oral oxycodone}}{\text{30 mg TDD oral oxymorphone}} = \frac{\text{20 mg equianalgesic factor of oral oxycodone}}{\text{10 mg equianalgesic factor of oral oxymorphone}}$$

Cross multiply:

(X)(10) = (20)(30)

10X = 600

X = 60

This calculation (going straight from oral oxymorphone to oral oxycodone) shows a TDD of **60 mg oral oxycodone** is approximately equivalent to a TDD 30 mg oral oxymorphone.

Whether you feel obligated to go to morphine first, and then to your opioid of choice, or take the short-cut and go directly to your opioid of choice, you get the same answer. Actually doing it both ways is a good check of your math.

Just for laughs, lets do the direct conversion (oxymorphone to oxycodone) using Method D.

As you recall, Method D is as follows:

$$\text{TDD current opioid} \times \frac{\text{equianalgesic factor of new opioid}}{\text{equianalgesic factor of current opioid}} = \text{TDD new opioid}$$

Let's plug and chug:

$$\text{30 mg TDD oral oxymorphone} \times \frac{\text{20 mg equianalgesic factor of oral oxycodone}}{\text{10 mg equianalgesic factor of oral oxymorphone}} =$$

$$\text{30 mg TDD oral } \cancel{\text{oxymorphone}} \times \frac{\text{20 mg equianalgesic factor of oral oxycodone}}{\text{10 mg equianalgesic factor of oral } \cancel{\text{oxymorphone}}} =$$

30 × 20/10 = 30 × 2 = **60 mg TDD oral oxycodone**

By gosh, I think we have a winner! BEFORE we individualize the dose for this patient, we have conclusively shown that a TDD of 30 mg oral oxymorphone is approximately equivalent to 60 mg TDD oral oxycodone.

Step 4—Because ZH has acceptable pain control on her current opioid regimen, and we know she will probably be more sensitive to the oxycodone due to incomplete cross-tolerance, it would be prudent to reduce our TDD of oral oxycodone. Using the one third rule, this reduces the TDD oral oxycodone to 40 mg.

Controlled-release oxycodone tablets are available as 10-, 15-, 20-, 30-, 40-, 60-, and 80-mg tablets. An appropriate order would be for 20 mg by mouth every 12 hours. The physiatrist could write the order for 20-mg tablets, or if he suspects the patient's pain will be improving fairly quickly, he may want to write for 10 mg tablets, and instruct the patient to take two 10-mg tablets by mouth every 12 hours, then reduce the dose to one tablet (10 mg) by mouth every 12 hours at some point later. Also, the physiatrist should write a prescription for oxycodone 5 mg short-acting tablets, one tablet every 4 hours as needed for break-through pain. ZH can begin the controlled-release oxycodone 12 hours after her last dose of controlled-release oxymorphone.

Step 5—It would be optimal for the physiatrist to switch ZH to the new regimen while she is still in the rehabilitation hospital to observe her response. In any case, ZH should keep a pain diary, and self-monitor her therapeutic response, and signs of toxicity. The nursing and physical therapy staff should assist in monitoring ZH's response to the oxycodone regimen if she is switched while still in the facility. If, for example, the patient finds that her pain has increased substantially after the switch, and she is requiring 4–6 doses of the short-acting oxycodone per day (e.g., 20 to 30 mg per day), it may be necessary to increase the extended-release oxycodone to 30 mg by mouth every 12 hours, and continue monitoring the patient.

 CASE 3.3
....
Switching from Oral Morphine to Parenteral Hydromorphone

BL is a 74 year old woman with a diagnosis of end-stage breast cancer, with diffuse bony metastasis, admitted to hospice several weeks ago. At the time of admission the patient was clinically stable, and receiving extended-release oral morphine 60 mg every 8 hours and oral naproxen 500 mg every 12 hours. Over the past 72 hours the patient has deteriorated rapidly; she has difficulty swallowing her tablets, her pain is increasing significantly, and she has become quite weepy with all that's transpired. BL is very clear that she does not want to die at home, and the hospice team feels that her time is near, therefore a decision is made to transfer her to the hospice's high-acuity facility.

Step 1—The hospice nurse made an unscheduled visit, at which time the decision was made to transfer BL. When the nurse asks BL about the pain she moans while crying and says "it's just awful, please make it stop." The patient is unable to describe precipitating and palliating factors. She says the pain is constant and everywhere and she describes it as throbbing, aching, and piercing. The patient is unable to rate the pain, but it is clear from observing her that it is severe.

Step 2—The family states that BL was able to get down her last scheduled doses of morphine and naproxen, although with significant difficulty.

Step 3—Upon arrival at the hospice facility, the attending physician decides to switch BL to subcutaneous injections of hydromorphone every 4 hours. Let's help the physician do this calculation.

Assuming BL did not miss any doses of oral morphine, her TDD was 180 mg (60 mg every 8 hours).

Using Method B we can set up the following ratio:

$$\frac{\text{``X'' mg TDD new opioid}}{\text{mg TDD current opioid}} = \frac{\text{equianalgesic factor of new opioid}}{\text{equianalgesic factor of current opioid}}$$

$$\frac{\text{``X'' mg TDD SQ hydromorphone}}{180 \text{ mg TDD oral morphine}} = \frac{1.5 \text{ mg parenteral hydromorphone}}{30 \text{ mg oral morphine}}$$

Cross multiply:

(X)(30) = (1.5)(180)

30X = 270

X = 9

This method shows the TDD parenteral (SQ) hydromorphone is 9 mg.

Step 4—We now need to decide whether to go with 9 mg SQ hydromorphone per day, to reduce it for incomplete cross-tolerance, or increase the TDD. Since BL is in severe pain, it would be reasonable to at least go no lower than 9 mg TDD SQ hydromorphone. Because hydromorphone is a relatively short-acting opioid, it should be dosed at least every 4 hours (and perhaps even every 3 hours). It we give the TDD of 9 mg on an every 4 hour basis, this would be 1.5 mg SQ hydromorphone every 4 hours. Given her severe pain, it would be reasonable to increase this to 2 mg SQ every 4 hours, and observe her response. The SQ hydromorphone can be started whenever clinically indicated; the last dose of extended-release oral morphine peaks about 3–4 hours after administration. If 3–4 hours have passed since BL took her last oral morphine tablet, and she is in pain, it would be appropriate to begin the SQ hydromorphone now.

Step 5—Parenterally-administered hydromorphone peaks in about 30 minutes, therefore, BL should be closely monitored, and given a repeat dose as clinically indicated. Alternately, BL could receive one or more IV or SQ injections of hydromorphone, and once made comfortable, switched to a continuous infusion of hydromorphone with a bolus option (will be discussed in Chapter 7).

 CASE 3.4

Switching from Oral Meperidine to Oral Oxycodone

CP is a 72 year old obese woman with a long-standing history of osteoarthritis of the hips and knees, and lower lumbar vertebrae. She presents in the Medication Refill Clinic for routine follow-up and a new prescription for oral meperidine (Demerol) 100 mg, which she takes four times daily. You are a recent hire at this hospital, and you are taken aback to see this prescription. Meperidine is not recommended because it is short acting, and with repeat dosing the metabolite normeperidine accumulates and can cause CNS excitation and possibly seizures. Meperidine should be especially avoided in patients with impaired renal function (because normeperidine is eliminated from the body by the kidneys), and you are keenly aware of the fact that renal function deteriorates as we age.

Step 1—CP describes her pain as widely spread in the lumbar area, made worse with standing more than 5 minutes (e.g., doing the dishes) and with activities that require bending (e.g., vacuuming, laundry). She tells you the pain is dull and aching, and she rates it as a 7 or an 8 on average (on a 0–10 scale) with no medication, and 4 or 5 with the meperidine. The pain does not affect her sleep (although she has more pain in the morning) or appetite, and while she is not happy about her pain status, she finds it bearable. CP has a past medical history of type 2 diabetes mellitus, hypertension and peptic ulcer disease. She has tried maximum doses of acetaminophen without relief, and NSAID therapy is contraindicated due to a past history of duodenal ulcer. She has been taking meperidine for several years. Her most recent serum creatinine was 1.4 mg/dL.

Step 2—CP does not take any extra doses of meperidine, nor does she miss any doses. She is very adherent to her regimen of 100 mg oral meperidine four times daily—with breakfast, lunch, dinner, and at bedtime.

Step 3—Although CP has been fortunate not to have suffered adverse effects from meperidine, as time goes by, she is at high risk, due to advancing age and reduced renal clearance (calculated creatinine clearance is approximately 36 mL/min; normal is 100 mL/min). Because morphine also has pharmacologically active metabolites which can also cause toxicity, morphine is not a great choice for CP. A better choice would be oxycodone, hydromorphone, oxymorphone, methadone or fentanyl. For educational purposes, let's choose oxycodone.

If you look at the Equianalgesic Opioid Dosing Table you will find meperidine listed. However, this does not imply that it is recommended patients be switched *to* meperidine—most contemporary pain management guidelines have eliminated meperidine from the list of recommended opioids due to its potential toxicity. Nevertheless, there are dose-equivalency studies with meperidine that can be used to develop an equianalgesic conversion *from* meperidine to another opioid. For purposes of saving CP from a potentially adverse outcome, let's look at the estimated equivalency data with meperidine:

Drug	Equianalgesic Doses (mg)	
	Parenteral	**Oral**
Morphine	10	30
Hydrocodone	NA	30
Hydromorphone	1.5	7.5
Oxycodone	10*	20
Oxymorphone	1	10
Meperidine	100	300

*Not available in the United States.

Let's use Method C to switch the patient to oxycodone:

$$\frac{\text{"X" mg TDD new opioid}}{\text{equianalgesic factor of new opioid}} = \frac{\text{mg TDD current opioid}}{\text{equianalgesic factor of current opioid}}$$

$$\frac{\text{"X" mg TDD oral oxycodone}}{20 \text{ mg oral oxycodone}} = \frac{400 \text{ mg TDD oral meperidine}}{300 \text{ mg oral meperidine}}$$

Cross multiply:

(X)(300) = (400)(20)

300X = 8000

X = 26.7 mg

This method shows an equivalent TDD of oral oxycodone would be 26.7 mg.

Step 4—Since the patient was content with her current level of pain control, it would be prudent to reduce the TDD of oral oxycodone. Since extended-release oxycodone tablets are available as 10 mg, it would be reasonable to switch her to 10 mg by mouth every 12 hours (TDD 20 mg oral oxycodone). You could also prescribe short-acting oxycodone 5 mg tablets for breakthrough pain if desired. This regimen may be started 3–4 hours or greater after the last meperidine dose.

Step 5—CP should keep a pain diary, recording her pain ratings, use of short-acting oxycodone tablets (if prescribed), signs or symptoms of toxicity, and ability to perform activities of daily living.

In this chapter you have learned how to switch from one opioid to another opioid, which may or may not be the same route of administration.

PRACTICE PROBLEMS

P3.1: Switching from Oral Acetaminophen/Hydrocodone to Oral Extended-Release Morphine

RD is 48 year old man who has residual pain from a motor vehicle accident. His pain is moderately controlled on Vicodin HP (10 mg hydrocodone and 650 mg acetaminophen), 1 tablet every 4 hours (he usually skips the middle of the night dose). He also receives desipramine 50 mg by mouth at bedtime, and gabapentin (Neurontin) 900 mg by mouth every 8 hours. RD rates his pain as 4–5/10 on average. RD is complaining about the need to take the Vicodin HP every 4 hours, and that when he wakes up each morning he is in pain. His pharmacy insurance plan covers generic extended-release morphine, and you are asked to recommend an appropriate dose.

P3.2: Switching from IV Hydromorphone to Oral Oxycodone

FA is a 62 year old man with colon cancer who underwent tumor debulking 3 days ago. Over the past 24 hours he has received 12 mg of IV hydromorphone. He has good pain control, and the attending physician would like to send him home on an equivalent regimen of long- and short-acting oxycodone. The physician anticipates FA will be able to taper down this dose significantly over the next few days.

P3.3: Switching from Oral Morphine to Oral Oxymorphone

SJ is an 84 year old woman with general debility, significant renal impairment, and generalized aches and pains. She has been receiving extended release morphine 30 mg by mouth every 12 hours for the past several months with good success. Over the past couple of weeks she has developed delirium, with both visual and auditory hallucinations. Other reversible causes have been ruled out, and the prescriber is concerned that the active metabolites of morphine are accumulating given SJ's renal function, and causing or contributing to the delirium. The prescriber asks that you calculate an equivalent regimen using oxymorphone (long- and short-acting). Just for fun, use all FOUR methods to calculate the oxymorphone regimen. That should keep you out of trouble for a while!

P3.4: Switching from Oral Acetaminophen/Codeine to Oral Morphine

KK is a 72 year old opioid-naive woman receiving rehabilitation services for a total hip replacement several weeks ago. KK had a stroke several years ago, and she has residual swallowing difficulties. She has an order for Tylenol with Codeine oral solution, 2 tablespoons every 4 hours as needed for pain (12 mg codeine phosphate and 120 mg acetaminophen per 5 mL). She has asked for the Tylenol with Codeine on several occasions, and it relieved the pain sufficiently, but she got so nauseated that she couldn't participate in therapy. You decide to switch her to oral morphine solution. What would be the appropriate dose to give an equivalent therapy effect?

PEARL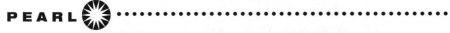

What Do You Mean You're "Allergic" to It?

It is not uncommon for patients to say they are "allergic" to an opioid, when in fact they are referring to an adverse effect. Codeine is a perfect example—it seems that everyone and their mother can experience nausea from codeine, which can be quite severe (think Linda Blair, the Exorcist, pea soup). A patient may be given too high a dose of an opioid such as morphine and experience delirium. When a patient says they are "allergic" to any medication, it is important to ask what happened when the patient took the medication, and how the event was handled by the health care team (discontinue medication vs. administer epinephrine).

SOLUTIONS TO PRACTICE PROBLEMS

P3.1

<u>Step 1</u>—Per the patient, his pain is fairly well controlled, but could stand to be improved a bit. He would like to switch due to the inconvenience of Vicodin HP dosing, and the fact that the Vicodin HP doesn't last all night, causing him to awaken with pain.

<u>Step 2</u>—Patient is taking 5 Vicodin HP tablets per 24-hour period, in addition to desipramine and gabapentin.

<u>Step 3</u>—RD would benefit from an extended-release opioid. His pharmacy insurance

plan covers long-acting oral morphine. RD's total daily dose of hydrocodone is 50 mg (5 doses × 10 mg per tablet).

Using Method D, we can determine the equivalent dose of morphine:

$$50 \text{ mg TDD oral hydrocodone} \times \frac{30 \text{ mg oral morphine}}{30 \text{ mg oral hydrocodone}}$$

$$50 \text{ mg TDD oral } \cancel{\text{hydrocodone}} \times \frac{30 \text{ mg oral morphine}}{30 \text{ mg oral } \cancel{\text{hydrocodone}}}$$

Completing the mathematics, we see the TDD oral morphine is also 50 mg. This is kind of a no-brainer since oral morphine and oral hydrocodone are equivalent on a mg:mg basis (30 mg oral morphine ~ 30 mg oral hydrocodone). Unsurprisingly, 50 mg TDD oral hydrocodone ~ 50 mg TDD oral morphine. Remember, though, this "equivalency" is *not* based on solid evidence. We could be over- or underestimating the equivalent amount of morphine.

The extended-release morphine can be started four or more hours after the last Vicodin HP tablet is taken.

Step 4—Given the 50 mg TDD oral morphine, we could use this number, increase or decrease for lack of cross tolerance. Since RD is not pleased with his level of pain control, it would not be reasonable to reduce the dose. Unfortunately, 50 mg TDD oral morphine does not divide well for every 12-hour dosing; our choices are reduce the morphine a bit and use Kadian 20 mg po q12h, or increase a bit and go with 30 mg extended release oral morphine, every 12 hours.

Step 5—Assuming we go with the higher dose, the patient needs to be counseled to avoid driving or operating machinery until he knows how he will react to the increased dose. He should maintain a pain diary and self-monitor his therapeutic and toxic response to the new regimen.

P3.2

Step 1—Per the physician, the patient's pain is well controlled.

Step 2—Patient's TDD IV hydromorphone is 12 mg.

Step 3—The physician has already asked that you calculate an equivalent dose of long- and short-acting oral oxycodone.

Using method B, we can set up the following ratio:

$$\frac{\text{"X" mg TDD oral oxycodone}}{12 \text{ mg IV hydromorphone}} = \frac{20 \text{ mg oral oxycodone}}{1.5 \text{ mg parenteral hydromorphone}}$$

Cross multiply:

(X)(1.5) = (20)(12)

1.5X = 240

X = 160

This method shows that the TDD oral oxycodone would be 160 mg.

Step 4—The patient's pain is well controlled, therefore it would be prudent to reduce the TDD of oral oxycodone by 25–50% (for a new TDD of 80–120 mg per day). Since the physician anticipates that the patient will be able to taper down the oxycodone dose significantly over the next few days, we can be more conservative with the long-acting oral oxycodone, and more liberal with the short-acting. For example, it would be reasonable to recommend extended-release oxycodone 40 mg by mouth every 12 hours, with short-acting oxycodone 10 mg every 2 or 4 hours as needed for break-through pain.

Step 5—The patient should maintain a pain diary, and the health care team should follow his therapeutic and toxic response to this regimen.

P3.3

Step 1—SJ has had good pain control per her prescriber with her analgesic regimen.

Step 2—SJ is receiving extended release oral morphine 30 mg every 12 hours, for a TDD of 60 mg oral morphine.

Step 3—The physician has asked that you calculate an equivalent dose of oxymorphone for SJ.

Use methods B, C, and D to calculate your answer, and compare. Let's take a look:

Method B

$$\frac{\text{"X" mg TDD oral oxymorphone}}{60 \text{ mg TDD oral morphine}} = \frac{10 \text{ mg oral oxymorphone}}{30 \text{ mg oral morphine}}$$

Cross multiply:
(X)(30) = (10)(60)
30X = 600
X = 20
This method shows that the TDD oral oxymorphone would be 20 mg.

Method C

$$\frac{\text{"X" mg TDD oral oxymorphone}}{10 \text{ mg oral oxymorphone}} = \frac{60 \text{ mg TDD oral morphine}}{30 \text{ mg oral morphine}}$$

Cross multiply:
(X)(30) = (10)(60)
30X = 600
X = 20
This method shows that the TDD oral oxymorphone would be 20 mg.

Method D

$$60 \text{ mg TDD oral morphine} \times \frac{10 \text{ mg oral oxymorphone}}{30 \text{ mg oral morphine}}$$

$$60 \text{ mg TDD oral } \cancel{\text{morphine}} \times \frac{10 \text{ mg oral oxymorphone}}{30 \text{ mg oral } \cancel{\text{morphine}}}$$

Multiplying through we see 60 × 10/30 = 20
This method shows that the TDD oral oxymorphone would be 20 mg.

As we can see, all three methods give us the same answer, a TDD of 20 mg oral oxymorphone.

Just to make SURE we're right, let's be brave and use *Method A*—your brain. Don't hurt yourself—here we go: If 30 mg oral morphine is about 10 mg oral oxymorphone, and the patient is on 60 mg oral morphine per day, it would be one third of that, or 20 mg oral oxymorphone. Clearly, the answer is a TDD of 20 mg oral oxymorphone!

<u>Step 4</u>—Now that everybody and their dog believes the TDD of oral oxymorphone should be 20 mg, we need to decide if we're going to go with this number, increase or decrease. Since the patient had good pain control, it's probably a good idea to reduce the dose. Because extended-release oxymorphone comes in 5-, 7.5-, 10-, 15-, 20-, 30-, and 40-mg strengths, we can recommend Opana ER 7.5 mg po every 12 hours. We can also order Opana IR, 5 mg by mouth as needed for breakthrough pain every 4 hours. If the patient consistently uses two doses per day of the short-acting oxymorphone, we can increase the extended-release to 10 mg by mouth every 12 hours.

<u>Step 5</u>—Monitor the patient for subjective and objective signs of therapeutic effectiveness and toxicity. Importantly, we should monitor the patient carefully for resolution of hallucinations.

P3.4

<u>Step 1</u>—Patient reports that the Tylenol with Codeine helped the pain, but she couldn't tolerate it (nausea).

<u>Step 2</u>—KK only uses the analgesic as needed. She has tried the Tylenol with Codeine several times.

<u>Step 3</u>—KK has not taken the Tylenol with Codeine consistently enough to calculate a TDD, but we can calculate an equivalent dose of a different opioid to be used "as needed" for pain. In this case, you have already decided to switch to morphine solution. We need to calculate an equivalent dose.

KK was prescribed 2 tablespoons (30 mL) of Tylenol with Codeine solution. How much codeine is she getting with every dose?

$$\frac{12 \text{ mg codeine}}{5 \text{ mL}} \times 30 \text{ mL}$$

$$\frac{12 \text{ mg codeine}}{5 \; \cancel{\text{mL}}} \times 30 \; \cancel{\text{mL}} = 12 \text{ mg codeine} \times 6 = 72 \text{ mg codeine}$$

Now we need to calculate a dose of oral morphine that is equivalent to 72 mg codeine. Let's use Method D.

$$\text{TDD 72 mg oral codeine} \times \frac{30 \text{ mg oral morphine}}{200 \text{ mg oral codeine}}$$

$$\text{TDD 72 mg } \cancel{\text{oral codeine}} \times \frac{30 \text{ mg oral morphine}}{200 \text{ mg } \cancel{\text{oral codeine}}}$$

$$72 \times 30/200 = 10.8$$

This method shows an equivalent dose of oral morphine is approximately 10.8 mg.

Step 4—Now we need to individualize the dose for the patient. As explained in the case, KK was opioid-naïve (she had not received opioids for some period of time post-operatively, before beginning rehabilitation). Ten milligrams of morphine is a high dose for an older adult—this could have been part of the nausea problem with the Tylenol with Codeine. This fact, along with incomplete cross tolerance would make a strong argument to recommend 5 mg of oral morphine as needed every 4 hours for pain, instead of 10 mg.

Step 5—The patient's pain level should be assessed prior to morphine administration, and 1 hour later. Signs and symptoms of toxicity should also be monitored and documented, and the opioid regimen adjusted as indicated.

CHAPTER 4

Titrating Opioid Regimens: Around the Clock and to the Rescue!

OBJECTIVES

After reading this chapter and completing all practice problems, the participant will be able to:

1. Recommend and initiate opioid therapy for opioid-naive patients with acute severe pain, and transition to around-the-clock opioid dosing.

2. Describe different types of break-through pain, and recommend and titrate an opioid regimen to treat these pains.

3. Determine an appropriate strategy to increase an opioid regimen, including both the regularly scheduled and rescue opioid.

4. Recommend a dosing strategy to wean or taper a patient from opioids when adverse effects occur, or when pain is otherwise alleviated.

INTRODUCTION

When crafting an opioid regimen for a patient with persistent pain, we generally have one opioid strategy for the baseline pain, and a different opioid strategy for breakthrough pain. In most cases the same opioid is used, although they may be different for various reasons. In the face of increasing pain, how does the astute health care practitioner know whether to increase the baseline opioid, or the rescue opioid? How much and how quickly can we increase the opioid? And how about the patient who needs to decrease their opioid dose due to the development of an adverse effect or implementation of an opioid-sparing intervention—how quickly can we decrease the dose and not cause opioid withdrawal symptoms? Even though this chapter is not specifically about *conversion* calculations, opioid titration is a critical calculation skill. We discussed the paradigm of safety and efficacy in Chapter 1—the same principles apply here. After reading this chapter, practitioners in the know will be able to calculate dosage increases (or decreases) that allow the patient to achieve pain relief as quickly as possible, while remembering "safety first!" Why does that sound like a Boy Scout doing drug math?

Initiating Opioid Therapy

There are several excellent review articles and consensus guidelines that will be of assistance as we consider the calculations in this chapter.[1-5] In this section we will discuss dose-finding strategies for patients moving from non-opioids, combination analgesics, or occasional opioid use to around-the-clock opioid therapy, as well as management of the opioid-naive patient with acute, severe sudden-onset pain. Calculations specific to methadone, fentanyl, and continuous opioid infusions will be addressed in subsequent chapters.

Acute Severe Pain in the Opioid Naive Patient

Most patients transition to opioid therapy after non-opioid or co-analgesic therapy fails to adequately control pain. Occasionally however, a patient who has not been taking opioids previously will experience acute onset severe pain. Examples include patients who suffer a pathologic fracture or nerve compression. The Cleveland Clinic guidelines for managing acute severe pain in opioid naive patients in a supervised inpatient setting (or very closely monitored outpatient setting) are as follows[1]:

- Morphine 1 mg intravenously (IV) every minute for 10 minutes, followed by a 5-minute respite, and repeated until pain is controlled. The health care practitioner (physician or licensed independent practitioner) should closely monitor (really closely, meaning park yourself by the bedside and don't leave!) sensorium and pain response. It is critically important to monitor level of arousal because sedation precedes respiratory depression. If the patient has not achieved pain relief after 30 mg of parenteral morphine has been administered, and/or the patient is sedated or respiratory rate is < 10 breaths/minute further investigation of the pain complaint should commence. Alternate opioids include fentanyl 20 micrograms (mcg) per minute or hydromorphone 0.2 mg per minute.

- If subcutaneous dosing is preferred, morphine 2 mg every 5 minutes (or fentanyl 40 mcg or hydromorphone 0.4 mg) until pain is managed. Monitoring and precautions discussed above are followed.

- Using the oral route of administration, 5 mg of immediate-release morphine (or 1 mg hydromorphone or 5 mg oxycodone) is given every 30 minutes until pain recedes.

░░▒▒▓▓ FAST FACT ▶ What Do You Mean "Until Pain Is Controlled?"

It is important to clearly describe what we mean by repeating doses of the opioid "until pain is controlled." How do you know when the pain is "controlled?" What you're looking for is an initial 2–4 point drop in the pain rating, not *complete* pain relief. If the practitioner continues to administer opioid until complete pain relief is achieved, this may result in over-administration of the opioid when all the drug administered achieves peak effect.

Another guideline we can draw on comes from the National Comprehensive Cancer Network Clinical Practice Guidelines in Oncology: Adult Cancer Pain.[6] These guidelines state that opioid-naive patients who experience moderate to severe pain should receive between one and five milligrams of morphine intravenously (or the equivalent with a different opioid) and reassess pain at 15 minutes. If the pain persists at 15 minutes, administer double the dose and reassess after 15 minutes. They advise considering an alternate strategy if the pain is not improved after two- or three-dose cycles as described.

It is critically important to recognize that the guidelines listed above pertain to patients in a **very closely monitored** environment, such as a hospital. In other words, an opioid antagonist such as naloxone (Narcan) is standing by if needed. These protocols would NOT be used for a home-based patient. For one thing, it would be unlikely that a home-based patient would have a parenteral opioid sitting around "just in case." However, patients admitted to hospice care may very well have a "starter kit" or "emergency kit" that contains a few doses of the most commonly used rescue medications, including an oral opioid. If this were the case, it would be appropriate for the prescriber to order the visiting nurse (not the patient or family of their own volition) to administer 5 mg of immediate-release morphine (e.g., oral morphine solution) every 30–60 minutes up to a total of 20 or 30 mg for an acute pain crisis. This may in fact be a stop-gap intervention pending inpatient admission to determine the cause of this sudden-onset severe pain. Let's look at a case of an opioid-naive patient who experiences sudden onset acute pain.

 CASE 4.1
• •
Acute Pain Management in an Opioid-Naïve Patient

HY is a 72 year old man diagnosed with colon cancer 8 years ago, diagnosed with prostate cancer two years ago, who is currently on hormone therapy for the prostate cancer. HY presents to the emergency department today complaining of sudden onset severe pain of the right proximal femur. He describes the pain as agonizing and rates it as a 10 on a 0 (no pain) to 10 (worst imaginable pain) scale. HY takes only naproxen 500 mg by mouth twice daily for pain; he has not taken an opioid since his prostate surgery two years ago. Before beginning diagnostic proceedings, it is imperative that HY's pain be treated. HY has no contraindications to opioid therapy (including any history of morphine allergy), and IV access is quickly established. The emergency department physician sits bedside and administers 1 mg IV morphine every minute for 10 minutes (total dose 10 mg). During this time, HY's respiratory rate decreases from 38 breaths per minute to 22 breaths per minute. He rates his pain as a 9 after the tenth injection. The ED physician waits 5 minutes, at which point the patient says his pain is now a 8; respiratory rate is 20 breaths per minute, patient is very much awake with a clear sensorium. The ED physician administers an additional milligram of IV morphine every minute for the next 5 minutes at which point the patient reports the pain is less than 6 and tolerable. The respiratory rate is now 16 breaths per minute and the patient has relaxed considerably. With 15 mg of morphine on board, the patient is able to tolerate an x-ray which confirms a fractured right femur, and a chest x-ray shows a solid mass in the hilum of his right lung. HY's fractured right femur was thought to be due to primary pulmonary cancer, and his fracture was surgically repaired.

Dose-Finding Around-the-Clock Opioid Therapy

Many patients transition from non-opioid therapy to opioid-therapy by the addition of an "as needed" order for an immediate-release (meaning, it's not "sustained release" or "long-acting"; see Sidebar, "Definitions"). An example is "Percocet (5 mg oxycodone/acetaminophen 325 mg per tablet), one tablet every 4 hours as needed for moderate to severe pain." If there is a concern about approaching or exceeding the maximum daily dose of the non-opioid component (e.g., acetaminophen), the prescriber could order "oxycodone 5 mg, one tablet every 4 hours as needed for moderate to severe pain."

Alternately, morphine 5 mg, hydromorphone 2 mg, or oxymorphone 5 mg could be ordered. Doses need to be reduced and adjusted accordingly for vulnerable populations such as pediatrics, frail elderly, and those with hepatic or renal impairment.

If the patient is having continuous or persistent pain (meaning pain around the clock, not just occasional pain) necessitating around-the-clock opioid therapy, many expert guidelines recommend using an immediate-release opioid regularly as a "dose-finding" tool.[2-3] For example, one recommendation by the Expert Working Group of the Research Network of the European Association for Palliative Care is to give immediate-release morphine (or an alternate opioid if desired) every 4 hours, with the same dose available for additional pain relief as needed every 1 or 2 hours.[3] It is important to have the patient maintain a pain diary so the practitioner can determine the total daily dose of opioid necessary to control the pain. Because morphine has an elimination half-life of 2-4 hours, the patient would be at "steady-state" (which is where the rate in of opioid equals the rate out [of the body], resulting in a steady serum concentration of the opioid) within 24 hours. Therefore, it would be permissible to increase the opioid dose every 24 hours. The guidelines further recommend that the patient can then be transitioned to oral sustained-release opioid therapy once good pain control is achieved using this dose-finding strategy. The rationale for this strategy (based on expert opinion) is to achieve steady-state as quickly as possible to optimize analgesia.

While many practitioners feel that it would be inappropriate to initiate therapy for persistent pain with a sustained-release opioid product in an opioid-naive patient, research has shown that in fact this strategy may be just as good or even better. Klepstad and colleagues randomized cancer patients who had continued pain despite treatment with codeine or propoxyphene to receive either 4-hourly doses of immediate-release morphine, or a once-daily sustained-release formulation of morphine (both with rescue doses available).[7] The primary end-point of their study was time needed to achieve adequate pain relief (2.1 days for immediate-release, 1.7 days for sustained-release); secondary end points included other symptoms, health related quality of life and patient satisfaction. Patients in the immediate-release morphine arm reported statistically significantly more tiredness after dosage titration, and no differences were shown in other secondary end-points. The authors pointed out that advantages of using sustained-release morphine from day one include increased patient convenience, less confusion about medication administration, and it eliminates the need to convert from immediate-release to sustained-release morphine subsequently. Of course, it is important to remember that vulnerable populations who would be started on a total daily dose of opioid *lower* than that which could be administered with commercially available sustained-release products cannot use this strategy. Let's look at a case illustrating these principles.

 CASE 4.2
• •
Switching an Immediate-Release Opioid to a Sustained-Release Opioid

VW is a 49 year old man diagnosed with lung cancer. He developed pain that increased over a several week period, to the point that he is using Tylenol #3 (acetaminophen and codeine) three to four tablets per day, and has significant persistent pain despite this. His prescriber wants to switch him to around-the-clock morphine. What are two potential dosing strategies you could recommend for VW?

DEFINITIONS

We use terms such as "immediate" and "sustained" release when we talk about opioid formulations, so it's important that we all have the same understanding about these terms.

An "immediate-release" opioid is an unmodified formulation, such as an oral solution or a plain film-coated tablet. Examples include oral morphine solution (e.g., Roxanol), generic morphine or oxycodone tablets or capsules, or hydromorphone tablets. An immediate-release tablet or capsule begins to dissolve after ingestion, or an oral solution delivers opioid readily available for absorption, and the opioid begins to work within 30 minutes or so. Morphine, hydromorphone, and oxycodone are examples of opioid that are widely used in "immediate-release" formulations, and they are generally dosed every 4 hours or more frequently when used for breakthrough pain. Oxymorphone is also available as a 5 mg immediate-release tablet; combination tablets and capsules such as hydrocodone/acetaminophen, oxycodone/acetaminophen and others are also available as immediate-release formulations.

A "sustained-release" opioid is a tablet or capsule that is used to control persistent, or "around-the-clock" pain. Sustained release oral formulations have been pharmaceutically altered to allow dosing every 12 or 24 hours. Examples include long-acting morphine (e.g., MS Contin, Kadian, Avinza), oxycodone (OxyContin) and oxymorphone (Opana ER). The transdermal fentanyl patch (Duragesic and generic versions) is another sustained-release product designed to maintain blood levels of fentanyl within the therapeutic range for 72 hours.

Knowing if a tablet or capsule is "immediate" or "sustained" release is an important consideration when treating persistent vs. breakthrough pain. If a patient took an extra dose of MS Contin for breakthrough pain, not only would the painful episode be over long before an analgesic effect could be realized, but it would place him at risk of overdose once peak levels were reached after several hours.

Within "immediate-release" opioid tablets and capsules, we can further break these products down into short-onset and rapid-onset. For example, oral morphine, oxycodone, oxymorphone and hydromorphone tablets or capsules are swallowed and start to act in about 30 minutes following dissolution and absorption. Fentanyl can be administered in the buccal cavity (known as transmucosal administration) and the onset of analgesia is 5-10 minutes. Therefore, transmucosal fentanyl would be considered "rapid-onset" and oral morphine, oxycodone, hydromorphone and oxymorphone would be considered "short-onset."

Methadone is an unusual beast compared to most of the other mu opioid agonists we have been discussing—it is rapid-onset (onset of analgesia in 10-15 minutes), but it's long-acting while not being a "sustained release" formulation. I know you've got your head cocked to the side re-reading that last sentence, but it's true! The long-lasting properties of methadone are not due to pharmaceutical manipulation of the oral dosage formulation; methadone (and levorphanol) are *inherently* long-acting, although the elimination half-life is highly variable. A further discussion on the use of methadone can be found in Chapter 6.

<u>Strategy 1</u>—Discontinue the Tylenol #3, and begin 5 mg oral morphine solution every 4 hours around the clock, and 5 mg oral morphine solution every 2 hours as needed for additional pain relief. Have VW keep a pain diary, documenting all doses of morphine taken. After 24 hours, calculate VW's total daily dose of morphine, and re-divide by 6. For example, if VW had taken his six scheduled doses, and three additional doses of morphine, this is a total daily dose of 45 mg oral morphine. On Day 2, VW's standing dose of morphine could be increased to 7.5 mg every 4 hours (his TDD of 45 mg divided into six equal doses), and either keep the "as needed" dose at 5 mg, or increase it to 7.5 mg every 2 hours. Continue with this strategy until VW has achieved good pain control with minimal use of the "as needed" doses of morphine, and then switch to sustained-release morphine. For example, 5 days later a review of VW's diary shows that an eventual increase to 10 mg oral morphine solution every 4 hours has controlled his pain with no need for additional morphine doses over the past 2 days. It would be appropriate to switch VW to a sustained-release morphine regimen based on this stable dose such as one of the following:

- MS Contin 30 mg by mouth every 12 hours, OR
- Avinza 60 mg by mouth once daily, OR
- Kadian 60 mg by mouth once daily, OR
- Kadian 30 mg by mouth every 12 hours

In all of these cases, you would also keep the immediate-release morphine for breakthrough pain, which we will discuss in the next section.

<u>Strategy 2</u>—VW was taking three or four Tylenol #3 tablets per day and had persistent pain despite this. If he was taking four tablets per day that would be 120 mg of oral codeine per day, which is approximately equivalent to 15 mg of oral morphine per day (refer to chapter 3 for an explanation of the mathematics involved). Minimally, VW needs a dosage increase (anywhere from 25-100% increase), therefore starting him at MS Contin 15 mg by mouth every 12 hours would be appropriate (the lowest strength of MS Contin, which is a 100% increase in the TDD of oral morphine). Of course you would also have an immediate-release oral morphine product available for additional pain, such as 5 mg oral morphine solution every 2 hours as needed. Again, you would ask VW to maintain a pain diary. If on day 2 you find that VW has taken four or five doses of the oral morphine solution (totally 20-25 mg oral morphine) in addition to the MS Contin 15 mg twice daily (30 mg oral morphine; total daily dose 50-55 mg oral morphine) it would be appropriate to increase his MS Contin to 30 mg by mouth every 12 hours. Similarly, you could have used Kadian or Avinza as well.

Breakthrough Pain

In the previous section, we discussed dosing opioids around the clock for "**persistent**" pain. Other terms used to describe this type of "always present" pain include "baseline, basal, continuous, intractable, and constant." On top of this, up to 90% of cancer and non-cancer pain patients have a different, or additional pain that comes and goes, referred to globally as "**breakthrough**" pain, presumably because it "breaks through" the persistent pain and around-the-clock analgesic the patient is taking (see Sidebar, "Characterizing Breakthrough Pain"). Breakthrough pain is also referred to as "episodic, incident, or transient" pain. Breakthrough pain is generally defined as a transitory flare of pain that occurs against a background of otherwise controlled pain.[8] An important point in this definition is that the background pain (the persistent or basal pain) is *controlled*. If the persistent pain is not controlled, then, by definition, the presence of breakthrough pain cannot be determined. Clearly the first order of business is to control the persistent pain, and that is what the focus of our exercises have been so far in this chapter, where the breakthrough dose of medication has been a "given." Now we will closely look at why ensuring breakthrough medication availability is essential in a good analgesic plan and how we magically determine the doses of the rescue opioid. On with the hunt!

Breakthrough pain can be classified as ***spontaneous pain*** (frequently idiopathic, occurring with no known stimulus), ***incident pain*** (secondary to a stimulus which the patient may or may not be able to control), or ***end-of-dose failure pain*** (pain at the end of the dosing interval of the long-acting opioid). A description of these terms and usual management options are shown in Table 4-1. Breakthrough pain can occur multiple times per day, lasting seconds to more than an hour, typically peaking within 10–30 minutes in patients with non-cancer pain.[9-10] The patient is unable to predict the occurrence of approximately half of all episodes of breakthrough pain.[10] Uncontrolled breakthrough pain has a negative impact on quality of life and makes patients fearful and sedentary, leading to further deconditioning and disability.[10]

Table 4-1
Types of Breakthrough Pain (BTP)

	Characteristics	Management Strategies
Spontaneous	Pain that requires no precipitating stimulus. Can occur without warning and be acutely severe. Spontaneous pain commonly has a neuropathic component.	Immediate-release opioid on an as-needed basis. Consider use of a co-analgesic (particularly if neuropathic)
Incident pain; volitional	Consistent temporal causal relationship with identifiable causes that are under the patient's control such as patient-precipitated movement, wound, or personal care.	Non-opioid or immediate-release opioid, on an as-needed basis prophylactically; rest; ice; patient education.
Incident pain; nonvolitional	Consistent temporal causal relationship with identifiable causes that are not under the patient's control such as sneezing, bladder spasm, or coughing.	Immediate-release opioid on an as-needed basis.
End-of-dose	Pain that recurs before the next scheduled dose of the around-the-clock analgesic. Likely due to a subtherapeutic dose of analgesic.	Increase in dose and/or frequency of around-the-clock analgesic.

CHARACTERIZING BREAKTHROUGH PAIN

Imagine you have advanced cancer, and a fairly complicated pain picture. Your health care team has switched your analgesics several times, which now provides you with fairly good pain control. You feel like you can't relax however, because you know that two to four times a day a lightening bolt of pain will hit you, leaving you tearful and shaken. How can you enjoy the time you have left living with this threat hanging over your head?

Portenoy and Hagen studied a cohort of patients with cancer pain, and showed that 64% of patients reported breakthrough pain, described as transient flares of severe pain.[8] The median number of breakthrough pain episodes was 4 per patient per day (range was 1–3600). A little less than half of these episodes were paroxysmal (the "out of the blue" experience; spontaneous pain) and the rest were more gradual in onset. Duration of pain was a median of 30 minutes (range 1–240 minutes). Not quite one third of the episodes were end-of-dose pain, 55% were precipitated by some event. Of these, most were volitional incident pain (e.g.,patient-initiated activity), and the remainder were nonvolitional incident pain (e.g., flatulence or coughing). The pain was thought to be somatic or neuropathic in about one third of the cases, and visceral or mixed in about 20% of the cases.

Looking at hospice patients specifically, Fine and Busch found that 86% of patients experienced breakthrough pain, averaging 2.9 episodes per day each.[11] Average pain intensity was 7 (compared to a baseline pain rating of 3.6 during the day and 2.6 at night on a 0 [no pain] to 10 [worst imaginable pain] scale), with an average of 30 minutes to pain relief. Zeppetella and colleagues found similar results in a hospice population, showing about half of episodes occurred suddenly, 59% were unpredictable, and 75% of patients were dissatisfied with their pain control.[12] Interestingly Gagnon and colleagues evaluated the impact of delirium on the circadian distribution of breakthrough analgesia in advanced cancer patients and found that patients without delirium used more breakthrough analgesics in the morning, while those with delirium used more in the evening and at night.[13]

The situation is just as grim with chronic pain patients. Seventy-four percent of opioid-treated chronic noncancer pain patients experience severe to excruciating breakthrough pain.[9] Half of the patients studied had low back pain, and the pathophysiology was characterized as somatic in a little more than one third of episodes, neuropathic in about 18%, visceral in 4% and mixed in 40% of events. The majority of these patients could identify a precipitating event for the pain, with 92% related to some activity. Looking at patients with chronic back pain specifically, Bennett and colleagues conducted a telephone survey of 117 patients with controlled baseline back pain.[14] Of these, 74% experienced breakthrough pain; median number of episodes was 2 per day, median time to maximum intensity was 10 minutes, and median duration was 55 minutes. The vast majority of these patients used short-acting opioids to manage the breakthrough pain, but many found these agents to be unsatisfactory in controlling these painful episodes.

It's easy to imagine how pain patients can become fearful and withdrawn, always waiting for the other shoe to drop. It is imperative that health care practitioners carefully characterize the nature of the patient's breakthrough pain(s) and strategize pre-emptive and reactive plans to address the pain. Questions used to assess the presence and nature of breakthrough pains are shown in Table 4-2.[15]

Table 4-2

Assessing the Presence of Breakthrough Pain (BTP)

- Do you have episodes of severe pain or BTP?

- How many episodes of BTP do you have each week? Each day?

- How long is it from the time the pain first occurs to when the pain is at its worst?

- How long does each episode of BTP last (minutes, hours)?

- On a scale of 0 to 10, with 0 being no pain and 10 being the worst pain you can imagine, how much does an episode of BTP hurt when it occurs?

- Describe where the BTP occurs. What does it feel like?

- Is the BTP similar to or different from your baseline persistent pain?

- Does your BTP occur with movement or other activity, spontaneously (not associated with any activity), or just before you are supposed to take your next dose of pain medicine?

- What impact does BTP have on your daily responsibilities at home/work? Are you able to do the things that you want/need to do?

- Are there any things that you avoid doing or that you are able to do only with severe pain?

- What do you do to relieve the BTP?

- What types of treatments have you used? How long did you use them? Were they effective? Are they still effective?

- What drugs have you used to relieve the BTP? What were the doses? Were they effective? Are they still effective?

Source: Reprinted with permission from reference 15.

Therapeutic Options for Breakthrough Pain

First, it is important not to overlook nonpharmacologic options that may be useful in treating breakthrough pain. This includes strategies such as pacing activities (not over-doing activities to the point of invoking pain), ice or heat applications, wraps/braces/corsets, physical therapy interventions, massage therapy, transcutaneous electrical nerve stimulation (TENS), and nerve blocks. Pharmacologic therapy will likely still be necessary, but these non-drug measures may reduce the frequency or amount of opioid required.

As stated earlier, one of the most important principles of treating pain is to assure that baseline persistent pain is controlled effectively with around-the-clock analgesics, usually with a sustained-release product. Non-opioid analgesics such as acetaminophen or a nonsteroidal anti-inflammatory agent may be used for breakthrough pain, but there are several disadvantages to this strategy. Most importantly, the patient will probably not achieve sufficient pain relief. Patients who require around-the-clock opioid therapy for persistent pain will likely need an opioid for breakthrough pain as well. Second, the non-opioid analgesics have a longer onset of action, a dose-related ceiling effect, and dose-related toxicities. Don't overlook the importance of co-analgesics (adjuvants) however. Spontaneous pain commonly has a neuropathic component and a co-analgesic may significantly reduces episodes of spontaneous breakthrough pain.

The opioids used most often for breakthrough pain include morphine, oxycodone, hydromorphone, and fentanyl. Oxymorphone is also available in an immediate-release formulation and may be used for breakthrough pain, and immediate-release combination analgesics (e.g., hydrocodone/acetaminophen or oxycodone/acetaminophen) may also be used, although practitioners must be mindful of the dose limitations of the non-opioid component.

Selecting the Best Opioid for Breakthrough Pain

There are several considerations that go into making the decision of *which* opioid to use for breakthrough pain. For example, since breakthrough pain tends to be fairly quick in onset and short-lived, it would be best to match the temporal characteristics of the pain with the onset and duration of opioid effectiveness. The pharmacokinetics of opioids (e.g., onset and duration of action) is partially related to the degree of water- or lipid-solubility of the opioid. The more lipid-soluble an opioid is (more "fat-soluble" such as fentanyl or methadone) the quicker the onset of action. The onset and duration of immediate release opioids used for breakthrough pain are shown in Table 4-3.

Most practitioners tend to use the same opioid for treating persistent, around-the-clock pain as they do for breakthrough pain (e.g., MS Contin with MSIR). This practice tends to make the calculation easier, and keeps things "cleaner." Patients may, however, end up on two different opioids for a variety of reasons. For example, a patient may be using a transdermal fentanyl patch for persistent pain, but oral morphine or oxycodone solution for breakthrough pain. Alternately, a patient may be receiving MS Contin around-the-clock, but using fentanyl buccal tablets for breakthrough pain due to quicker onset of action. A bit more controversial is the use of two different opioids based on the concept of genetic polymorphism of opioid receptors. We already know that there are a *bunch* of mu opioid receptors (probably 25 or more), and different opioids (e.g., morphine vs. oxycodone) may bind or activate receptors slightly differently, giving a different therapeutic effect. For the most part, if the patient can swallow oral tablets, capsules or solutions, it is probably easier to use the same opioid for persistent pain and breakthrough pain, unless the pain is not optimally controlled, and usual and customary interventions do not rectify the situation.

Table 4-3

Pharmacokinetic Properties of Immediate-Release Opioids Used for Breakthrough Pain

Solubility	Immediate-release opioid	Onset of analgesia	Duration of effect
Hydrophilic	Morphine (oral)	30–40 minutes	4 hours
	Oxycodone (oral)	30 minutes	4 hours
	Oxymorphone (oral)	30 minutes	4–6 hours
	Hydromorphone (oral)	30 minutes	4 hours
	Methadone (oral)	10–15 minutes	4–8 hours
Lipophilic	Fentanyl (transmucosal)	5–10 minutes	1–2 hours

Source: Adapted from reference 16.

Determining the Dose of Rescue Opioid

There are many suggested guidelines for determining the dose of an opioid for break-through pain, but assuming the patient is receiving an oral long-acting opioid (e.g., morphine, oxymorphone or oxycodone) for the baseline pain, a reasonable rule of thumb is to offer 10–15% of the total daily dose of the same opioid for rescue. For example, if a patient were receiving MS Contin 30 mg po q12h, the total daily dose of *scheduled* morphine is 60 mg. Ten percent of 60 mg is 6 mg, and 15% is 9 mg. Both 6 and 9 are goofy numbers for a dose, so it would be likely we'd recommend either 5 mg or 10 mg. Therefore, a sample order would be MS Contin 30 mg po q12h, and morphine oral solution 10 mg po every 1–2 hours as needed for breakthrough pain. Bear in mind, however, that this rule of thumb is NOT evidence-based. Also, accrediting organizations (e.g., Joint Commission) dislike "range" orders for dose or dosing interval (e.g., take every 1–2 hours). Also, if the patient can take the breakthrough opioid every hour, the "every 2 hours" part of the order becomes meaningless.

If the patient were receiving their around-the-clock opioid as an immediate-release product dosed every 4 hours, additional opioid could be offered for break-through pain in between doses (e.g., every 1–2 hours). The dose should be 25–50% of the scheduled 4-hourly around-the-clock dose. For example, if the patient were receiving oxycodone 10 mg every 4 hours around the clock, an additional 2.5 or 5 mg of oxycodone could be made available for breakthrough pain, including volitional incident pain (such as physical therapy) administered pre-emptively.

The dose of the rescue opioid should be adjusted based on patient response. For example with volitional incident pain, the best way to assess the appropriateness of the rescue dose is to assess the pain rating *before and after* the incident. For example, if Mrs. Smith knows that jumping into the passenger side of the Buick to go to Wendy's drive-through for a Frosty causes pain, she could pre-medicate with morphine about 30–45 minutes before leaving home. Hmmmm…a Frosty with morphine beads sprinkled on top! Add some Senna sprinkles and you're all set! If Mrs. Smith were able to go to Wendy's after taking 10 mg of oral morphine and her pain never exceeded a 3 (on a 0–10 scale) and she was content with her pain control, that's an appropriate dose. On the other hand, if she says despite 10 mg of oral morphine, the pain increased to a very un-comfortable 6 or 7, it might be appropriate to increase the dose of opioid to perhaps 15 or even 20 mg. The goal is patient comfort, short of adverse effects. It is not uncommon for the dose of opioid used to prevent volitional incident pain to be disproportionately higher than what may be required for spontaneous pain (e.g., greater than the 10–15% of the total daily dose, or perhaps equivalent to the 4-hourly standing dose of opioid).

A word about the dosing interval for opioid rescue dosing: as briefly discussed previously, most short-acting opioids generally have a duration of 4 hours. Unfortu-nately, many practitioners will order a short-acting opioid such as morphine, hydro-morphone or oxycodone as every 4–6 hours. In the majority of patients these three opioids do not provide pain relief for 6 hours and the pain may recur and last until the next dose may be administered. Even giving a short-acting opioid every 4 hours may result in the pain recurring. It is probably best to allow administration of the rescue short-acting opioid every 1–2 hours. In the case of volitional incident pain, the patient will be administering the short-acting opioid 30–45 minutes before the event that trig-gers the pain.

The best way to assess the appropriateness of the rescue dose of opioid for non-volitional incident pain or spontaneous pain is to compare the pain rating before taking the rescue opioid dose, and one hour after administering the rescue dose. For example, let's suppose Mr. Johnson tells you his background persistent pain is usually an acceptable 2 or 3 (on a 0–10 scale), and the spontaneous pain he experiences several times a day shoots it up to a 7 or 8. If he tells you his pain comes back down to a 3 or 4 one hour after taking 10 mg of oral morphine, and he is content with this, then your dose is appropriate. On the other hand, if he tells you the pain one hour after administration is still a 5 or 6 you would want to increase the dose of breakthrough analgesic by 50–100%. A rule of thumb is if the rescue dose relieves less than 50% of the pain, double the rescue dose. If 50–100% of the pain is relieved, increase the rescue dose by 50%. Close to 100% pain relief (or otherwise acceptable to the patient) indicates no change is necessary.

What about patients who require a more lipid-soluble opioid to treat breakthrough pain that comes on very quickly? As mentioned above, two possibilities are methadone and fentanyl. Methadone is an extremely useful opioid to have in our arsenal, and the onset of analgesia is 10–15 minutes. However, the duration of effect is 4–8 hours, which is probably longer than needed for breakthrough pain. However, methadone has been used successfully in this manner, and will be discussed in greater detail in a subsequent chapter.

Fentanyl administered by the transmucosal route has an onset of analgesia of 5–10 minutes, and a short duration of action (1–2 hours). This includes both the oral transmucosal fentanyl citrate (OTFC) lozenge (Actiq, generics) and the effervescent transmucosal tablet (Fentora). Unfortunately, the dose of oral transmucosal fentanyl cannot be determined as a percentage of the around-the-clock opioid the patient is receiving, whether it's a fentanyl product or not. A Cochrane Review on the use of opioids for the management of breakthrough pain in cancer patients found no meaningful relationship between the successful dose of OTFC and the around-the-clock oral or transdermal opioid medication.[17] The authors recommended determining the most appropriate dose of oral transmucosal fentanyl by appropriate titration to determine the most successful dose. Table 4-4 shows recommendations for the dosing and titration of oral transmucosal fentanyl (both the OTFC and effervescent tablet) as well as information on how to switch from OTFC to Fentora.[18-19]

 PITFALL •
Fentora Precautions

In September 2007 the FDA reported receiving reports of death and life-threatening side effects in patients who have taken Fentora. According to this Public Health Advisory, Fentora was prescribed for patients who were not appropriate candidates, received unapproved doses, and were inappropriately switched between oral transmucosal fentanyl citrate (OTFC, Actiq) and Fentora. In response to these reports, the FDA issued the following Public Health Advisory:

- "Fentora should only be used for breakthrough pain in opioid-tolerant patients with cancer.
  - Fentora should not be used to treat any type of short-term pain including headaches or migraines, postoperative pain, or pain due to injury.

- Fentora should not be used by patients who only take narcotic pain medications occasionally.

■ The dosage strength of fentanyl in Fentora is NOT equal to the same dosage strength of fentanyl in other fentanyl-containing products.
   - Healthcare professionals must not directly substitute Fentora for other fentanyl medicines, including Actiq (e.g., on a mcg-per-mcg basis; see prescribing information).
   - Doctors must select the Fentora dose carefully for each patient.

■ Patients who take Fentora and their caregivers must understand how to use it safely and follow the directions exactly. Directions for taking Fentora are provided in the Medication Guide for patients.

■ Healthcare professionals who prescribe Fentora and patients who use Fentora and their caregivers should be aware of the signs of fentanyl overdose. Signs of fentanyl overdose include trouble breathing or shallow breathing; tiredness, extreme sleepiness or sedation; inability to think, talk or walk normally; and feeling faint, dizzy or confused. If these signs occur, patients or their caregivers should get medical attention right away."[20]

● ●

Types of Breakthrough Pain

As discussed previously, there are several types of breakthrough pain. Incident pain that the patient can control and/or predict is best treated with a pre-emptive strike. The patient can use a more cost-effective short-acting opioid such as morphine, oxycodone, oxymorphone or hydromorphone, taking a dose 30-60 minutes before the painful activity. The dose is usually 10–15% of the total daily dose of their around-the-clock opioid, but the dose should be increased or decreased to keep the patient comfortable.

Non-volitional incident pain and spontaneous breakthrough pain should be treated by administering the dose as soon as the breakthrough pain is experienced, or pain begins to worsen. If the pain is very rapid in onset, it may be appropriate to use a more rapid-onset opioid such as transmucosal fentanyl. This is a considerably more expensive option, and formulary considerations may limit this option. However, for patients with very quick-onset severe pain that significantly impacts their quality of life, use of a more expensive medication may be appropriate. One other strategy is to increase the around-the-clock opioid dose above that required to control baseline pain. Mercadante and colleagues demonstrated this with 25 patients with movement-related episodic pain due to bone metastases.[21] The dose of opioid was escalated beyond that required for pain control at rest, but short of adverse effects. This approach was successful and only a small minority of patients required treatment of opioid-induced adverse effects or a decrease in opioid dose.

The last type of breakthrough pain, end of dose failure, may be treated with the use of rescue opioid doses, by giving the around-the-clock opioid more frequently, or by increasing the dose of the regularly scheduled (around-the-clock) opioid. Fewer doses per day is preferred, therefore it would be worth a trial of an increased dose using the original dosing schedule.

A final word about titrating the around-the-clock opioid regimen based on the use of rescue medication. If a patient is *routinely* using their rescue medication, it is important to do a careful reassessment of the pain complaint. Perhaps a co-analgesic

Table 4-4

Dosing and Titration of Oral Transmucosal Fentanyl for Breakthrough Pain

Fentanyl Buccal Tablet (FBT; Fentora)

Initial dose and titration instructions	■ For opioid-tolerant patients ONLY (patients taking at least 60 mg of oral morphine/day, at least 25 mcg of transdermal fentanyl/hour, at least 30 mg of oxycodone daily, at least 8 mg of oral hydromorphone daily, or an equianalgesic dose of another opioid for a week or longer)
	■ Initial dose of FBT is 100 mcg
	■ If breakthrough pain is not relieved within 30 minutes of the first dose, *one* additional 100 mcg FBT may be administered.
	■ If breakthrough pain is not relieved with this second dose, patient must wait *at least 4 hours* before treating the next breakthrough pain episode with FBT
	■ If the initial one or two doses were insufficient to treat the breakthrough pain, the next higher dose of FBT may be administered (available as 100-, 200-, 300-, 400-, 600-, and 800-mcg tablets).
	■ Patients titrating above 100 mcg may use two 100-mcg tablets (one on each side of the mouth in the buccal cavity). If this dose is not successful in controlling the breakthrough pain episode, the patient may be instructed to place two 100 mcg tablets on each side of the mouth in the buccal cavity (total of four 100-mcg tablets).
	■ For doses above 400 mcg, titration can continue by 200-mcg increments. NOTE: Using more than 4 tablets simultaneously has not been studied.
	■ To reduce the risk of overdose during titration, patients should have only one strength of FBT available at any one time.
Maintenance dosing	■ Once titrated to an effective dose, patients should generally use only ONE FBT per breakthrough pain episode.
	■ On occasion, when the breakthrough pain episode is not relieved within 30 minutes, patients may take ONLY ONE additional tablet of the same strength for that episode.
	■ Patients MUST wait *at least 4 hours* before treating another breakthrough pain episode with FBT

Table 4-4 (contd.)
Dosing and Titration of Oral Transmucosal Fentanyl for Breakthrough Pain

Fentanyl Buccal Tablet (FBT; Fentora)

Switching from OTFC to FBT	■ For opioid-tolerant patients switching from oral transmucosal fentanyl citrate (Actiq), use the following dosing conversion. The doses of Fentora in this table are starting doses and not intended to represent equianalgesic doses to Actiq.

Current Actiq dose (OTFC) in mcg	Initial Fentora (FBT) dose in mcg
200	100-mcg tablet
400	100-mcg tablet
600	200-mcg tablet
800	200-mcg tablet
1200	2 × 200-mcg tablets
1600	2 × 200 mcg tablets

Oral Transmucosal Fentanyl Citrate Lozenges (OTFC; Actiq)

Initial dose and titration instructions	■ For opioid-tolerant patients ONLY (patients taking at least 60 mg of oral morphine/day, at least 25 mcg of transdermal fentanyl/hour, at least 30 mg of oxycodone daily, at least 8 mg of oral hydromorphone daily, or an equianalgesic dose of another opioid <u>for a week or longer</u>) ■ Initial dose of OTFC is 200 mcg ■ If breakthrough pain is not relieved 15 minutes after completing the previous dose (30 minutes after the start of the previous dose), an additional 200 mcg dose may be used. No more than two units should be taken for each individual breakthrough cancer pain episode. ■ If several episodes of breakthrough pain require more than one OTFC lozenge, consider increasing dose to next higher available strength (available as 200-, 400-, 600-, 800-, 1200-, and 1600-mcg lozenges)

would be appropriate to add to the regimen. Or, the patient could be experiencing disease progression and more opioid is required. When the patient is consistently using two, three, or four doses of rescue opioid per day, it would be appropriate to recalculate the total daily dose of opioid necessary to keep the patient comfortable (standing dose and rescue doses used on average per day) and increase the regularly scheduled dose. It is likely that you will need to readjust the rescue dose as well (to keep the same ratio that already worked for the patient; for example, 15% of the total daily dose of scheduled opioid to be available for breakthrough pain). These principles will be illustrated in the next section of this chapter as we continue on this amazing mathematical journey!

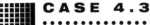

CASE 4.3
••
Pre-empting Volitional Incident Pain

EY is an 82 year old woman with end-stage dementia and multiple pressure ulcers. She has a long-standing history of severe osteoarthritis pain for which she receives Kadian 30 mg po q12h. Although EY is not able to provide a pain rating due to her dementia, the nurse observes that when she is doing a dressing change EY moans and cries out, and becomes very tense, holding her body very stiffly. The nurse clearly suspects that the dressing change is causing EY additional pain.

Clearly this is volitional incident pain. It's volitional in that the pain is caused by an activity that *could* be anticipated and controlled; obviously EY herself cannot prevent the dressing change, but it's not an incident beyond *everyone's* control (e.g., coughing or sneezing). With volitional incident pain the best strategy is to administer a dose of rescue opioid 30–45 minutes before the precipitating event. Our rule of thumb is 10–15% of the total daily dose of the regularly scheduled ("around the clock") opioid. In this case the patient is receiving 60 mg of oral morphine per day. Ten to fifteen percent would be 6–9 mg; the RN recommends starting with 5 mg of morphine prior to dressing changes and allowing a repeat dose if ineffective, which the prescriber approves.

During the next dressing change, 5 mg of morphine was administered 45 minutes beforehand, and it had little to no effect on EY's behavior, so the procedure was stopped until the additional 5 mg was given. This was the ticket—EY did not exhibit the behaviors previously associated with the dressing change, and she took a short nap afterwards, but was easily arousable.

CASE 4.4
••
Dosing Transmucosal Fentanyl

MJ is a 42 year old man with lung cancer, who is using a transdermal fentanyl (TDF) patch 75 mcg every 3 days to control his pain. The TDF mostly controls his pain, but several times a day he unexpectedly experiences an unprovoked "grabbing" sensation in his lower back that feels like a hot poker branding him that is exquisitely painful. The pain lasts for about 15 minutes, leaving him completely drained for the next 30 minutes or so. He has morphine oral solution 20 mg every 2 hours available for breakthrough pain, which MJ says he takes, but it doesn't kick in quickly enough to address the pain. As a matter of fact, the morphine actually makes the post-episode exhaustion worse. MJ is extremely anxious about this situation, because he feels like he's on "pins and needles" all day long waiting for this lightning bolt.

To better match the onset of analgesia with the temporal nature of the pain, you decide to switch MJ to the fentanyl buccal tablet (FBT; Fentora). Because there is no consistent correlation between the around-the-clock opioid dose and FBT, you prescribe the lowest dose, 100 mcg FBT, and advise MJ to insert one tablet between his cheek and upper molar the instant the pain occurs. If the pain has not resolved 30 minutes after inserting the tablet in the buccal cavity, MJ can take one additional 100 mcg tablet. After several days, MJ tells you that this approach has been more successful, but he is requiring two tablets every time he has the breakthrough pain. To make things simpler for MJ, you prescribe the 200 mcg FBT for future episodes of this spontaneous breakthrough pain.

FAST FACT Determining Rescue Dosing with Transdermal Fentanyl

In the case of MJ above (Case 4.4) how did the prescriber come up with the dose of morphine oral solution for breakthrough pain? As you will learn in Chapter 5, most practitioners consider 2 mg per day of oral morphine to be approximately equivalent to 1 mcg per hour of transdermal fentanyl. Therefore, a TDF 75 mcg patch would be approximately equal to oral morphine 150 mg per day. Using our 10–15% rule for rescue opioid dosing, this would be 15–22.5 mg of oral morphine. The 20 mg oral morphine dose is right in the middle of the range; this dose would be adjusted (up or down) per patient response.

Opioid Dose Escalation Strategies

Surprisingly, there is not much evidence-based research on opioid dose escalation. This primarily leaves us with the standard of practice as a guideline. An important part of the rule of thumb commonly used in practice is the recognition that the analgesic effect is a logarithmic function of the opioid dose, therefore dosage increases are done as a percentage of the current total daily dose, not increasing by a specific milligram amount. Practitioners routinely use this strategy when increasing from one to two tablets of a combination product—for example, "Increase from one Percocet tablet every 4 hours to two Percocet tablets." This represents a 100% increase in the regularly scheduled opioid dose. When put in those terms, you're probably holding your head thinking, "Whoa…" But if you think about it, as Dr. David Weissman has said, practitioners don't increase a furosemide dose from 10 mg to 11 mg, but that's what practitioners like to do with opioids, especially parenteral infusions (increase from 4 mg/hour to 5 mg/hour).[22] Dr. Weissman further points out that patients generally do not notice a change in analgesia when dose increases are less than 25% above baseline. Going from 4 mg/hour to 5 mg/hour of parenteral morphine is only a 20% dosage increase. So where does this leave us? Let's consider oral opioids and parenteral opioids separately. Methadone, fentanyl and continuous opioid infusions will be discussed in later chapters.

Oral Opioid Regimens

Many patients are receiving an oral long-acting opioid plus an immediate-release opioid for breakthrough pain. A rule of thumb that is commonly followed in clinical practice for patient who continue to have pain despite their opioid regimen is as follows[22]:

- For moderate to severe pain, increase opioid total daily dose by 50–100%, regardless of starting dose

- For mild-moderate pain increase opioid total daily dose by 25–50%, regardless of starting dose

- Short-acting, immediate-release single-ingredient opioids (e.g., morphine, oxycodone, hydromorphone) can be safely dose-escalated every 2 hours

- Long-acting, oral sustained-release opioids can be increased every 24 hours (except for transdermal fentanyl and methadone, which will be discussed in later chapters).

These guidelines assume the patient has normal renal and liver function; if this is not the case dosage escalation recommendations should be reduced.

Let's consider a patient on MS Contin plus MSIR (morphine sulfate immediate release) for breakthrough pain. If the patient has acceptable pain control but finds he needs to use the MSIR multiple times per day, it would be reasonable to determine his *total* daily dose of morphine, which keeps him comfortable, and administer *that* dose as MS Contin. A few caveats however. First, the Cleveland Clinic guidelines recommend *not* including rescue doses taken for volitional incident pain; after all the patient controls the events that cause that pain so if the patient chooses not to participate in those pain-precipitating activities, then including the MSIR taken in response to those activities may result in an overdose. Second, we have all seen patients who seem to be *emotionally attached* to their short-acting opioid. You get the feeling you could increase their MS Contin to a million milligrams every 12 hours, and they would still feel the need to take their short-acting MSIR. If this is the case or if the patient doesn't clearly understand the purpose and intended outcome of increasing the MS Contin you may be better off leaving the regimen as is.

Wells and colleagues evaluated a variation of the above guidelines by designing a standard opioid titration order sheet to be used to manage pain in ambulatory cancer patients, and implemented by nurses.[23] The protocol was as follows:

- For patients with <u>controlled pain</u> (pain rated as 4 or less with four or fewer rescue doses per 24 hours, and meeting these criteria for three consecutive days), their long-acting opioid was adjusted by an amount equal to the daily rescue dose to decrease the frequency of short-acting opioid administration.

  - Example: MS Contin 30 mg po q12h plus MSIR 10 mg q2h prn, using 3 doses per day for 3 days → change to MS Contin 45 mg po q12h and continue MSIR 10 mg q2h prn

- Patients with <u>moderate pain</u> (5–6) had their long-acting opioid increased to 125% of their average total daily dose (long-acting opioid plus short-acting opioid) over the past 3 days.

  - Example: OxyContin 40 mg po q12h plus OxyIR 15 mg q2h, using 3 doses per day for three days (pain average 5–6) → change to OxyContin 80 mg po q12h plus OxyIR 20 mg po q2h prn

- Patients with <u>severe pain</u> (≥ 7) had their long-acting opioid increased to 150% of their average total daily dose (long-acting opioid plus short-acting opioid) over the past 3 days.

  - Example: Avinza 90 mg po q24h plus MSIR 10 mg q2h, using 3 doses per day for three days (pain average ≥ 7) → change to Avinza 180 mg po q24h plus MSIR 20 mg po q2h prn

Results from this study included 39 study nurse titration interventions in 17 patients over the four week trial. No adverse effects were observed in any of the dosage increases, and opioid toxicities, worst pain, usual pain and pain-related distress declined from baseline to the end of the study.[23]

Parenteral Opioid Regimens

We can use the same strategies discussed above for patients receiving regular doses of an opioid by the IV or SQ route of administration. For example, around-the-clock and rescue doses (not counting those for volitional incident pain) given over the past 24 hours can be totaled, and the new every 4 hourly, or continuous infusion hourly dose determined accordingly. For moderate pain, this new 24-hour dose could be increased by 25%; for severe pain the new 24-hour dose could be increased by 50%. For very acute severe pain, we can following the dosing guidelines presented at the beginning of this chapter (Acute Severe Pain in the Opioid Naive Patient) and adjust the dose as appropriate. Again, please refer to Chapter 7 for a complete review of parenteral opioid administration and titration.

 CASE 4.5

•••
Opioid Dosage Escalation

HB is a 54 year old woman who works as an administrative assistant to the Dean at the local community college. HB has significant osteoarthritis pain and was referred to you for evaluation of her analgesic regimen. She was receiving Percocet (7.5 mg oxycodone/325 mg acetaminophen), 1 tablet every 4 hours as needed (taking 5 tablets per day), gabapentin 300 mg po three times daily, and Celebrex 200 mg po qd. She told you that her pain rating ranged between a 4 and 6 during the day while she was at work, and when she took a walk in the evening with her dog. You decided to start her on OxyContin 20 mg po q12h, and keep the Percocet for breakthrough. After 2 weeks she returns to your office and tells you that when she takes an additional 3 tablets of Percocet during the day, she has an average pain rating of 2 or 3, which she finds acceptable. She asks you if there is a way she can stop taking the Percocet however, because she doesn't like taking analgesics while at work.

She is taking oxycodone 40 mg per day from the long-acting OxyContin, and an additional 22.5 mg from the Percocet, for a total daily dose of 62.5 mg. It would be reasonable to increase the OxyContin to 30 mg po q12h, and keep the Percocet for breakthrough pain, although it is less likely she will need to take it during the work day.

Decreasing Opioid Doses

Occasionally we are able to reduce a patient's opioid dose either due to the introduction of an opioid-sparing co-analgesic, or use of a non-pharmacologic intervention (e.g., radiation, neural block) that has a significant positive effect on the pain. Sometimes we also need to reduce the opioid dose due to the development of unacceptable adverse effects. How quickly can we reduce the dose of the opioid, and how can we clinically monitor the patient to determine if we are being too aggressive?

Again, unsurprisingly, there is little data to guide us in this quest. The Cleveland Clinic offers the following guidelines[1]:

- For patients with good pain control, but experiencing dose-related excessive side effects on an oral opioid regimen, it would be appropriate to reduce the around-the-clock opioid dose by 30%, but keep the rescue dose unchanged.

- For patients with continued pain but experiencing an opioid-induced adverse effect, consider adding a co-analgesic, and reducing the around-the-clock opioid by 30–50%. Of course switching to an entirely new opioid is also a consideration.

- If the patient undergoes a definitive pain-relieving procedure it would be appropriate to reduce the regularly scheduled opioid dose by 50% immediately, and continue dose reductions every third day until the opioid is entirely discontinued. The rescue dose should remain available during this downward titration period for unexpected breakthrough pain.

How can we tell if the taper is too rapid? Certainly the first clue would be pain out of control. If the patient finds he is using the rescue medication consistently, it may be prudent to go back up on the dose of the regularly scheduled opioid a bit, and resume decreasing the opioid dose with a slower/lower taper. The second indication is the development of signs or symptoms of the opioid withdrawal syndrome, including any combination of the following: restlessness/irritability/agitation/dysphoric mood, abdominal pain/cramping, pupillary dilatation, lacrimation, rhinorrhea, piloerection (goosebumps), yawning, sneezing, anorexia, nausea, vomiting and diarrhea.[23] There are several instruments used in clinical practice to diagnose physical dependence and assess opioid withdrawal, including the Objective Opioid Withdrawal Scale (OOWS), the Subjective Opioid Withdrawal Scale (SOWS) (can be viewed at www.aodgp.gov. au/resourcekit/b4/handout6_opioids.pdf), and the Clinical Opiate Withdrawal Scale (COWS) (can be viewed at www.pcssmentor.org/pcss/resources_clinicaltools.php).[24] The COWS scale for example, assigns a numerical rating to resting pulse rate, sweating, restlessness, pupil size, bone or joint aches, runny nose or tearing, GI upset, tremor, yawning, anxiety or irritability and gooseflesh skin. When tapering opioids it is probably not necessary to rate the patient using one of these scales, but instead to be mindful of the presenting symptoms of opioid withdrawal.

CASE 4.6
• •
Opioid Dosage Reduction

EK is a 72 year woman with chronic back pain who has failed several non-opioid analgesics, and was recently started on morphine 5 mg po q4h. She was eventually titrated to Oramorph 45 mg po q8h, but she complained that this made her too sleepy and nauseated. She was switched to OxyContin 30 mg po q12h with OxyIR 10 mg po q2h prn breakthrough pain, but the sedation and nausea have persisted. Several antiemetics and methylphenidate have been tried with minimal success. You have decided to reduce her opioid regimen to see if this helps alleviate her complaints.

Using the guideline described above, it is worth reducing the regularly scheduled opioid by 30%. When you reduced the OxyContin to 20 mg po q12h (keeping the OxyIR 10 mg po q2h prn), her nausea was reduced to an acceptable level, and the sedation clearly completely. EK is content with this regimen, and she knows she can use the OxyIR if she has a flare in the pain.

This has certainly been an action-packed chapter! You've been putting out fires all over the place! We've discussed how to manage acute severe pain in an opioid-naive patient, how to perform dose-finding for a regularly-scheduled opioid regimen, how to design an opioid regimen for breakthrough pain, and how to increase and decrease opioid regimens. You might want to take a nap before you go on to the next chapter!

P4.1: Acute Severe Pain in an Opioid-Naive Patient

JK is a 62 year old woman with adenocarcinoma of the descending colon, who presented to the ER several days before her scheduled colon resection surgery complaining of sudden onset, severe supra-clavicular swelling and pain. JK takes only an occasional acetaminophen, and is not receiving opioids. She rates this pain as the worst imaginable pain possible (she says it's "at least" 10 out of 10), and states it started abruptly at this intensity. The pain started about an hour and a half ago, and her physician directed her to the Emergency Room. JK tells you she has a history of itching when given morphine, but she has taken hydromorphone successfully in the past. How would you go about controlling JK's pain? What would you monitor?

P4.2: Switching from an Immediate-release to Sustained-release Oral Opioid

WM is an 82 year old woman living in a long-term care facility, with advanced osteoarthritis pain that has made it difficult for her to ambulate. Non-opioid medications do not provide any degree of significant relief, however she has responded to 2.5 mg oral oxycodone in the past. WM despises taking medication, and says "if I can't take it just once a day, I'm not going to take it." When WM was given 5 mg of oxycodone it made her very somnolent, leaving her fairly distrustful of opioids in general. However, WM complains constantly about her persistent pain. WM also has mild hepatic impairment. What do you recommend?

P4.3: Calculating Oral Opioid Rescue Doses

LP is a 64 year old man with end-stage lung cancer. He is receiving MS Contin 200 mg po q12h and naproxen 500 mg po q12h, as well as Percocet (5 mg oxycodone/325 mg acetaminophen), 1–2 tablets every 4 hours as needed for breakthrough pain. LP tells you that when he experiences unanticipated, unprovoked breakthrough pain, he takes 2 Percocet tablets, but they are not particularly effective (bringing pain rating down from an 8 to about a 6). LP is growing weaker, and is now experiencing shortness of breath occasionally as well. Your formulary has immediate-release oxycodone, morphine and hydromorphone available. What do you recommend?

P4.4: Switching from OTFC Lozenges to Fentanyl Buccal Tablets

FM is a 24 year old man with a glioblastoma, receiving methadone 20 mg po q8h around the clock for persistent pain. He had been using an oral transmucosal fentanyl citrate lozenge (OTFC; Actiq), 600 mcg as needed for spontaneous breakthrough pain. He was originally able to correctly use the lozenge, continuously moving it through his cheeks coating the mucosal tissues to optimize absorption giving him good pain relief. Now, however, he has grown too weak to do so, and his pain relief from each lozenge is not as great. You've heard about the new fentanyl buccal tablets (FBT; Fentora), which do not require this kind of physical manipulation. The prescriber is agreeable and asks what the starting dose should be, since she heard that there is no consistent correlation between the around-the-clock opioid, and the starting dose of Fentora. What do you recommend?

P4.5: Parenteral Opioid Dosage Escalation

QN is 47 year old woman with end-stage breast cancer admitted to your inpatient Hospice unit for pain control. She was taking three or four Lortab tablets (5 mg hydrocodone bitartrate/500 mg acetaminophen) per day and was complaining of moderate to severe pain. On admission she was switched to parenteral hydromorphone, and is now receiving 4 mg every 4 hours with 2 mg every 2 hours for breakthrough pain. QN has been getting approximately five extra doses of the 2 mg hydromorphone, and her pain persists between a 7 and an 8. She has been examined and her complaint carefully assessed, and you do not feel any additional coanalgesics would provide additional relief. How should you adjust her parenteral hydromorphone? Assuming this does the trick, what dose of oral hydromorphone should you send her home on assuming she is NOT using the breakthrough hydromorphone (I know, tricky, asking you to do drug math from previous chapters!)?

P4.6: Opioid Dosage Reduction

RR is a 49 year old man diagnosed with pancreatic cancer. He has failed chemotherapy and has been referred to hospice. He is complaining of severe pain, which he describes as a sharp pain between shoulder blades that radiates straight through his back, as well as pain in both the right and left upper quadrant. His opioid regimen was increased over a week to MS Contin 90 mg po q12h with minimal relief. The physician has decided to send RR for a celiac plexus block. Over the 12–24 hours after receiving the block, RR cries "It's a miracle—the pain is gone! I have my life back. Now I don't need this morphine!" You interrupt RR as he's doing the happy dance to inform him that he cannot stop the morphine cold, because it would most likely cause symptoms of opioid withdrawal. How should you taper RR off this morphine regimen?

REFERENCES

1. Walsh D, Rivera NL, Davis MP, et al. Strategies for pain management: Cleveland Clinic Foundation guidelines for opioid dosing for cancer pain. *Support Cancer Ther.* 2004;1(3):157–164.

2. Mercadante S. Opioid titration in cancer pain: a critical review. *Eur J Pain.* 2007;11:823–830.

3. Hanks GW, de Conno F, Cherny N, et al. Morphine and alternative opioids in cancer pain: the EAPC recommendations. Expert Working Group of the Research Network of the European Association for Palliative Care. *Br J Cancer.* 2001;84(5):587–593.

4. Davis MP, Weissman DE, Arnold RM. Opioid dose titration for severe cancer pain: a systematic evidence-based review. *J Palliat Med.* 2004;7(3):462–468.

5. Davis MP, Lasheen W, Gamier P. Practice guide to opioids and their complications in managing cancer pain: what oncologists need to know. *Oncology.* 2007;21(10):1229–12.

6. National Comprehensive Cancer Network. NCCN Clinical Practice Guidelines in Oncology. Adult Cancer Pain, v.1.2007. Accessed online at 222.nccn.org, March 29, 2008.

7. Klepstad P, Kaasa S, Jystad A, et al. Immediate- or sustained-release morphine for dose finding during start of morphine to cancer patients: a randomized, double-blind trial. *Pain.* 2003;101:193–198.

8. Portenoy RK, Hagen NA. Breakthrough pain: definition, prevalence and characteristics. *Pain.* 1990;41:273–281.

9. Portenoy RK, Bennett DS, Rauck R, et al. Prevalence and characteristics of breakthrough pain in opioid-treated patients with chronic noncancer pain. *J Pain.* 2006;7:583–591.

10. Portenoy RK, Payne D, Jacobsen P. Breakthrough pain: characteristics and impact in patients with cancer pain. *Pain.* 1999;81:81:129–134.

11. Fine P, Busch MA. Characterization of breakthrough pain by hospice patients and their caregivers. *J Pain Symptom Manage.* 1998;16:179–183.

12. Zeppetella G, O'Doherty CA, Collins S. Prevalence and characteristics of breakthrough pain in cancer patients admitted to a hospice. *J Pain Symptom Manage.* 2000;20:87–92.

13. Gagnon B, Lawlor P, Mancini IS, et al. The impact of delirium on the circadian distribution of breakthrough analgesia in advanced cancer patients. *J Pain Symptom Manage.* 2001;22:826–833.

14. Bennett DS, Simon S, Brennan M, et al. Prevalence and characteristics of breakthrough pain in patients receiving opioids for chronic back pain in pain specialty clinics. *J Opioid Mang.* 2007 Marc–Apr;3(2):101–6.

15. Bennett D, Burton AW, Fishman S, et al. Consensus panel recommendations for the assessment and management of breakthrough pain. Part I: Assessment. *P&T.* 2005;30:296–301.

16. Bennett D, Burton AW, Fishman S, et al. Consensus panel recommendations for the assessment and management of breakthrough pain. Part II: Management. *P&T.* 2005;30:354–361.

17. Zeppetella G, Ribeiro MDC. Opioids for the management of breakthrough (episodic) pain in cancer patients. Cochrane Database of Systematic Reviews 2006, Issue 1, Art. No.: CD004311. DOI: 10.1002/14651858.CD004311.pub2.

18. Fentora Prescribing Information. Available online at: http://www.fentora.com/2000-hcp-homepage.aspx, Accessed May 25, 2008. Also on FDA web page at: http://www.fda.gov/cder/foi/label/2008/021947s006lbl.pdf, accessed May 25, 2008.

19. Actiq Prescribing Information. Available at: http://www.actiq.com/pdf/actiq_package_insert_4_5_07.pdf. Accessed May 25, 2008.

20. FDA Public Health Advisory. Important information for the safe use of fentora (fentanyl Buccal tablets). Available online at: http://www.fda.gov/cder/drug/advisory/fentalyn_buccal.htm. Accessed May 25, 2008.

21. Mercadante S, Villari P, Ferrera P, et al. Optimization of opioid therapy for preventing incident pain associated with bone metastases. *J Pain Symptom Manage.* 2004;28:505–510.

22. Weissman DE. Fast Fact and Concept #20; Opioid Dose Escalation, 2nd edition. Available online at: http://www.eperc.mcw.edu/fastFact/ff_020.htm. Accessed May 26, 2008.

23. Prommer E. Opioid withdrawal: creating more problems. *J Pain Symptom Manage.* 2007;33(2):114–115.

24. Methadone Research Web Guide, NIDA International Program. Available online at: http://international.drugabuse.gov/collaboration/guide_methadone/partc_question2.html, Accessed May 26, 2008.

ADDITIONAL SUGGESTED READINGS

Davis MP, Weissman DE, Arnold RM. Opioid dose titration for severe cancer pain: a systematic evidence-based review. *J Palliat Med.* 2004;7:462–468.

Driver LC. Case studies in breakthrough pain. *Pain Med.* 2007;8(S1):S14–S18.

Moryl N, Coyle N, Foley KM. Managing an acute pain crisis in a patient with advanced cancer: "This is as much of a crisis as a code." *JAMA.* 2008;299(12):1457–1467.

Payne R. Introduction: The scope of breakthrough pain in clinical practice. *Pain Med.* 2007;8(S1):S1–S2.

Payne R. Recognition and diagnosis of breakthrough pain. *Pain Med.* 2007;8(S1):S3–S7.

McCarberg BH. The treatment of breakthrough pain. *Pain Med.* 2007;8(S1):S8–S13.

William L, MacLeod R. Management of breakthrough pain in patients with cancer. *Drugs.* 2008;68(7):913–924.

SOLUTIONS TO PRACTICE PROBLEMS

P4.1: Establish IV access and administer hydromorphone 0.2 mg every minute for 10 minutes. The prescriber should be bedside monitoring the patient's sensorium (level of alertness/sedation), respiratory rate and pain rating. After 10 injections, the prescriber should wait 5 minutes and continue to assess patient. If pain is still not controlled after the 5 minute respite, continue administering hydromorphone 0.2 mg every minute for up to 10 additional minutes while monitoring the therapeutic and potential response. This cycle can be repeated one more time (for a total of 30 doses of hydromorphone 0.2 mg); if pain still is not relieved the patient should be further evaluated as to the cause of the pain. In this case, after controlling JK's pain subsequent imaging and cytology of the lesion showed it to be a metastasis to the right clavicle that resulted in this pathological fracture.

P4.2: Clearly WM would benefit from around-the-clock opioid therapy given her complaint of persistent pain. She is sensitive to the effects of opioids (e.g., 5 mg oral oxycodone made her very somnolent), and she doesn't want to take medication frequently. WM has almost tied your hands—but you're smarter than the average bear, and you recommend Kadian 10 mg by mouth once daily. This is the lowest strength sustained-release oral morphine product available (equivalent to 1.7 mg oral morphine every 4 hours). You could also recommend she continue the 2.5 mg oral oxycodone if needed (although it's unlikely she'll take it). Given WM's history of mild hepatic impairment it would be prudent to wait at least 1 week before considering a dosage increase. Since WM probably won't take the "prn" oral oxycodone, it would be best to assess her complaint of pain and her functional status after 1 week on the Kadian 10 mg once daily, and if she is tolerating it well but there is room for improvement, recommend increasing to Kadian 20 mg by mouth once daily (the equivalent of 3.3 mg every 4 hours). Don't forget the bowels, or WM will *really* get cranky!

P4.3: Let's consider why 2 Percocet tablets aren't giving LP sufficient relief. He is taking 400 mg per day of oral morphine. Ten to fifteen percent of this would be 40–60 mg of oral morphine as breakthrough. This is approximately equivalent to 27–40 mg of oral oxycodone. Two Percocet (5 mg oxycodone/325 mg acetaminophen) tablets only provide 10 mg oral oxycodone. Sherlock Holmes rides again—it's not enough opioid! Your formulary options for immediate-release oral opioids include morphine, oxycodone and hydromorphone. We have no reason to suspect that LP wouldn't respond to morphine (since it's working for the persistent pain), plus morphine has a very strong track record in treating dyspnea, which LP is starting to experience. An appropriate dose of rescue morphine would be 40–60 mg. Oral morphine is available as a 15- and 30-mg tablet, or a variety of oral solutions. You decide to use the oral concentrated solution, 20 mg/mL, and recommend a starting dose of 40 mg (2 mL) for breakthrough pain or dyspnea. If LP becomes too weak to swallow the oral concentrated solution, it can be instilled in the buccal cavity (perhaps 1 mL in each side of the buccal cavity).

P4.4: The prescriber is correct that there is no consistent correlation between the dose of the regularly scheduled opioid and the appropriate dose for the FBT, however we do have conversion guidelines between OTFC and FBT (see Table 4-4). FM was using a 600 mg OTFC lozenge, and the recommended dose to convert to FBT is 200 mcg.

The prescriber orders six 200 mcg FBTs with instructions to insert one tablet in between the cheek and gum when the patient experiences breakthrough pain. If the pain has not resolved 30 minutes later, FM may administer a second 200 mcg FBT. If this is not sufficient, FM must wait 4 hours before using FBT again, at which time he can use two 200 mcg FBT (one on each side of the mouth in the Buccal cavity). If 400 mcg of FBT is the appropriate dose, the prescriber should order the 400 mcg FBT for FM.

P4.5: The first thing to do is calculate QN's total daily dose of IV hydromorphone. She is getting 4 mg every 4 hours, plus five doses per day of the 2-mg dose, for a total daily dose of 34 mg. She is rating her pain as severe (7 or 8), therefore it would be appropriate to increase her total daily dose by 50%, which would be 51 mg. If we continue giving the hydromorphone every 4 hours this is 8.5 mg. We would recommend 8 mg hydromorphone every 4 hours with 4 mg every 2 hours as needed for breakthrough pain.

If the 8 mg every 4 hours controls QN's pain, this is a total daily dose of 48 mg. Consulting our Equianalgesic Opioid Dosing Table, we see that 1.5 mg parenteral hydromorphone is approximately equivalent to 7.5 mg oral hydromorphone. Therefore, her total daily dose of oral hydromorphone would be 240 mg, or 40 mg every 4 hours (with 20 mg every 2 hours as needed for breakthrough pain).

P4.6: Using the guideline presented in this chapter, we can reduce RR's morphine dose by 50% every third day. On Day 1 we can reduce it to MS Contin 45 mg po q12h. On Day 4 we can reduce it to MS Contin 30 mg po q12h. On Day 7 we can reduce it to MS Contin 15 mg po q12h, then discontinue the MS Contin on Day 10. Meanwhile, we will continue his MSIR 20 mg po q2h as needed for breakthrough pain, or even lower the dose as the days pass. As the week progresses, you would monitor RR for recurrent pain (and encourage use of the rescue dose) and for signs or symptoms of opioid withdrawal. Don't forget to reduce/discontinue any bowel regimen RR is receiving when you discontinue the opioid (if appropriate).

CHAPTER 5

Transdermal and Parenteral Fentanyl Dosage Calculations and Conversions

OBJECTIVES

After reading this chapter and completing all practice problems, the participant will be able to:

1. Describe the pharmacokinetics of transdermal fentanyl, and variables that can influence dosing.

2. Recommend an appropriate dose of transdermal fentanyl when switching from other opioids, including rescue opioid dosing. The participant will be able to describe the appropriate timing of this conversion.

3. Recommend a strategy for switching from transdermal fentanyl to another opioid regimen, including dosing and appropriate timing.

4. Describe how to transition between intravenous (IV) fentanyl and transdermal fentanyl.

INTRODUCTION

Fentanyl is a synthetic pure mu opioid agonist with pharmacologic properties similar to morphine, hydromorphone, oxycodone and other opioids. Important differences about fentanyl include its high degree of potency (about 75–100 times more potent than morphine on a mg-to-mg basis), and greater lipid solubility than morphine. The lipophilic nature of fentanyl facilitates rapid diffusion across the blood-brain barrier, resulting in a quick onset of action once the drug is absorbed from the administration site. Fentanyl is available in several dosage formulations, and may be administered by the following routes for a variety of pain-related indications:

- *Parenteral*—fentanyl may be given by intravenous (IV) injection, IV infusion, subcutaneous (SQ) infusion or intramuscular (IM) injection (although we already agreed that an IM analgesic is an oxymoron, and this practice is discouraged). It is used parenterally preoperatively, intraoperatively and postoperatively, and is occasionally used for the management of severe acute and chronic pain in other clinical situations. Preservative free fentanyl has been injected or infused epidurally or intrathecally by specialist practitioners.

- *Transdermal*—we have had transdermal fentanyl patches (TDF; also referred to as "fentanyl transdermal system") available for many years; this formulation relies on passive diffusion (drug moving from an area of higher concentration [the transdermal patch] to an area of lower concentration [the skin]); this formulation is indicated for the management of cancer and non-cancer pain for patients whose pain cannot be controlled with less intensive analgesic therapy (e.g., non-opioids, or intermittent dosing with short-acting opioids), and who are opioid-tolerant.

- *Buccal* and *transmucosal* fentanyl, as discussed in the previous chapter, are immediate release dosage forms approved to treat breakthrough pain in cancer patients.

- Other rapid-acting fentanyl products are in various stages of development. A *"fentanyl iontophoretic transdermal system"* has been developed for the short-term management of acute post-operative pain in adults, although it is not clear if this product will make it to market. The drug is delivered on patient demand, with an electrical charge driving the drug into the skin. Another transdermal fentanyl electrical enhancement delivery system under development uses *electroporation* technology. With this delivery system high voltage electric pulses of extremely short duration enhance skin permeability and consequently, fentanyl absorption.

In this chapter we will focus on conversion calculations involving switching to and from transdermal fentanyl, and conversion calculations involving IV fentanyl.

Transdermal Fentanyl

Transdermal fentanyl patches were designed to provide long-lasting opioid therapy (three days) for patients with stable chronic pain. Because fentanyl has a low molecular weight and high solubility in both fat and water, the drug is a good candidate for transdermal administration. There are 5 patch strengths currently available: 12 mcg/h (actually it delivers 12.5 mcg/h, but is referred to as 12 mcg/h to avoid a medication error by mistaking the intended dose to be 125 mcg/h), 25 mcg/h, 50 mcg/h, 75 mcg/h and 100 mcg/h. The dose is determined by the surface area of the patch, therefore the patches are larger as the dose increases.[1]

Pharmacokinetics

Transdermal fentanyl is formulated as both a gel-containing reservoir and a drug-in-adhesive matrix patch (see Sidebar: Transdermal Fentanyl Patch Formulations). Manufacturer's guidelines state that the TDF patch should be applied to an intact, non-irritated and non-irradiated flat skin surface such as the chest, back, flank or upper arm. If necessary, hair should be clipped (not shaved) at the site of application. Fentanyl is absorbed through the skin, producing a drug depot in the upper skin layers, then diffusing into the systemic circulation. On average minimally effective blood concentrations of fentanyl are seen in about 12 hours, and the time to maximum concentration is approximately 36 hours.[1] It may take up to 3 to 6 days to ultimately reach steady-state serum concentrations with TDF.

It is important to recognize that transdermal drug delivery is fraught with variability from patient to patient. Even when considering any given patient, there are variables that can affect fentanyl absorption. For example, an elevated body temperature (e.g., 40°C [104°F]) increases fentanyl absorption by about one third.[1,2] So when you hear that a patient has been tucked into bed, "snug as a bug in a rug" you might want to think about increased body temperature. This also applies to use of electric blankets, heating pads, tanning beds, sunbathing, hot baths, hot tubs, saunas and heated

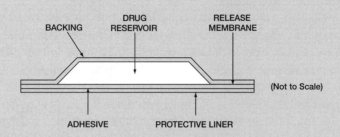
water beds.[3] In one recent case example, a patient on TDF for residual hip pain after a nasty construction accident (who insisted he had to apply his patch directly over the site of the pain) accidentally discovered the "bonus dose" effect of applying a heating pad directly over the patch. Obviously this practice should be strictly discouraged. There have been several fatalities reported due to nonadherence to this warning.

Another variable that is frequently talked about is the use of TDF in cachectic, low body weight patients. The Duragesic® package insert states "Duragesic® should be used with caution in elderly, cachectic, or debilitated patients as they may have altered pharmacokinetics due to poor fat stores, muscle wasting or altered clearance."[4] Many practitioners claim that cachectic patients do not respond as well as expected to TDF, and may report little or no improvement in pain when increasing the patch strength. Unfortunately there is no evidence base currently to support this claim. Despite the lack of evidence, opioid conversion calculations skills while mostly science, still have an artful component. If a cachectic patient has not responded to recent dosage increases in TDF, it may be wise to use the *last* effective patch strength upon which to base conversion calculations and be liberal with rescue opioid dosing (more on this later).

Another important pharmacokinetic parameter to consider when doing opioid conversion calculations involving TDF is how slowly the fentanyl serum concentration falls after patch removal. After removal, serum levels fall gradually; about half the drug has been eliminated after 17 hours.[4] Obviously it takes longer for the fentanyl serum concentration to fall after patch removal as compared to ending an IV infusion of fentanyl, since fentanyl continues to be absorbed from the depot in the upper layers of the skin continuing to diffuse into the systemic circulation even after the patch is removed. Knowledge of this pharmacokinetic parameter is of particular importance when converting a patient *from* TDF to another opioid. For example, it would be prudent to wait 24 hours or longer before starting the full replacement dose of a different long-acting opioid after removing the TDF patch. Rather, the practitioner would encourage use of the rescue opioid during that time period.

Other Important Considerations

We have seen that there are many misconceptions about the appropriate use of TDF among health care providers, occasionally resulting in avoidable morbidity and mortality. One recent survey questioned physician knowledge of TDF dosing strategies including initial dosing, use of rescue opioids with the patch, converting to and from TDF, and how to manage escalating pain in a patient receiving TDF.[7] Physicians who routinely prescribed TDF were more knowledgeable than less frequent prescribers about the appropriate use of TDF, but overall knowledge and confidence in using TDF was poor. The bad news is that failure to completely understand these dosing principles may result in patient harm, including death. The good news is that they will probably want to buy this book!

The Food and Drug Administration has released two public health advisories in recent years with safety warnings about TDF due to increased serious side effects and deaths from fentanyl overdose. Some precautions listed in the Healthcare Professional Advisory released in December 2007 are as follows[8]:

"Recommendations and Considerations for Healthcare Professionals:

- The fentanyl patch is indicated for the management of persistent, moderate to severe chronic pain in opioid-tolerant patients 2 years of age or older who require a total daily opioid dose at least equivalent to fentanyl transdermal system 25 mcg/h. Opioid-tolerant patients are those who have been taking daily, for a week or longer, at least 60 mg of oral morphine, 30 mg of oral oxycodone, or at least 8 mg of oral hydromorphone or an equianalgesic dose of another opioid. Fentanyl patch use in non-opioid tolerant patients has resulted in fatal respiratory depression.

- Consult the prescribing information to determine the initial fentanyl patch dose. Overestimating the dose when converting patients from another opioid analgesic can result in fatal overdose with the first dose.

- The fentanyl patch is contraindicated in the management of post-operative pain, mild pain, or intermittent pain (e.g., use on an as needed basis) because of the risk for serious or life-threatening respiratory depression. Fatalities from fentanyl overdose have occurred in these situations.

- Concomitant use of the fentanyl patch with any cytochrome P450 3A4 inhibitors (such as ketoconazole, erythromycin, nefazodone, diltiazem, or grapefruit juice) may result in an increase in fentanyl plasma concentrations, which may cause potentially fatal respiratory depression. Carefully monitor patients concomitantly taking cytochrome P450 3A4 inhibitors and using the patch for an extended period of time and adjust the fentanyl dose if necessary."[8]

As shown above, the FDA recommends starting a TDF patch of 25 mcg/h or greater only in patients who are opioid tolerant. The Duragesic® package insert states that TDF is contraindicated[4]:

- "In patients who are not opioid-tolerant [NOTE: Prescribing information does *not* exclude the 12 mcg/h TDF patch from this contraindication)
- In the management of acute pain or in patients who require opioid analgesia for a short period of time
- In the management of post-operative pain, including use after out-patient or day surgeries (e.g., tonsillectomies)
- In the management of mild pain
- In the management of intermittent pain (e.g., use on an as needed basis [prn])"

Probably the two big "take-home" messages from these warnings are that TDF is inappropriate for acute pain management, for intermittent or mild pain management, and should not be used in opioid-naïve patients. Therefore, our discussion of "starting doses" of TDF will focus on conversion calculations from other opioid regimens.

Regarding the 12 mcg/h TDF patch, the package labeling states that there have been no systematic evaluation of Duragesic as an initial opioid analgesic in managing chronic pain, including the 12 mcg/h patch. The package labeling states once again that TDF should only be used in patients who are opioid-tolerant.

 PITFALL ••
Transdermal Fentanyl—Too Much of a Good Thing?

The Duragesic® prescribing information warns about death and serious medical problems that have occurred when people were accidentally exposed to TDF.[4] Examples of accidental exposure include transfer of a TDF patch from an adult's body to a child while hugging, accidentally sitting on a patch and possible accidental exposure of a caregiver's skin to fentanyl in the patch while applying or removing a patient's patch. One reported case of caregiver toxicity involved the mother of a 40 year old patient receiving 600 mcg/h of TDF every 36 hours.[9] Due to skin irritation, the caregiver sprayed the patient's skin with the corticosteroid fluticasone propionate prior to patch application and applied beclomethasone cream, another corticosteroid, to the application site when the patch was removed. The author hypothesized that the effects of opioid intoxication experienced by the caregiver were likely exacerbated by the use of corticosteroids which may have enhanced transdermal fentanyl absorption, the caregiver's application technique, and the high dosage involved.

It is also important to counsel patients, families and caregivers on the appropriate disposal of used and unused TDF patches. The manufacturer of Duragesic brand transdermal fentanyl recommends that unused patches should be folded in half so the adhesive side adheres to itself, and immediately flushed down the toilet after removal from the skin. Unused patches should be similarly disposed of. Simply folding the patch in half and discarding in the trash does not preclude a child or pet retrieving and playing with the patch, potentially leading to fatality. Practitioners should be aware of, and adhere to any local or state guidelines regarding disposal of discontinued medications such as TDF, especially if they differ from the recommendations described here.

•••

Converting TO Trandermal Fentanyl—Equivalent Dosing
When converting to TDF, it is important that the patient's pain be under relatively stable control prior to the conversion. It is too difficult to chase increasing pain with a drug delivery system (such as a transdermal patch) that can take up to 6 days

to achieve steady state serum levels. Initial dose-finding with TDF takes longer to achieve pain relief and carries a greater risk of adverse effects as compared to using a short-acting oral opioid.

Given a patient with stable pain control that we want to convert to TDF, what is the process we use? As you will see in the next few paragraphs, there are many approaches that are used. We will start by examining what is reported in the manufacturer's insert and then review selected literature which support the conversion ratio most practitioners use today. Hang in there with me and you'll be a pro in no time at all!

Let's look at the conversion process suggested in the Duragesic package insert[4]:

- Determine the patient's 24-hour opioid requirement (don't forget to add in rescue medication consistently use for non-volitional incident and spontaneous pain)

- If the patient was not already receiving oral morphine, convert their 24-hour opioid to oral morphine equivalents using a conversion chart and process as explained in previous chapters and shown in Chapter 1, Table 1-1. (Note: do *not* reduce the morphine equivalent amount to account for lack of complete cross-tolerance).

- Consult a conversion table that provides an equianalgesic recommendation from oral morphine to TDF. The conversion chart provided by the manufacturer's of Duragesic is shown in Table 5-1.[4]

- Initiate treatment with the recommended dose, and titrate dosage upward no more frequently than every 3 days after administering the initial dose or every 6 days thereafter until analgesic efficacy is reached.

Sounds so straightforward, doesn't it? Well, you wouldn't be reading this chapter if it was *that* easy!

Table 5-1

Conversion from Oral Morphine to Duragesic[4]

Recommended Initial Duragesic® Dose Based on Daily Oral Morphine Dose

Oral 24-hour morphine (mg/day)	Duragesic® dose (mcg/h)
60–134	25
135–224	50
225–314	75
315–404	100
405–494	125
495–584	150
585–674	175
675–764	200
765–854	225
855–944	250
945–1034	275
1035–1124	300

In the package insert for Duragesic® the manufacturers are clear that the starting TDF dose determined from using the table above is likely too low for 50% of patients. This manufacturer-provided conversion guideline has been criticized for having morphine ranges that are too broad, and for being based on opioid conversions that have also been criticized.[10] For example, the guidelines shown above convert oral to parenteral morphine at a 6:1 ratio (which is based on single-dose studies) instead of the more accepted 3:1 ratio associated with chronic administration. Other cited inaccuracies include an oral morphine to oral hydromorphone ratio of 8:1, and an assumption that methadone is 3 times the potency of morphine and equipotent when given parenterally.[10] The consequences of underestimating the correct TDF strength are more than just merely an inconvenience necessitating increased use of the rescue medication. There have been at least four published case reports of patients experiencing a withdrawal syndrome when converting from oral opioids to TDF.[11] You would not be *wrong* to use this conversion guideline to switch to TDF, just recognize that it is extremely likely the TDF dose will be too low to meet patient needs. On the other hand, if a patient is taking a cytochromic P450 3A4 inhibiting medication (e.g., ketoconazole, erythromycin, nefazodone, diltiazem or grapefruit juice) use of this conversion chart may result in a TDF starting dose that will require less titration to achieve pain relief because the interacting drug will reduce fentanyl metabolism, resulting in an increased fentanyl serum level. Last, the manufacturer's guidelines are very clear that the table shown above, which is admittedly conservative, should *not* be used to convert *from* TDF to oral morphine.[4] If the table is purposefully conservative going *to* TDF, it would be too *aggressive* converting *from* TDF.

We know that fentanyl is 75–100 times more potent than morphine.[12] Keep your eye on the ball as we think this through:

- 100 mg oral morphine per day ~ 1 mg (1000 mcg) fentanyl per day (transdermal or IV)

- Therefore, 60 mg oral morphine per day ~ 0.6 mg (600 mcg) fentanyl per day

- 0.6 mg (600 mcg) fentanyl per **day** (24 hours) = 25 mcg per **hour** (25 mcg/h) fentanyl (transdermal or IV)—we just divided the TDD by 24 to determine the hourly dose of fentanyl

Therefore, **60 mg oral morphine per day** is about equivalent to **25 mcg/h of TDF** Donner and colleagues evaluated this ratio in 98 cancer patients who were on sustained-release oral morphine and whose pain was stable, using the morphine:TDF equivalencies shown in Table 5-2.[12]

Table 5-2

Donner Recommended Conversion from Oral Morphine to Duragesic

Recommended Initial Fentanyl Doses Based on Daily Oral Morphine Dosage[12]

24-Hour oral morphine dose (mg/day)	Transdermal fentanyl dose (mcg/h)
30–90	25
91–150	50
151–210	75
211–270	100
Every additional 60 mg per day	An additional 25 mcg per hour

Patients were converted to transdermal fentanyl patches, which were changed every 72 hours and titrated to pain relief. Oral morphine solution was used for breakthrough pain. Their results showed that pain control was equivalent between sustained release morphine and TDF, but that patients on TDF used more oral morphine solution for breakthrough pain. Slightly more than 40% of patients achieved sufficient pain relief with the initial TDF dose. The remainder required a dosage increase. The authors concluded that using the 100:1 (oral morphine:transdermal fentanyl) ratio is safe and effective, but that the actual ratio is probably closer to 70:1.

Are you still with me—here comes the best part! Building on the model that 60 mg oral morphine is approximately equivalent to 25 mcg/h of TDF, and having research that shows even this is a bit conservative (although no where near as conservative as the manufacturer's recommendations), it was a small leap to the conversion that most practitioners (including this author) use today, which is:

- Use a 2:1 ratio → every 2 mg oral morphine per ***day*** ~ 1 mcg per ***hour*** TDF

- Another way to word this is the number of mcg per ***hour*** of TDF should be about half the number of milligrams of oral morphine per ***day***

- For example, 50 mg per day of oral morphine ~ 25 mcg/h TDF

Breitbart and colleagues popularized this recommendation, offering the following process to convert to TDF[13]:

- Determine the total daily dose of oral morphine required to control patient's pain (or the equivalent based on their current opioid regimen; refer to Table 1-1).

- Use a conversion of 2:1 (mg oral morphine per day to mcg/h of TDF) to calculate the mcg/h dose of fentanyl.

- Once an approximate mcg/h dose for fentanyl is calculated, round up or down based on the available patch strengths (12 mcg/h, 25 mcg/h, 50 mcg/h, 75 mcg/h or 100 mcg/h) and based on the patient's pain level and overall clinical status. If the patient's pain is well controlled, round down to the next patch strength. If the current opioid regimen is not adequately controlling the pain, consider rounding up to the next patch strength.

The American Academy of Hospice and Palliative Medicine Fast Fact on "Converting To/From Transdermal Fentanyl"[14] also cites Breitbart and colleagues. They further recommend that the 2:1 (mg oral morphine per day to mcg/h of TDF) may be excessive in opioid-naïve patients and/or the elderly. (Note: we're not supposed to be starting TDF in opioid-naïve patients! Thought you had me, didn't you!). When in doubt, they recommend rounding down to the closest patch strength, and being liberal with rescue medication. While we have not described how these folks calculated an appropriate rescue opioid dose, we will do so during our case exercises. You didn't think I'd leave you hanging, did you?

Well I can't speak for you, but I'm exhausted after thinking all that through! Let's look at a case!

CASE 5.1

. . . .

Switching from Oral Long-acting Morphine to TDF

JR is a 72 year old woman with esophageal cancer. Her pain has been well controlled on MS Contin 60 mg by mouth every 12 hours, with morphine oral solution 20 mg every 2 hours as needed for breakthrough pain. She has been using about two doses per day of the morphine oral solution, and this regimen has kept her comfortable. Unfortunately she is having increased difficulty swallowing the MS Contin tablets. How would we convert her to TDF? Let's take a closer look—step by step, inch by inch...

Step 1—Assess the patient's pain: We have assessed JR's pain, and it's well-controlled. We are only switching her to TDF because of swallowing difficulties.

Step 2—Determine the patient's total daily dose of their current opioid: JR is taking MS Contin 60 mg po q12h (120 mg oral morphine) plus two doses of morphine oral solution 20 mg (an additional 40 mg) for a grand total of 160 mg oral morphine per day.

Step 3—Decide which opioid to switch to, and consult conversion chart: we already know we're switching to TDF. Using our guidelines of 2:1 oral morphine mg per day : TDF mcg per hour, we calculate a dose for TDF of 80 mcg/h.

Step 4—Individualize the dosage and ensure adequate access to breakthrough pain medication: Because TDF is not available as 80 mcg/h, we must either round down to 75 mcg/h or round up to 100 mcg/h. JR is elderly, and her pain is well controlled, therefore it seems prudent to round down to the 75 mcg/h strength. Let's discuss the issue of break-through pain in a moment.

Step 5—Patient follow-up and reassessment: We will discuss the timing of switching to and from TDF below, but we must always remember to monitor our patient carefully dur-ing and after the transition. But we're not done with JR! This case raises several addi-tional issues. First, how do we time the transition from MS Contin to TDF? Also, what do we do for breakthrough pain?

Because it takes 12–16 hours to achieve therapeutic fentanyl serum levels, we must pro-vide the patient with opioid coverage during the conversion period. In cases such as JR, she should take one last dose of MS Contin (60 mg) at the same time the TDF is applied. This last dose of sustained release morphine (which lasts 8–12 hours) will be tapering off as the TDF is kicking in. JR should also continue to have the same dose of short-acting morphine available for breakthrough pain, as this dose has been effective for her.

If JR is too weak to swallow one last sustained-release morphine tablet prior to applica-tion of the TDF, she should receive at least two to three doses of short acting morphine after the TDF is applied. In other words, instead of taking one last MS Contin 60 mg tablet, if she can't swallow it, instead she would be given MSIR 20 mg at time zero (time of patch application), 4 hours after patch application, and 8 hours after patch application. These three 20-mg doses equal the 60-mg dose she would have received from that one last MS Contin tablet.

This same principle should be followed for any patient who was receiving only short-act-ing opioids around-the-clock prior to TDF conversion. Let's look at a patient taking MSIR

10 mg q4h around the clock, with MSIR 5 mg every 2 hours for additional pain, being switched to TDF 25 mcg/h. When the 25 mcg/h TDF patch is applied, the patient should continue to receive their regularly scheduled MSIR 10 mg every 4 hours for at least two or three more doses. Keep the "prn" MSIR 5 mg q2h order in place for additional pain relief.

This brings us to the question of *which* opioid to use for breakthrough pain when patients are using TDF for persistent pain. We discussed this at length in the previous chapter—our options are buccal or transmucosal fentanyl, or short-acting/immediate-onset morphine, oxycodone, hydromorphone, or oxymorphone. There is no compelling reason why we *must* use the same opioid for the persistent pain and the breakthrough pain, and the rapid-acting fentanyl products are fairly expensive compared to the more traditional opioids. However, if you decide the use of a rapid-acting fentanyl product is appropriate, following the dosing guidelines as discussed in the previous chapter. Remember, there is *no* reliable correlation between the TDF patch strength and the appropriate starting dose of rapid-acting fentanyl. You must begin with the lowest available rapid acting fentanyl dose and titrate per recommended guidelines.

If the patient had been using a short-acting opioid for breakthrough pain successfully prior to conversion to TDF, they can continue taking the same opioid at the same dose once they convert to TDF. This is permissible because the patient's pain is stable and we are not increasing or decreasing the total daily dose of oral morphine (or equivalent dose of another opioid) other than to accommodate patch strength availability. However, if the patient did not have a short-acting opioid available we can still calculate a ballpark starting dose for breakthrough pain. For example, if a patient had been receiving Kadian 100 mg po per day prior to conversion to TDF, a reasonable dose of short-acting morphine would have been 10–15 mg (using our 10–15% of the TDD rule to determine the dose for breakthrough pain). If the patient was switched to TDF 50 mcg/h, it would be appropriate to also recommend MSIR 15 mg po q2h prn breakthrough pain. Of course you would follow the same guidelines as discussed in the previous chapter to determine if this were an appropriate dose or not. Let's look at another case, shall we?

 CASE 5.2
. . . .
Switching from Multiple Opioids to TDF

KG is a 52 year old woman with a history of pancreatic cancer, admitted to your hospital with a complaint of significant nausea with oral ingestion of food or medications, and occasional vomiting. Her analgesic regimen is as follows:

- TDF 25 mcg/h
- OxyContin 20 mg po q12h
- Hydromorphone 4 mg po q2h prn breakthrough pain, using on average 6 doses per day

You would like to roll all of this into TDF due to the nausea. What's the first step? As I'm sure you recall, the first step is to do a careful assessment of the pain and determine if an opioid is the best treatment of KG's pain. Perhaps she needs a co-analgesic added. Let's assume we've done the assessment and feel that switching entirely to TDF is the best plan. Step 2 is to perform an accurate accounting of how she has been taking her opioids. Importantly, with a complaint of nausea and occasional vomiting, it is important to determine how much of her opioid regimen she has received over the past 24–48 hours (e.g., to be alert for possible opioid withdrawal, etc.). Let's assume she has experienced only very occasional vomiting, and it doesn't significantly affect her total daily opioid use.

Step 2 is to convert her OxyContin and hydromorphone to an equivalent dose of oral morphine. Her total daily dose of oxycodone is 40 mg—how much oral morphine is this approximately equivalent to? Using Method A (e.g., simple ratio) we know that the oral oxycodone:oral morphine ratio is 20:30 (see Table 1-1: Equianalgesic Opioid Dosing Table). Using this we calculate that 40 mg oral oxycodone is equivalent to 60 mg oral morphine. You can also use Method B:

Actual Drug Doses: **Equianalgesic Data from Chart:**

$$\frac{\text{“X” mg TDD new opioid}}{\text{mg TDD current opioid}} = \frac{\text{equianalgesic factor of new opioid}}{\text{equianalgesic factor of current opioid}}$$

Let's fill in the numbers:

$$\frac{\text{“X” mg TDD new opioid}}{\text{40 mg oral oxycodone}} = \frac{\text{30 mg oral morphine}}{\text{20 mg oral oxycodone}}$$

We cross multiply:

$(30) \times (40) = (X) \times (20)$

$1200 = 20X$

$X = 60$

This method also shows that 40 mg oral oxycodone per day is approximately equivalent to 60 mg oral morphine per day.

Now we need to do the same exercise with the oral hydromorphone the patient has been using for breakthrough pain. She is taking on average six doses of hydromorphone 4 mg, which gives us a total daily dose of 24 mg oral hydromorphone. How much oral morphine is this approximately equivalent to?

$$\frac{\text{“X” mg TDD new opioid}}{\text{24 mg oral hydromorphone}} = \frac{\text{30 mg oral morphine}}{\text{7.5 mg oral hydromorphone}}$$

Cross multiply:

$(30) \times (24) = (X) \times (7.5)$

$720 = 7.5X$

$X = 96$

We see that 24 mg oral hydromorphone per day is approximately equivalent to 96 mg oral morphine per day.

If we add the oral morphine equivalent we got from the oxycodone calculation (60 mg) to the oral morphine equivalent from the hydromorphone calculation (96 mg) we have determined the patient is receiving an equivalent dose of 156 mg of oral morphine per day.

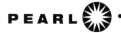

PEARL ·

A Critically Important Point to Note at This Juncture Is as Follows

When switching from one opioid to another, we discussed how we usually reduce the dose of the new opioid by 25–50% to allow for incomplete cross-tolerance. **We do not do this** *when doing the calculation for the purposes of converting to TDF. The incomplete cross tolerance factor has already been taken into account when making the jump from oral morphine (or oral morphine equivalent) to TDF. You will see this same concept discussed in the next chapter on methadone dosing. The converse holds true as well; when we convert* **from** *TDF to oral morphine, the "lack of cross tolerance" factor has already been considered.*

· ·

OK, back at the ranch—the patient is receiving approximately the equivalent of 156 mg oral morphine per day. Half of this is 78—which would represent 78 mcg/h TDF. Obviously we don't have a 78 mcg/h TDF patch, so we would round down to 75 mcg/h (this is Step 4—individualization for the patient). Also, don't forget the goal of this exercise was to combine all the opioids the patient was receiving into one opioid—TDF. She's already on TDF 25 mcg/h. If we add 75 mcg/h based on the calculations we've just done, we could discontinue the OxyContin and hydromorphone, and increase the TDF from 25 mcg/h to 100 mcg/h.

The next burning question is, "How do we time all this?" If she is able to swallow it, the patient should receive her last OxyContin 20 mg tablet at the same time the TDF patch is changed from 25 mcg/h to 100 mcg/h (or a 75 mcg/h patch added), if she is able to swallow it. If she is too nauseated to take anything by mouth, discontinue both the OxyContin and hydromorphone, and switch to TDF 100 mcg/h. You will then need to rely on a non-oral route of administration to provide a rescue opioid. Your options are parenteral or rectal. How do we calculate the dose for both routes assuming we want to use morphine? This is hurting your head to use skills you learned in previous chapters isn't it? I know you can do it—keep the faith!

OK, let's recap. We have calculated that TDF 100 mcg/h will probably maintain the level of comfort she had initially on her three-opioid regimen (OxyContin, TDF 25 mcg/h and hydromorphone for breakthrough pain). TDF 100 mcg/h is approximately equivalent to 200 mg per day of oral morphine. Ten to fifteen percent of this is 20–30 mg, therefore we could offer morphine rectal suppositories 20 mg q2h prn breakthrough pain, and increase to 30 mg rectal morphine as needed. Alternately, if you want to provide a SQ injection of morphine as needed, we need to convert the 200 mg TDD oral morphine to parenteral morphine. As you recall, 10 mg parenteral morphine is equivalent to 30 mg oral morphine, therefore her TDD of parenteral morphine would be about 66 mg. Ten to fifteen percent of 66 mg is 6.6–10 mg, therefore an appropriate dose of SQ morphine would be 7.5 or 10 mg q2h prn breakthrough pain.

One last note about the timing of this conversion. Let's say the patient had her current 25 mcg/h TDF patch placed 24 hours ago. You have two options when converting to TDF 100 mcg/h. You could add a 75 mcg patch now, and at the end of 48 additional hours you could remove *both* the 25 and 75 mcg/h patches (which is technically a day earlier than when we would have to change the 75 mcg/h patch) and replace with a 100 mcg/h

TDF patch. Or, you could remove the 25 mcg/h TDF patch when you admitted the patient and switch immediately to a 100 mcg/h TDF. As stated earlier, it will take a minimum of 12 hours to see a clinically meaningful increase in fentanyl serum concentrations with the new patch addition, and at least 36 hours (if not 3–6 days) to achieved maximum steady-state concentrations.[1] The last step is to carefully monitor the patient during and after this transition to assure an optimal therapeutic outcome.

 P I T F A L L •

"Set and Forget" Method Akin to "You Snooze, Your Patient May Lose"

Many providers feel that once a TDF patch is "set" in place on the patient, you can walk away and "forget" about the patient for 3 days. Wrong-O! You MUST continue to use good clinical judgment and monitor your patient regularly. If the patient is becoming overmedicated on fentanyl, you will need to take special precautions to reverse the opioid intoxication for hours and hours after patch removal. Similarly, TDF is not a cure-all; patients still need to be monitoring for responsiveness and use rescue medications appropriately.

• •

Titrating Transdermal Fentanyl

Once we have switched a patient to TDF, how do we titrate the dose up—let's consider both the dose and the timing. Let's start with how quickly we can increase the patch strength. According to the guidelines in the prescribing information for Duragesic® "the initial Duragesic® dose may be increased after 3 days based on the daily dose of supplemental opioid analgesics required by the patient in the second or third day of the initial application. Physicians are advised that it may take up to 6 days after increasing the dose of Duragesic® for the patient to reach equilibrium on the new dose. Therefore, patients should wear a higher dose through two applications before any further increase in dosage is made on the basis of the average daily use of a supplemental analgesic."[4] It makes sense that we cannot gauge the efficacy of the TDF dose within the first 24 hours after initial patch application (or dosage increase) because the serum fentanyl continues to rise during this period. One reference states TDF absorption is 47% complete at 24 hours, 88% complete at 48 hours and 94% complete at 72 hours.[15] Therefore, we should look at average use of the rescue medication on days 2 and 3, and let that guide our titration decision making. Generally speaking, if the patient requires more than three doses of their rescue medication for spontaneous pain in a 24-hour period to achieve good pain control, the patch strength should be increased. Titrating with TDF is challenging and often cumbersome due to the long onset and duration of action. The best rule of thumb is to change the dose when the pain is stable (note I didn't necessary say the pain was *controlled*, but *stable*), but not more quickly than described above.

How much should we increase the patch strength? There are two ways you can do this—first, calculate how much of the rescue opioid the patient was using per day on average, and calculate the conversion to TDF. For example, consider a patient who was switched from an oral opioid regimen to 50 mcg/h TDF with 15 mg MSIR q2h for breakthrough pain. Assume the patient took 4 doses of MSIR on both days 2 and 3, for a total daily dose of 60 mg oral morphine. Half of this is 30 mcg/h, therefore it would be appropriate to increase the TDF to 75 mcg/h. You can also use a rule of thumb to increase the TDF by 25 mcg/h when at lower doses, but increase by 50 mcg/h if the patient is using a greater amount of rescue medication, their pain is severe, and a 50 mcg/h increase is within reason. For example, you would *not* increase from 25 mcg/h to 75 mcg/h—this would be a 200% increase. We discussed in a previous chapter that we increase by 25–50% for moderate pain, or 50–100% for severe pain. Therefore in the face of more severe pain, you can comfortably increase by up to 100% while not exceeding the absolute increase by 50 mcg/h. For example, a patient on 50 mcg/h TDF who is using around the clock rescue medication and continues complain of pain (assuming an opioid remains the appropriate analgesic) may be increased to 100 mcg/h on day 4. It may also be reasonable to increase the dose of the rescue medication, and observe the patient's response over the next 6 days before considering an additional dosage increase of TDF.

Transdermal fentanyl patches are approved for use for 3 continuous days (72 hours). Clinical practice and research have shown that about 20% of patients may require a shorter application interval to 48 hours.[16] If possible, an increase in the TDF dose is preferred (to be able to maintain the q72h dosing interval), but if the patient consistently has more breakthrough pain during the last 24 hours of each cycle (e.g., using more than 4 doses of rescue opioid), changing to q48h dosing would be appropriate. Dosage intervals less than 48 hours in duration are inappropriate and should not be used in any patient, regardless of the circumstances.

Converting FROM Transdermal Fentanyl—Equivalent Dosing

Occasionally we have a clinical situation where it would be in the patient's best interests to switch *from* TDF to a different opioid or route of administration. Alternately, it may be a formulary consideration driving this decision. In any case, what guidelines do we use to switch off TDF?

The manufacturer's guidelines offer the following recommendations for discontinuation of Duragesic®[4]: "To convert patients to another opioid, remove Duragesic® and titrate the dose of the new analgesic based upon the patient's report of pain until adequate analgesia has been attained. Upon system removal, 17 hours or more are required for a 50% decrease in serum fentanyl concentrations." Can we use our 2 mg oral morphine:1 mcg fentanyl guideline in reverse? Probably, but timing is everything. Let's look at the following case.

 CASE 5.3
• •
Switching Off TDF: Timing Considerations

BL is a 52 year old man admitted to your hospice program with a diagnosis of lung cancer; he is receiving 50 mcg/h TDF with MSIR 15 mg po q2h prn breakthrough pain. He is able to swallow tablets and capsules, and TDF is not on your formulary. BL is agreeable to switching to sustained release morphine tablets. You use the 2 mg oral morphine:1 mcg TDF rule, and calculate an approximate total daily dose of oral morphine of 100 mg. But how do we make this switch—how do we time taking off the patch, and beginning the morphine therapy? An important part of answering this question is knowing the rate at which the fentanyl is eliminated from the body after patch removal, as follows:

- 17 hours after patch removal, 50% of fentanyl is eliminated from the body
- 34 hours after patch removal, 75% of fentanyl is eliminated from the body

- 51 hours after patch removal, 87.5% of fentanyl is eliminated from the body
- 68 hours after patch removal, 93.5% of fentanyl is eliminated from the body

Remember, even though fentanyl is a quick-onset, short-acting opioid, when administering by transdermal patch it takes many hours for the drug to completely be absorbed from the site of application (the skin), enter the systemic circulation, be metabolized, and eliminated from the body.

One guideline published in the literature to prevent pain recurrence when switching from TDF to a different opioid/route of administration is as follows[17]:

- Calculate your new opioid regimen. (Note: if you're working with a home-based patient, make *sure* the new opioid is *in* the home before removing the patch; don't gamble on the time of delivery because if you're wrong the patient may end up in a pain crisis!)
- Remove the TDF patch.
- For the first 12 hours after patch removal, use *only* the previously prescribed rescue opioid only for pain that occurs.
- Twelve hours after patch removal, begin with 50% of the calculated scheduled opioid regimen, and continue to offer the rescue opioid as needed.
- Twenty-four hours after patch removal, increase to 100% of the calculated scheduled opioid regimen, and continue to offer the rescue opioid as needed.

In the case of BL, even though we have a good idea that TDF 50 mcg/mL is equivalent to 100 mg/day of oral morphine, you decide to move first to using the oral morphine solution he has in the home on an around the clock basis before ultimately switching him to oral sustained-release morphine tablets. So, let's take a look at how we do this.

After removing the patch, you instruct the patient to wait 12 hours before taking *scheduled* doses of oral morphine, however he is welcome to use the morphine 15 mg every 2 hours as needed for *breakthrough* pain. Based on our rule of thumb of TDF 50 mcg/hour is equivalent to 100 mg oral morphine per day, we determine the 4-hourly dose of oral morphine to be 15 mg. Twelve hours after the patch is removed we instruct BL to take 50% of the calculated dose of morphine, which would be MSIR 7.5 mg po q4h (with rescue opioid still available). After 24 hours BL is instructed to increase to MSIR 15 mg po q4h around the clock. After two days of this regimen, he is switched to sustained-release oral morphine 45 mg po q12h, keeping the MSIR 15 mg po q2h prn breakthrough pain.

Transdermal Fentanyl in Older Adults and Cachectic Patients

As previously discussed, many variables affect the absorption of fentanyl from a transdermal system and age is no exception. By determining the amount of fentanyl left in the transdermal patch after 72 hours, Solassol and colleagues determined that patients > 75 years of age absorbed 50% of fentanyl while patients < 65 years of age absorbed 66% (difference was statistically significant).[18]

As briefly discussed earlier in this chapter, some practitioners who care for patients with advanced illnesses have noticed that cachectic patients occasionally seem to get less relief from TDF than expected.[19] There is no published data to support this finding, but just as we know it makes no sense to actually try to teach a pig to whistle, it would be imprudent to ignore this perceived lack of response. Let's look at a case that illustrates this point.

CASE 5.4

● ●

TDF and Cachetic Patients

SW is a 92 year old woman (5'5", 82 lb) admitted to hospice with a diagnosis of failure to thrive. She has a long-standing history of osteoarthritis, affecting her knees, hips and spine. She has painful diabetic neuropathy and a range of general aches and pain. Her pain did not adequately respond to non-opioid analgesics, therefore she was started on morphine 2.5 mg po q4h, over time increasing to 15 mg po q4h. Her pain was fairly well controlled on this regimen, but the morphine made her nauseated. Her physician switched her to 50 mcg/h TDF with good response for about 10 days. When she complained of increased pain, her physician increased the TDF to 75 mcg/h, then to 100 mcg/h 6 days later. Neither dosage increase had any appreciable effect on her pain. You decide to switch her to subcutaneous injections of morphine around the clock. This brings up to our burning question—which strength patch do you base your calculations on? The 50 mcg/h patch, the 75 mcg/h patch or the 100 mcg/h patch?

Since SW did not show a response to either the 75 mcg/h or 100 mcg/h TDF, it would be prudent to base your calculations on the 50 mcg/h patch. Therefore, a 50 mcg/h TDF patch is about equal to 100 mg oral morphine, which is about equal to 33 mg parenteral morphine per day. If we decide to give the SQ injection every 4 hours, this calculates to a 5-mg dose. In addition, you could even get an order for morphine 2.5 or 5 mg SQ every 2 hours as needed for breakthrough pain on top of the regularly scheduled doses of SQ morphine. Using the guidelines discussed above, for the first 12 hours after removing the patch, you would rely solely on the "prn" order; during the next 12 hours you could begin with morphine 2.5 mg SQ every 4 hours (plus the 5 mg q2h prn dose). After 24 hours you would move to your full dose of morphine 5 mg SQ every 4 hours. After 24–48 hours of therapy you will determine if this regimen is sufficient or not.

Importantly, this is not an evidence-based recommendation, it's based more on a violent objection to being thrown in jail for overdosing a LOL (little old lady) on opioids. As we have discussed from the beginning of this book, "Safety First" is our mantra. The second mantra is to make sure the patient has adequate rescue opioid available.

Parenteral Fentanyl

As described in the beginning of the chapter, fentanyl may be administered by several routes of administration. Use of parenteral fentanyl includes IV injection, IV infusion, IM injection (no, no, bad dog!), and SQ injection or infusion. In the hands of skilled practitioners, fentanyl has also been administered epidurally and intrathecally. The remainder of this chapter will be devoted to conversion calculations regarding parenteral fentanyl.

IV Fentanyl

In Chapter 7 we will be discussing advanced opioid therapy including continuous infusions and neuraxial opioid therapy. But since we're talking about fentanyl, let's look at a conversion from oral morphine to a continuous IV (or SQ) fentanyl infusion. As we discussed earlier in the chapter fentanyl is approximately 70–100 times more potent than morphine on a mg-to-mg basis, but there is some debate over the exact morphine~fentanyl equivalency (of course, life would be too simple if that were not the case!). Let's take a look at a case:

CASE 5.5

Switching from an Oral Opioid to IV Fentanyl

MB is a 48 year old man with a history of a work-related injury resulting in chronic low back pain. His pain is currently being treated with sustained-release morphine 120 mg po q12h with MSIR 30 mg every 4 hours as needed for breakthrough pain (which he takes on average twice a day) with good pain control. He has been admitted to the hospital for back surgery and the surgeon has asked you to convert his oral morphine regimen to a continuous IV fentanyl infusion prior to surgery. No pressure there! Let's take a look at how we do this:

Our first step is to assess the patient's pain; he has told you his current oral morphine regimen controls his pain. Second, we need to calculate his total daily dose of oral morphine. He is getting a total of 300 mg oral morphine per day (120 × 2 plus 30 × 2 = 240 + 60 = 300). Step 3 is the conversion calculation, followed by Step 4, which is individualizing the dose for the patient. Three hundred milligrams a day of oral morphine is equivalent to 100 mg per day of parenteral morphine. If we were going to put him on a continuous IV morphine infusion, we would divide by 24 to get the hourly infusion rate, which would be about 4 mg/hour. Using the equivalency shown in the table in Chapter 1 (10 mg parenteral morphine ~ 0.1 mg parenteral fentanyl), we determine that 4 mg parenteral morphine ~ 0.04 mg fentanyl. We can convert 0.04 mg fentanyl to mcg, which comes out to 40 mcg IV fentanyl/hour. However, as explained in the footnote on that table, many practitioners consider the 1:100 equivalency far too conservative and instead consider 4 mg/hour of IV morphine to be equivalent to 100 mcg/hour of IV fentanyl (a 1:40 equivalency). Using this rule of thumb, MB's *300 mg of oral morphine per day* is approximately equivalent to *100 mg of parenteral morphine per day*, which is equal to *4 mg/hour of parenteral morphine*, which would be equivalent to *100 mcg/hour of IV fentanyl*. So the answer to the question "what hourly dose of parenteral fentanyl is equivalent to 300 mg a day of oral morphine?" is somewhere between 40 mcg/hour and 100 mcg/hour (of IV fentanyl). Based on what we see clinically, the correct answer is closer to the 100 mcg/hour, but if you want to be conservative you could start lower and allow for a generous bolus dose. For example, you could start the patient at 60 mcg/hour of IV fentanyl with a 30 mcg bolus every 15 minutes. Step 5 is closely monitoring your patient; within a few hours you will be able to determine how many doses of breakthrough fentanyl the patient requires, and you can adjust your infusion rate accordingly. Because we are stopping a sustained release oral opioid, we will allow MB to use the fentanyl bolus option for the first 6 hours, then begin the continuous IV infusion of fentanyl.

Converting from Transdermal to IV Fentanyl

As stated earlier, the dose of TDF and IV fentanyl is the same. When you really think about it, transdermal drug delivery technically *is* parenteral drug delivery (it's not enteral)! While you're wrapping your head around that, just recognize that 25 mcg/h of TDF is equivalent to 25 mcg/h of IV fentanyl, and 100 mcg/h of TDF is equivalent to 100 mcg/h of IV fentanyl, and so forth.

So if the dosing equivalency is such so straight forward, why are we taking time to discuss how to switch patients from TDF to IV fentanyl. Funny you should mention "time"—it's all in the timing! As stated earlier, once you remove a TDF patch, it takes about 17 hours to see a 50% decrease in the fentanyl serum concentration. Clearly we don't want to wait 17 hours to start our IV fentanyl, so what is an appropriate way to work out this timing? Most practitioners would use the following technique:

- Remove the TDF patch.

- For the next 6 hours, use "as needed" IV fentanyl for pain management.

- Six hours after TDF patch removal, being an infusion of IV fentanyl at 50% the anticipated dose (in other words, 50% of the TDF patch strength). The "as needed" dose of IV fentanyl is still available.

- Twelve hours after TDF patch removal, increase the IV fentanyl infusion to 100% the anticipated dose (which should be equivalent to the TDF patch strength). The "as needed" dose of IV fentanyl continues to remain available.

On occasion patients receiving transdermal fentanyl experience rapidly escalating pain picture than cannot be managed with a transdermal system. In these cases, the practitioner may chose to switch the patient to intravenous fentanyl. Kornick and colleagues described their protocol for this conversion in patients with acute cancer-related pain.[20] Their protocol was as follows: all transdermal patches were removed from the patient, and a continuous infusion of IV fentanyl was begun at an equivalent hourly rate (1:1, transdermal:IV) at the time of patch removal. A patient-demand bolus of 50–100% of the hourly infusion rate was available every 15–20 minutes. In this published case series, ten patients were switched from transdermal to IV fentanyl, the results of nine were reported. Eight of the nine patients reported pain in excess of 8 on a 0-10 scale on presentation; seven of the nine had a significant decrease in pain intensity at 24 hours. One of the nine patients reported sedation 24 hours after starting IV fentanyl, which resolved by the next day. As discussed by the authors, during the initial hours after the switch from transdermal to IV fentanyl, the patient was actually receiving approximately twice as much fentanyl as the prescribed IV dose due to the continued absorption of fentanyl from the skin depot despite TDF patch removal. In the cases they described, this was useful because all the patients were in pain crisis. This would *not* be appropriate for a patient who was *not* in acute pain crisis.

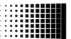 **CASE 5.6**
• •
Switching from TDF to Parenteral Fentanyl

AL is a 62 year old man with history of prostate cancer, admitted to the hospital for a course of radiation. To have increased flexibility in treating his pain while hospitalized, the palliative care team has been asked to switch him from his current 50 mcg/h TDF to a continuous IV infusion of fentanyl. AL's pain is currently well controlled on TDF along with a nonsteroidal anti-inflammatory agent. How should we convert AL to a continuous IV fentanyl infusion?

Based on the discussion above, AL is not is pain at this time, so clearly this is not a crisis situation. It would be appropriate to remove the TDF patch, establish IV access and have a 25 mcg fentanyl bolus available every 20 minutes for the first 6 hours. At 6 hours, the continuous IV infusion of fentanyl should begin at 25 mcg/h, and the bolus option is still available. Twelve hours after TDF patch removal, the IV infusion of fentanyl should be increased to 50 mcg/h, and the bolus options remains in place. Should AL's pain increase or decrease over the next few days, the continuous infusion can be adjusted accordingly.

Converting from IV to Transdermal Fentanyl

When a patient's pain has been stabilized on a continuous infusion of fentanyl, it is common practice to want to switch the patient to a more convenient dosage formulation, such as TDF. Our friends Kornick et al have kindly provided guidance in this area as well![21] They report on a series of adult patients with cancer-related pain who had been treated with continuous infusion fentanyl (with a patient-demand bolus at 50-100% of the hourly infusion rate, available every 15–20 minutes). All patients reported stable and acceptable pain control in the 12 hours prior to conversion to TDF. The protocol they used was to round the effective hourly infusion rate to the closest TDF patch strength, and apply the patch(es). Six hours after TDF patch application, the continuous fentanyl infusion rate was decreased by 50%, and was discontinued 6 hours thereafter. The demand bolus option remained in place at the same dose and lockout interval for at least 24 hours after TDF patch application. Fifteen patients were evaluated in this case series; only one patient reported unsatisfactory pain control at 6 and 12 hours, but acceptable pain control at 18 and 24 hours. Overall, all 15 patients had acceptable pain control using this two-step taper without significant increases in sedation or demand fentanyl bolus use.

 CASE 5.7
• •
Switching from Parenteral Fentanyl to TDF

AL, our 62 year old man with prostate cancer from case 5.6, has completed his course of radiation and is ready for discharge home. He is being maintained on a fentanyl continuous infusion at 70 mcg/hour; he has only used his bolus dose (35 mcg) once in the past 24 hours. He would like to resume TDF therapy. How do we handle this transition?

Per the research from Kornick et al., we round the patient's continuous hourly infusion rate to the closest TDF patch strength. The patient is receiving 70 mcg/h, therefore the 75 mcg/h TDF patch seems reasonable. We apply the patch at 8 a.m., and continue the continuous infusion at 70 mcg/h and the bolus dose (35 mcg q20 minutes) remains available to the patient. At 2 p.m. (6 hours later) we reduce his continuous infusion to 35 mcg/h (and continue the demand bolus dose at 35 mcg/h). At 8 p.m. (12 hours after patch application) we discontinue the continuous infusion, but keep the demand bolus dose (35 mcg) available until 8 a.m. day 2 (an additional 12 hours). We will of course be vigilant in monitoring AL for pain control and adverse effects, particularly over-sedation. At 24 hours after patch application if all is well we can discontinue the IV altogether, and order an oral short-acting opioid for breakthrough pain (e.g., MSIR 15 mg po q2h prn pain).

In this chapter we have explored conversions in the land of fentanyl—to and from transdermal fentanyl, and to and from parenteral fentanyl. All that converting to and fro has left me a bit dizzy—hopefully you'll find Table 5-3 helpful. In this summary table you will find all the "pearls" we discussed when converting to and from TDF, and how to adjust the TDF dose. What's not to love about a good cheat sheet?

Table 5-3

Rules of Thumb with Fentanyl Conversions

- **Converting from an oral long-acting opioid to TDF**

  - If patient is not taking oral morphine, convert to oral morphine

  - Using the 2 mg oral morphine/day ~ 1 mcg/h TDF rule, calculate TDF patch strength

  - Advise patient to take one last dose of the oral long-acting opioid at the same time the first TDF patch is applied

  - Increase TDF if necessary in 3 days, and every 6 days thereafter as needed

- **Converting from an around-the-clock oral short-acting opioid to TDF**

  - If patient is not taking oral morphine, convert to oral morphine

  - Using the 2 mg oral morphine/day ~ 1 mcg/h TDF rule, calculate TDF patch strength

  - Advise patient to take two or three scheduled doses of their oral short-acting opioid after TDF patch application: one dose at the time of application, another dose 4 hours later, and if needed, a third dose 4 hours later. Rescue opioid should be available throughout.

  - Increase TDF if necessary in 3 days, and every 6 days thereafter as needed

- **Titrating TDF upward**

  - After initiation of TDF therapy, evaluate use of rescue opioid on days 2 and 3. If patient using more than three doses of rescue opioid, calculate TDD of rescue opioid, and increase TDF patch strength in an equivalent amount.

  - Increase by 25–50 mcg/h, but not to exceed a 100% increase. Also, no dosage increase should exceed 50 mcg/h

    - Increase from 25 mcg/h to 50 mcg/h

    - For patients on 50 mcg/h or higher, increase by 50 mcg/h

- **Converting from TDF to an oral opioid**

  - Based on TDF patch strength, calculate oral morphine equivalent (or other opioid equivalent). If converting to oral morphine, use the 2 mg oral morphine/day ~ 1 mcg/h TDF rule

  - Once the new opioid product is in the patient's home, remove the TDF patch

  - For the first 12 hours after patch removal, use only the previously prescribed rescue opioid

  - Twelve hours after patch removal begin with 50% of the calculated scheduled opioid regimen; rescue opioid continues to be available

  - Twenty-four hours after patch removal, increase to 100% of the calculated scheduled opioid regimen; rescue opioid continues to be available

- **Converting from TDF to IV fentanyl**

  - Remove the TDF patch

  - Establish IV access and allow an "as needed" bolus dose of fentanyl

  - Six hours after TDF patch removal, begin 50% of IV fentanyl infusion (which should be 50% of the TDF patch strength); bolus option remains in place

  - Twelve hours after TDF patch removal, increase IV fentanyl infusion to 100% of prescribed amount (which should be equal to the TDF patch strength); bolus option remains in place

Table 5-3 (contd.)
Rules of Thumb with Fentanyl Conversions

■ **Conversion from IV fentanyl to TDF**

- Apply TDF patch in same strength as IV fentanyl infusion.

- Six hours after application of TDF, reduce IV fentanyl infusion by 50%; bolus option remains in place

- Twelve hours after application of TDF, discontinue IV fentanyl infusion; bolus option remains in place.

- Twenty-four hours after application of TDF, discontinue IV fentanyl bolus

PRACTICE PROBLEMS

P5.1: Switching from oral morphine to TDF

TS is a 72 year old man with severe osteoarthritis pain. His prescriber has him on a regimen of morphine oral solution, 20 mg every 4 hours around the clock. When TS remembers to take all six doses of morphine per day his pain is very well controlled. Unfortunately, when he forgets to take doses he ends up in pain crisis. His prescriber asks your help in converting TS to TDF. What do you recommend, and specifically how should the switch be timed?

P5.2: Switching from oral long-acting oxycodone to TDF

HH is a 62 year old woman with chronic low back pain, currently taking OxyContin 40 mg po q12h with OxyIR 10 mg every 2 hours (takes about 4 times per day). This reduces HH's pain to about a 4 on a 0–10 scale. Unfortunately, HH complains that she cannot afford the OxyContin tablets, and she would like to switch to generic TDF. What do you recommend?

P5.3: Switching from TDF to oral morphine

DW is a 48 year old man who just moved to the area for a new job. He has a 10-year history of chronic low back pain for which he receives 100 mcg/h TDF. Unfortunately his new prescription plan does not cover TDF and he has been referred to you for conversion to oral morphine. What do you recommend?

P5.4: Switching from TDF to IV fentanyl

TJ is a 58 year old man with end-stage lung cancer, who has been admitted to your inpatient hospice unit for uncontrolled pain. He is currently receiving 75 mcg/h TDF with MSIR 15 mg po q2h for breakthrough pain. He rates his pain as a 9 out of 10, where it has been for the past 24 hours. He has taken several doses of the MSIR but tells you "that stuff doesn't work, so I quit taking it." You would like to switch him to a continuous IV infusion of fentanyl. What is your dosing strategy?

P5.5: Switching from IV fentanyl to TDF

TJ, the 58 year old man with end-stage lung cancer described in case P5.4, was admitted and switched to a continuous fentanyl infusion. Several days later his pain is very well controlled on 120 mcg/h of fentanyl with a 40 mcg bolus every 15 minutes as needed for breakthrough pain. He has used 4 doses of the rescue fentanyl over the past 24 hours. He would now like to be transitioned back to TDF so he can return home. What do you recommend and how do you make a smooth transition?

REFERENCES

1. Muijsers RBR, Wagstaff AJ. Transdermal fentanyl: An updated review of its pharmacological properties and therapeutic efficacy in chronic cancer pain control. *Drugs.* 2001;61(15):2289–2307.

2. Carter KA. Heat-associated increase in transdermal fentanyl absorption. *Am J Health-Syst Pharm.* 2003;60:191–2.

3. McLean M, Fudin J. Optimizing pain control with fentanyl patches. Medscape Pharmacists 2008. Available at: www.medscape.com/viewarticle/576398. Accessed online July 27, 2008.

4. Duragesic (Fentanyl Transdermal System) Prescribing Information. Available at http://www.duragesic.com/duragesic/shared/pi/duragesic.pdf#zoom=100. Accessed July 27, 2008.

5. Marquardt KA, Tharratt RS, Musallam NA. Fentanyl remaining in a transdermal system following three days of continuous use. *Ann Pharmacother.* 1995;29:969–971.

6. Freynhagen R, von Giesen HJ, Busche P, et al. Switching from reservoir to matrix systems for the transdermal delivery of fentanyl: a prospective, multicenter pilot study in outpatients with chronic pain. *J Pain Symptom Manage.* 2005;30:289–297.

7. Welsh J et al. Physicians' knowledge of transdermal fentanyl. *Palliat Med.* 2005;19:9–16.

8. U.S. Food and Drug Administration. Information for Healthcare Professionals—Fentanyl Transdermal System (marketed as Duragesic and generics). Available at http://www.fda.gov/cder/drug/InfoSheets/HCP/fentanyl_2007HCP.htm, Accessed July 27, 2008.

9. Gardner-Nix J. Caregiver toxicity from transdermal fentanyl. *J Pain Symptom Manage.* 2001;21:447–8.

10. Anderson R, Saiers JH, Abram S, et al. Accuracy in equianalgesic dosing: conversion dilemmas. *J Pain Symptom Manage.* 2001;21:397–406.

11. Skaer TL. Practice guidelines for transdermal opioids in malignant pain. *Drugs.* 2004;64:2629–2638.

12. Donner B, Zenz M, Tryba M, et al. Direct conversion from oral morphine to transdermal fentanyl: a multicenter study in patients with cancer pain. *Pain.* 1996;64:527–534.

13. Breitbart W, Chandler S, Eagel B, et al. An alternative algorithm for dosing transdermal fentanyl for cancer-related pain. *Oncology.* 2000;14:695–705.

14. Weissman DE. Converting To/From Transdermal Fentanyl, 2nd ed. Fast Fact and Concept #2: July 2005, End-of-Life Palliative Education Resource Center, www.eperc.mcw.edu.

15. Portenoy RK, Southam MA, Gupta SK, et al. Transdermal fentanyl for cancer pain. Repeated doses pharmacokinetics. *Anesthesiology.* 1993;78:36–43. Abstract.

16. Donner B, Zenz M, Strumpf M, et al. Long-term treatment of cancer pain with transdermal fentanyl. *J Pain Symptom Manage.* 1998;15:168–175.

17. Abrahm JL. A Physician's Guide to Pain and Symptom Management in Cancer Patients. 2nd ed. Baltimore: The Johns Hopkins University Press; 2005:249.

18. Solassol I, Caumette L, Bressole F, et al. Inter- and intra-individual variability in transdermal fentanyl absorption in cancer pain patients. *Oncol Rep.* 2005;14:1029–1036.

19. Abrahm JL. A Physician's Guide to Pain and Symptom Management in Cancer Patients. 2nd ed. Baltimore: The Johns Hopkins University Press; 2005:167.

20. Kornick CA, Santiago-Palma J, Schulman G, et al. A safe and effective method for converting patients from transdermal to intravenous fentanyl for the treatment of acute cancer-related pain. *Cancer.* 2003;97:3121–3124.

21. Kornick CA, Santiago-Palma, Khojainova N, et al. A safe and effective method for converting cancer patients from intravenous to transdermal fentanyl. *Cancer.* 2001;92:3056–3061.

ADDITIONAL SUGGESTED READING

Kornick CA, Santiago-Palma J, Moryl N, et al. Benefit-risk assessment of transdermal fentanyl for the treatment of chronic pain. *Drug Safety.* 2003;26:951–973.

SOLUTIONS TO PRACTICE PROBLEMS

P5.1: Importantly, TS's pain is well controlled when he takes all the morphine prescribed for him, which is 120 mg per day (morphine 20 mg po q4h around the clock). Using our 2 mg oral morphine:1 mcg TDF guideline, this works out to be 60 mcg/h TDF. Our decision at this point is to either round up to 75 mcg/h TDF or down to 50 mcg/h TDF. Given TS's age and the fact that his pain was very well controlled (when he took the morphine), it would be appropriate to round down to 50 mcg/h TDF. Specific timing would be as follows:

> 8 a.m.—apply 50 mcg/h TDF patch
> 8 a.m.—take oral morphine 20 mg
> 12:00 p.m.—take oral morphine 20 mg
> Offer oral morphine 20 mg q2h prn from 8 a.m. onward

P5.2: First, we calculate HH's total daily dose of oral oxycodone. OxyContin 40 mg po q12h = 80; plus OxyIR 10 mg × 4 doses per day = 40 mg, for a TDD of 120 mg oral oxycodone. Using one of our ratio equations, we determine that 120 mg oral oxycodone is approximately equivalent to 180 mg oral morphine. Using our 2 mg oral morphine:1 mcg TDF rule of thumb, this works out to be 90 mcg/h TDF. Therefore we must either round down to 75 mcg/h TDF or increase to 100 mcg/h TDF. Since HH's pain control could be improved, it would be appropriate to increase to 100 mcg/h TDF. For breakthrough we can continue to use the OxyIR, giving 10-15% of the TDD (120 mg oxycodone)—15 mg every 2 hours as needed for breakthrough pain would be appropriate. HH should take one last OxyContin tablet when she applies the 100 mcg/h TDF patch, and use her rescue opioid as needed.

P5.3: DW is using a 100 mcg/h TDF patch, which is approximately equivalent to 200 mg per day of oral morphine. If we gave the oral morphine using the short-acting formulation this would be 30 mg every 4 hours, and a rescue dose of 20 mg every 2 hours as needed. We recommend the following conversion plan for DW:

- Remove 100 mcg/h TDF patch at 8 a.m.

- For the next 12 hours use short-acting morphine 20 mg every 2 hours as needed for pain

- For the next 12 hours (hours 13–24) patient should take oral morphine 15 mg every 4 hours, and an extra 15 mg as needed every 2 hours

- Starting at 24 hours take oral morphine 30 mg every 4 hours around the clock, and an extra 15 mg as needed every 2 hours

After 3 days on oral morphine 30 mg every 4 hours around the clock, he had good pain control (rated as a 3 or 4 on a 0–10 scale) and did not need any rescue doses. He was switched to MS Contin 100 mg q12h

P5.4: As was described in the Kornick study, because TJ is in pain crisis, it would be appropriate to remove the 75 mcg/h TDF patch, and immediately begin a continuous IV infusion of fentanyl at 75 mcg/h. The patient should also have a demand bolus available at 50–100% of the continuous infusion hourly rate, therefore it would be appropriate to offer 40 mcg every 20 minutes as needed. Of course the palliative care practitioners will have to closely monitor TJ for sedation, as well as pain control and other adverse effects. TJ will also have to be carefully assessed to determine why he is having a pain crisis (e.g., pathological fracture, etc.).

P5.5: TJ's pain is well controlled on 120 mcg/h of IV fentanyl, therefore we will apply one 100 mcg TDF and one 25 mcg/h TDF patch at 8 a.m.. We will continue the infusion at 120 mcg/h and keep the bolus option in place. At 2 pm (6 hours after patch application) we reduce the continuous infusion to 60 mcg/h, but keep the same bolus option in place. At 8 pm (12 hours after patch application) we discontinue the continuous infusion, but keep the same bolus option in place. At 8 a.m. on Day 2 we discontinue the bolus option and convert TJ to an oral short-action opioid for breakthrough pain, such as MSIR 30 mg po q2h prn pain.

CHAPTER 6

Methadone: A Complex and Challenging Analgesic, But It's Worth It!

OBJECTIVES

After reading this chapter and completing all practice problems, the participant will be able to:

1. Describe the pharmacodynamics and pharmacokinetics of methadone.

2. Explain the mechanism of pharmacodynamic and pharmacokinetic drug interactions with methadone, list medications that commonly induce or inhibit methadone metabolism, and describe strategies for dealing with these interactions.

3. Describe appropriate and inappropriate candidates for methadone therapy.

4. Determine a starting dose of methadone for an opioid-naïve patient, as well as a recommendation for rescue medication.

5. Given an actual or simulated patient receiving methadone, describe a monitoring plan designed to detect methadone toxicity.

6. List variables that increase the risk for methadone-induced QTc prolongation.

7. Calculate an appropriate dose of methadone for a patient converting to and from another opioid regimen.

8. Describe the conversion process to and from oral to parenteral methadone, and recommended dosing parameters for methadone delivered via patient-controlled analgesia.

INTRODUCTION

Ah methadone, magical, mystical, mischievous methadone! Dosing of no other opioid fuels controversy and heated debate as does methadone, yet one has to admire methadone's sheer cheekiness. Many are drawn to the cost-effectiveness of oral methadone, but methadone is clearly not for the uninitiated or uneducated practitioner. From an intellectual point of view, we could probably teach students in pharmacy school for four years just using methadone as the example drug. We have drama (the pharmacodynamics of methadone), we have intrigue (why DO we have so many conversion charts), excitement (wow—look at all those drug interactions) and we have danger (QT interval prolongation?). Despite, or in spite of, the good, the bad, and the ugly sides of methadone, its use for chronic cancer and non-cancer pain is growing. Despite the lack of well-designed clinical trials, evaluation of the literature that is available on using methadone for chronic noncancer pain shows that the majority of patients achieve effective pain control.[1] In this chapter we will review the pharmacodynamics and pharmacokinetics of methadone, dosing of methadone in opioid-naïve patients, conversion calculations to and from methadone, and a look at the use of intravenous methadone. That should keep us out of trouble!

Pharmacodynamics of Methadone

Methadone is a synthetic opioid agonist developed almost 50 years ago, best known (sometimes to our disadvantage in pain management) for its use in treating opioid dependence. Thanks to the long duration of action, efficacy, and low cost, methadone is enjoying increased popularity in the treatment of chronic pain.

Methadone is a racemic mixture of R- and S-methadone; R-methadone is 8–50 times more potent than S-methadone and is responsible for most of its action.[2] Methadone is a mu-opioid receptor agonist (like morphine, oxycodone, hydromorphone), and it also binds to the kappa and delta opioid receptors. Additional mechanisms of action include inhibiting the re-uptake of serotonin and norepinephrine (which is how antidepressants act to treat pain), and it works as an antagonist at the N-methyl-D-aspartate (NMDA) receptor, thought to prevent central sensitization and reduce opioid tolerance, and possibly increase its effectiveness in treating neuropathic pain as compared to other opioids.

Pharmacokinetics of Methadone

Absorption
Methadone may be given by a variety of routes of administration with different dosage formulations. Routes of administration include oral, rectal, intravenous (IV), intramuscular (IM; no, no, bad dog!), subcutaneous (SQ), epidural, and intrathecal (spinal administration is not FDA approved).

Methadone is a basic and lipophilic drug that is detected in the blood 15–45 minutes after oral administration with peak plasmas concentrations achieved in 2.5–4 hours.[3] Oral bioavailability is approximately 70–80% (range 36–100%), and absorption of oral methadone tablets and solution is equivalent.[2] Studies in healthy normal subjects who received methadone rectally, orally, and intravenously showed an absolute bioavailability of 76%, and 86% respectively.[4]

Distribution
Being highly lipophilic (fat-soluble), methadone is widely and quickly distributed throughout the body to the brain, gut, kidney, liver, muscle and lung. Methadone is retained in these tissues and slowly released back into the plasma during redistribution and elimination. Due to these properties, methadone has a very long half-life (time it takes for half the drug to be eliminated from the body) in the body. Methadone binds to alpha 1-acid glycoprotein, as well as albumin and globulin to a lesser degree. The portion of drug that is "free" or "unbound" is that which results in the pharmacologic actions of the drug; this portion varies four-fold among patients.[2] The range in protein-binding could partially explain the extreme variability in patient responsiveness to methadone. For example, methadone 5 mg twice a day prescribed for me may result in a different response than methadone 5 mg twice a day prescribed for you.

Metabolism
Methadone is extensively metabolized, primarily by N-demethylation, to pharmacologically inactive metabolites which are eliminated in the urine and feces.[3] Metabolism takes place primarily in the liver, with some also occurring in the gut. There is significant variation in how methadone is metabolized among individuals. The cytochrome

P450 (CYP450) enzymes responsible for the metabolism of methadone in the liver include CYP3A4, 2B6, 2C8, 2C9, 2C19, and 2D6.[2] The metabolism of methadone is significantly influenced by medications that alter the activity of some of these enzyme systems, resulting in either increased or decreased methadone metabolism in many cases. Drugs metabolized by the 2D6 enzyme system are also subject to genetic variability. Finally, methadone even induces its own metabolism in the liver (OK, that's pretty wild!). We will discuss drug interactions with methadone more extensively later in the chapter.

Elimination

As discussed above, the inactive metabolites of methadone are eliminated in the urine and feces. Because the metabolites are inactive, methadone is a useful opioid in patients with renal impairment. Methadone has a very long elimination half-life, ranging from 5 to 130 hours, with a mean of about 20–35 hours.[3] The long half-life of methadone can result in toxicity due to accumulation in the body. Given this long and variable half-life, it can take 4 to 10 days to achieve a steady-state concentration of methadone in the serum. Steady-state is where *the rate of drug in* = *the rate of drug out* and the serum concentration is fairly steady. If the dose of methadone is increased or decreased, or a new medication is started that increases or decreases methadone metabolism, it will take *another 4–10 days* to achieve the new steady-state. Some of the variables that influence (and alter) the metabolism and elimination of methadone have been discussed above. Additional variables worth mention are patient gender (e.g., women metabolize methadone faster than men), and urine pH.[5]

Drug Interactions with Methadone

A "drug interaction" describes a clinical scenario where one drug alters the pharmacologic effect of another drug given at the same time (e.g., in the same drug regimen).[6] Drug interactions can alter the pharmacokinetics or pharmacodynamics of a drug.

When we talk about a pharmacodynamic drug interaction, we are referring to one medication increasing or decreasing the therapeutic effectiveness or adverse effects of another drug. Giving methadone with other opioids would be a pharmacodynamic drug interaction—we will see increased analgesia (which is a good thing), but it could be *too* much of a good thing due to the additive toxicities such as respiratory depression and sedation. We may see increased CNS depression when alcohol, neuroleptics, or other psychoactive medications (e.g., benzodiazepines, antidepressants) are used with opioids, including methadone. Another example of a pharmacodynamic drug interaction is administering methadone along with another medication that may prolong the QTc interval, such as an antiarrhythmic or antipsychotic agent, and selected antibiotics and antidepressants.[6]

Pharmacokinetic drug interactions affect or alter the absorption, distribution, metabolism or elimination of the target drug. For example, there are some medications that compete with methadone for protein binding sites. If methadone has a lower affinity for the protein-binding site than does the competing drug, methadone will be less likely to bind to the protein (because protein binding is competitive), resulting in a higher percentage of methadone that is "unbound" or "free." This will result in a greater pharmacologic effect, both therapeutic and possibly toxic. The tricyclic antidepressants and neuroleptic medications can compete with methadone for binding on alpha 1-acid glycoprotein.[6] This represents a pharmacokinetic drug interaction affecting the distribution (and ultimately pharmacodynamics) of methadone.

As described previously, methadone is extensively metabolized in the intestines and liver by the CYP enzyme system. The primary enzyme responsible for the metabolism of methadone is CYP3A4 with less involvement of the other enzymes mentioned above. Even without the influence of interacting medications, the level of activity of the 3A4 enzyme varies significantly among individuals—with up to a 30-fold difference in the liver 3A4 enzymes, and an 11-fold difference in the intestinal 3A4 enzymes.[3,7] Next we must consider the influence of medications that can *induce* (increase) the activity of enzymes, and those that *inhibit* (reduce) the activity of enzymes, thus affecting the serum level of the object drug being metabolized (methadone in this case), known as the *substrate*. Enzyme induction usually takes 1–2 weeks, while enzyme inhibition occurs much more quickly.[6] This means you may see an increase in methadone serum levels and adverse effects within a day or two of the patient starting a new medication that reduces methadone metabolism (an inhibitor). Conversely, it may take 1–2 weeks to see a decrease in methadone serum levels and an increase in pain after introducing a medication that induces methadone metabolism. Table 6-1 to help you understand the effect of giving methadone along with another medication known to be an enzyme *inhibitor* or enzyme *inducer*:

Table 6-1

Effect of Enzyme Inhibitors and Inducers on Methadone Metabolism

What's the situation?	What happens in this situation?	What does this mean for my patient?	What should you do about it?
Taking methadone with medications known to be enzyme *inhibitors*.	The enzyme inhibiting medication will slow the metabolism of methadone, resulting in an *increased* methadone serum level.	The patient may become toxic from a methadone overdose.	When converting to methadone and patient is already taking a medication known to inhibit methadone metabolism, reduce your calculated methadone dose by 25% or more. Encourage use of the rescue opioid as needed.
Taking methadone with medications known to be enzyme *inducers*.	The enzyme inducing medication will *increase* the metabolism of methadone, resulting in a *decreased* methadone serum level.	The dose of methadone may be insufficient and the patient can experience increased pain.	Because this effect cannot be easily quantified, go with your calculated methadone dose but strongly encourage use rescue opioid. Methadone dosage increase may be appropriate after patient achieves steady-state.

Table 6-2 lists selected medications known or thought to interact with methadone.[3,6] Practitioners are strongly encouraged to use a drug interaction program to screen for potential interactions with any patient in whom methadone is going to be used. One example is at the Indiana University School of Medicine web page (http://medicine. iupui.edu/flockhart/).[8] To be safe, it would be prudent to empirically reduce the calculated methadone dose by 25% or more for patients whose drug regimen contains a medication known to inhibit methadone metabolism. However, clinicians are encouraged to review the drug interactions literature in order to make their own determination regarding proactive dose reduction specific to a given CYP enzyme inhibition.

Table 6-2

Selected Drug Interactions with Methadone (Enzyme Inducers and Inhibitors)[6]

Enzyme Inducers

Rifampicin/rifampin/rifabutin	The enzyme inducing medication will *increase* the metabolism of methadone, resulting in a *decreased* methadone serum level. The dose of methadone may be insufficient and the patient can experience increased pain.	Encourage use of rescue medication.
Phenobarbital		
Phenytoin		
Spironolactone		
Nevirapine		
Efavirenz		
Amprenavir		
Nelfinavir		
Ritonavir		
Carbamazepine		
St. John's Wort		

Enzyme Inhibitors

Fluconazole	The enzyme inhibiting medication will slow the metabolism of methadone, resulting in an *increased* methadone serum level. The patient may become toxic from a methadone overdose.	Empirically reduce projected methadone dose by 25% or more and encourage use of rescue medication.
Fluoxetine		
Paroxetine		
Sertraline		
Ciprofloxacin		
Fluvoxamine		
Amitriptyline		
Ketoconazole		
Erythromycin		
Troleandomycin		
Citalopram		
Desipramine		
Clarithromycin		
Telithrymycin		
Itraconazole		

Candidates for Methadone Therapy

So, for whom should methadone therapy be considered? Some proposed indications for methadone treatment include the following:

- Patients with true morphine allergy (or other pure mu opioid agonists)
- Patients with significant renal impairment
- Presence of neuropathic pain
- Opioid-induced adverse effects (e.g., hallucinations)
- Pain refractory to other opioids or uncontrolled pain
- In cases where the cost of the opioid is an issue
- Patients who would benefit from an oral long-acting opioid, particularly those who require an oral solution
- Potentially any patient who requires opioid therapy, such as opioid-naïve patients

Patients for whom methadone may *not* be an appropriate therapeutic option includes the following:

- Patients with a very limited prognosis (e.g., less than a week to live)
- Numerous drugs in the medication regimen that interact with methadone, including those that prolong the QTc interval
- Individuals with a history of syncope or arrhythmias
- Patient lives alone, has poor cognitive functioning, is unreliable or noncomprehending of instruction
- Patients with a history of unpredictable adherence to therapy (e.g., taking more or less opioid that prescribed)

Methadone in Opioid-Naïve Patients

While there are mixed feelings about using methadone as a first-line opioid, there are some advantages to doing so. Methadone is the only opioid available in a solution that is inherently long-acting. For patients who cannot swallow tablets or capsules, or who have a feeding tube, methadone oral solution is an attractive option. Methadone can even be used as an initial opioid in older, frail patients at a very low dose (e.g., 1 mg a day), with close observation after initiation of therapy for potential accumulation and adverse effects.

   The dosage recommendation for opioid non-tolerant (naïve) patients per the prescribing information for Dolophine® Hydrochloride (Roxane Laboratories) is 2.5 to 10 mg every 8 to 12 hours, slowly titrated to effect.[9] Most pain practitioners consider this to be too aggressive and broad a dosing range (e.g., could be anywhere from 2.5 mg po q12h [5 mg total daily dose] to 10 mg po q8h [30 mg total daily dose]). The College of Physicians and Surgeons of Ontario published guidelines for the treatment of nonmalignant pain in 2000. They recommend an initial dose of 2.5 mg methadone by mouth every 8 hours; they further recommend starting with a lower dose, such as 2.5 mg once a day, in frail older patients, and 2.5 mg once or twice daily in patients who are taking medications known to inhibit the metabolism of methadone (see Table 6-2).[10] Let's look at a typical case example.

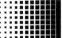

CASE 6.1

• •
Starting Methadone in an Opioid-Naïve Patient

FA is an 89 year old man admitted to hospital with a terminal diagnosis of failure to thrive, and he's complaining of general aches and pains. FA is still ambulatory but somewhat frail. He has a recent history of a bleeding ulcer, therefore his primary care provider (PCP) does not want to begin non-steroidal anti-inflammatory (NSAID) therapy. FA has not responded with any degree of significance to acetaminophen, and his description of the pain is not suggestive of neuropathic pain. The PCP would like to start methadone; what dose would you recommend? FA is not taking any other medications known to interact with methadone.

The starting dose recommended by the College of Physicians and Surgeons of Ontario is 2.5 mg one to three times per day. Given FA's frail state, it would be reasonable to begin with 2.5 mg by mouth at bedtime. The PCP may or may not choose to provide rescue medication for FA. Some practitioners would be even more conservative and start at 1 mg a day—perhaps even dosing in the morning for better observation during the dayshift. Let's take a look at another case.

CASE 6.2

• •
Starting Methadone in an Opioid-Naïve Patient

BL is a 54 year old woman with a 20 year history of type 2 diabetes mellitus. She has complained of painful diabetic neuropathy in her feet for the past 5 years. Unsurprisingly the pain did not respond to acetaminophen or NSAIDs. Her physician tried gabapentin, but the patient complained of excessive somnolence and dizziness. She tried duloxetine (Cymbalta) but complained of excessive nausea. Her physician would like to start methadone and asks your help in suggesting a starting dose. BL is not taking any other opioids, and is not receiving any medications known to interact with methadone. What do you recommend?

BL is considerably younger than the patient we discussed in Case 6.1, therefore we can safely recommend methadone 2.5 mg by mouth every 12 hours. Also, it would be acceptable to go right to 2.5 mg by mouth every 8 hours. Many times, especially early in therapy, we find that patients do better with a shorter dosing interval such as every 8 hours. When they achieve steady state, they can receive their total daily dose divided into two equal amounts (every 12 hours). Cancer pain patients have been shown to require 2.4 doses of methadone per day to achieve good pain control (e.g., which we can interpret to mean that half of this population take their methadone q12h, and the other half take it q8h).[11]

⬛ FAST FACT ▶ Oral Methadone Dosage Formulations

Oral methadone is available as a 5 and 10 mg tablet (which may be cut in half). There is also a 40-mg dispersible tablet (Methadone Disket), which is only available to substance abuse treatment programs. There are three different concentrations of methadone oral solution including 5 mg/5 mL, 10 mg/5 mL and the oral concentrated solution 10 mg/mL. It is important to counsel patients, families, caregivers carefully about accurate dosing and administration of all oral solutions, but particularly the concentrated 10 mg/mL solution.

Monitoring the Methadone Regimen in Opioid-Naïve Patients

As we discussed at the beginning of this chapter, I promised you "edge-of-the-seat" excitement with methadone. One of the more interesting facts about methadone is its duration of analgesic action. For single doses methadone is effective for about 4-8 hours. With chronic dosing, as steady-state is approached the duration increases. As we discussed earlier, the elimination half-life is considerably longer than the half-life of analgesia. Because of this discrepancy, it takes days to achieve the full analgesic effect of methadone (see Figure 6-1). What are the implications of these findings? First, we must carefully explain to the patient that it takes several days to achieve the full analgesic effect of methadone (several days to achieve steady state serum levels). Second, it is vital that health care professionals, patients, families and caregivers work together closely to monitor the patient's response to methadone while on the road to steady-state. Let's take a closer look at this important implication.

You don't just start a patient on methadone (either as their first opioid, or converted from a different opioid) and walk away. The prescribing information states "Respiratory depression is the chief hazard associated with methadone hydrochloride administration. Methadone's peak respiratory depressant effects typically occur later, and persist longer than its peak analgesic effects, particularly in the early dosing period. These characteristics can contribute to cases of iatrogenic overdose, particularly during treatment initiation and dose titration."[9]

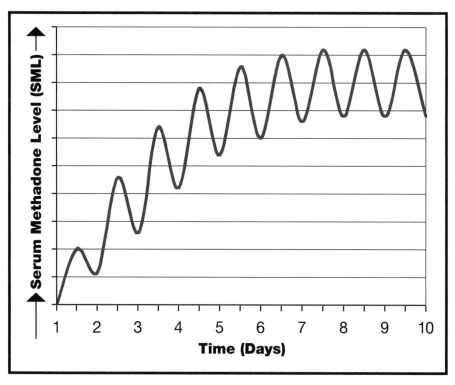

Figure 6-1. Methadone serum concentration increases gradually over five or more days while continuing the same daily dose. Source: adapted from Payte JT. Opioid agonist treatment of addiction. Slide presentation at ASAM Review Course in Addiction Medicine, 2002. See: http:www/jtpayte.com. Used with permission.

What is very important, however, is understanding that a patient doesn't go from sitting in their easy chair watching a re-run of "Law and Order" to cessation of breathing. What happens in between? Specifically, central nervous system depression, namely drowsiness, occurs first. Families, caregivers and case managers need to know to monitor the patient's level of arousal. We want the patient to be able to wake up easily if they doze off when their name is called, or if given a firm shake.

Signs of methadone overdose from acute intoxication include evident euphoria, ataxia, and slurred speech. Late signs include unconsciousness, loud snoring and brown pulmonary edema secretion from mouth or nose.[12] While these symptoms are associated with a 5–6 hour period after an acute ingestion of methadone, we can use this information to suggest a monitoring plan for the initiation of methadone when used for pain management. Specifically, to prevent more serious toxicity, it is important to monitor the following during methadone initiation and titration:

- Excessive drowsiness/level of arousal (see Modified Ramsay Scale in Chapter 2)
- Slowed respiration or periods of apnea, more rapid respiration, shallow breathing
- Slurring of speech
- Loud snoring
- Pinpoint pupil size

Since patients are not taking one large dose (as in an overdose situation), it is important to monitor for these signs and symptoms of toxicity over a 5–7 day period after initiation of methadone therapy or a dosage change.

The vigilance with which we monitor the patient depends partially on the clinical situation. For ambulatory outpatients who are otherwise in good physical condition, and are being started on a low dose of methadone, it is probably sufficient to educate the patient and family members who live in the home about what to keep an eye out for and monitor. For example, ask the spouse to purposefully assess the patient's level of arousal/drowsiness twice a day (or more frequently if there are concerns). For patients with more advanced illness (such as hospice patients), some programs have the nurse call or visit the patient every day for the first 5 days, specifically assessing for signs and symptoms of methadone toxicity. Thorough education of the patient and family will help significantly, such as not missing or taking extra doses of methadone.

Another important consideration is understanding the variables that increase the risk for methadone toxicity. These include starting at too high a dose, increasing the dose too quickly, forgetting to consider the influence of interacting medications (particularly those that inhibit methadone metabolism), and co-administration of medications such as benzodiazepines, alcohol, cocaine, cannabis, and other opioids. Co-administration of benzodiazepines with methadone has actually been shown to cause sleep apnea.[13]

 CASE 6.3
• •
Importance of Determining Previous Total Daily Opioid Dose

Let's consider a case from this author's practice. A hospice nurse called for advice on an elderly patient experiencing significant pain. After discussing the case, we agreed that switching the patient from her current regimen of long- and short-acting morphine to methadone was a good plan. I added the standing dose and breakthrough opioid doses given, did the calculation, and made a recommendation which was accepted and implemented on Day 1. The morning of Day 2 the nurse case manager called me to tell me I was a rock star—the patient was tearfully grateful with her level of pain control. (Note: I get very nervous when I'm a rock star on Day 2—when this happens it generally means I'm in big trouble down the road). On Day 3 the nurse called to say all was well, but the patient was sleeping a bit more than normal. In retrospect, we should have intervened at this point. On Day 4 the nurse called to say the woman was increasingly sedated and "acting like a drunk monkey." I couldn't believe I had miscalculated so badly! Assailed by personal self-doubt, I instructed the nurse to hold the methadone for 24 hours, then resume at a significantly lower dose. The patient made it through Day 5, and on Day 6 the nurse called to say the patient was back to a good state of pain control and she was awake. Then she told me that the patient's son confessed that he actually had never given his mother all the rescue morphine he'd originally claimed; he didn't want the nurse to think he was a bad son!

What are the morals of this story? First, be alert when you have saved the universe on Day 2 of methadone therapy. Second, don't believe the patient/family when they say "I swear, she's been getting that liquid morphine stuff EVERY 2 hours around the clock!" Third, be vigilant in monitoring your patient to prevent an outcome no one wants! I don't want *you* saying one day "my bad!"

Breakthrough Pain Management in Methadone-Treated Patients

There are two schools of thought as to whether or not to use methadone for breakthrough pain in patients getting methadone for their baseline pain: yes and no. There are some proposed dosing strategies (particularly with conversion from other opioids) that recommend using methadone around-the-clock and letting patients use their "prn" methadone as a way to self-titrate to pain relief. More practitioners probably do *not* use methadone for rescue dosing. If we use morphine, oxycodone, oxymorphone or hydromorphone instead, we have a much greater comfort level knowing that the rescue opioid is not affecting the time to steady-state of methadone, or absolute methadone steady-state serum concentration (e.g., when using methadone as the "around the clock" opioid). Let's say you decide to go with morphine for breakthrough pain; you would choose a dose of that is appropriate for an opioid-naïve patient (e.g., morphine 2.5 to 5 mg po every 2–4 hours as needed, etc.).

If you chose to use methadone for breakthrough pan, you could use 50–100% of the scheduled methadone dose, and offer it every 3 hours for additional pain (usually recommended not to exceed 30 mg of oral methadone). Make sure to ask the patient to maintain a pain diary documenting use of the methadone.

Titrating the Methadone in Opioid-Naïve Patients

The speed with which we titrate (increase) methadone depends to some extent on the patient's clinical situation and how closely the patient can be monitored. For outpatients, methadone should be titrated cautiously, based on patient response, signs of toxicity and our knowledge of time to steady-state. Most practitioners adhere to the recommendation that the dose of methadone should not be increased until the patient has received five or seven days of the same dose.[14] As discussed earlier, a phone call or visit to the patient daily is highly recommended during the titration period. Any card-carrying hospice nurse will tell you it's no coincidence that both "Monday" and "methadone" begin with "M"— this gives the nurse the workweek to assess the potential for potential toxicity!

The optimal dosage increase is not clear with methadone. If you are using morphine or another short-acting opioid for breakthrough pain, one strategy is to evaluate how much rescue opioid they are using on days 5, 6, and 7. Average that amount, and convert it to methadone (conversion calculations in next section). Alternately, the VA/DoD (Veterans Administration/Department of Defense) recommends increasing by 2.5 mg per dose every 5–7 days.[15] For example: starting dose 2.5 mg po q12h; week 2 increase to 5 mg po q12h; week 3 increase to 7.5 mg po q12h; week 4 increase to 10 mg po q12h, etc. As you get to larger doses it would probably be acceptable to increase a bit more (by 5 mg/dose), for example week 5 increase to 15 mg po q12h.

In situations where opioid-naïve patients are in a controlled, monitored environment, methadone may be started at a higher dose (e.g., 2.5 mg po q6 or 8 hours) and increased more aggressively. The VA/DoD guidelines recommend a 2.5 mg increase/dose, as often as every day, over about 4 days.[15] Shir and colleagues describe their experience using epidural and oral methadone in hospitalized patients for severe pain.[16] For opioid-naïve adult patients, the initial dose of methadone did not exceed 5–10 mg two or three times daily, and the dose was increased in increments of 20–30%. They reported no incidents of respiratory depression or severe mental obtundation, although minor side effects (e.g., mild-moderate mental obtundation, itching, nausea, urinary retention) were reported in 13% of patients. This is a fairly aggressive titration schedule and it is important to know that these hospitalized patients were generally titrated off methadone prior to discharge. If this wasn't the case, it would be very important to monitor the patient for 4–5 days *after* the last dosage change (e.g., monitor until you are at or close to steady-state) before discharging the patient.

:::::::⬛⬛⬛ FAST FACT ⟩ **Recommendations for Cardiac Safety Monitoring with Methadone**

A multidisciplinary panel of experts met in late 2007 to review the cardiac effects of methadone, and to develop cardiac safety recommendations for methadone prescribers. Their recommendations are as follows:

"Recommendation 1 (Disclosure): Clinicians should inform patients of arrhythmia risk when they prescribe methadone.

Recommendation 2 (Clinical History): Clinicians should ask patients about any history of structural heart disease, arrhythmia, and syncope.

Recommendation 3 (Screening): Obtain a pretreatment electrocardiogram for all patients to measure the QTc interval and a follow-up electrocardiogram within 30 days and annually. Additional electrocardiography is recommended if the methadone dosage exceeds 100 mg/d or if patients have unexplained syncope or seizures.

Recommendation 4 (Risk Stratification): If the QTc interval is greater than 450 ms but less than 500 ms, discuss the potential risks and benefits with patients and monitor them more frequently. If the QTc interval exceeds 500 ms, consider discontinuing or reducing the methadone dose; eliminating contributing factors, such as drugs that promote hypokalemia; or using an alternative therapy.

Recommendation 5 (Drug Interactions): Clinicians should be aware of interactions between methadone and other drugs that possess QT interval-prolonging properties or slow the elimination of methadone."[22]

METHADONE PUBLIC HEALTH ADVISORY

In November 2006 the Food and Drug Administration issued a public health advisory titled "Methadone use for pain control may result in death and life-threatening changes in breathing and heart beat."[17] They described patient deaths from the use of methadone in both opioid-naïve patients and those converted to methadone. This public health advisory actually lead to a change in the product labeling of methadone. Specific speaking points included the following:

- **"Patients should take methadone exactly as prescribed.** Taking more methadone than prescribed can cause breathing to slow or stop and can cause death. A patient who does not experience good pain relief with the prescribed dose of methadone, should talk to his or her doctor.

- **Patients taking methadone should not start or stop taking other medicines or dietary supplements without talking to their health care provider.** Taking other medicines or dietary supplements may cause less pain relief. They may also cause a toxic buildup of methadone in the body leading to dangerous changes in breathing or heart beat that may cause death.

- **Health care professionals and patients should be aware of the signs of methadone overdose.** Signs of methadone overdose include trouble breathing or shallow breathing; extreme tiredness or sleepiness; blurred vision; inability to think, talk or walk normally; and feeling faint, dizzy or confused. If these signs occur, patients should get medical attention right away."

We have discussed earlier in this chapter the need to monitor the patient closely for over-sedation and respiratory depression. The other important message in this FDA Public Health Advisory is the admonition to be mindful of methadone's ability to cause QTc (e.g., QT interval corrected for heart rate) interval prolongation. Prolongation of the QT interval is a surrogate marker for the risk of developing a potentially fatal ventricular arrhythmia called torsades de pointes. A study by Ehret and colleagues evaluated QT interval prolongation in former and current IV drug users admitted to the hospital over a 5-year period; half of the subjects were receiving methadone maintenance therapy and half were not.[18] The QT interval in healthy cardiac tissue is 400 milliseconds (msec) or less. International regulatory guidelines suggest a gender-independent threshold for QTc (QT corrected for heart rate) prolongation of 450 msec and a QTc interval greater than 500 msec as the threshold for significant arrhythmia risk.[19, 20] The study by Ehret showed that 16.2% of patients receiving methadone had a QTc of 500 msec or longer on at least one ECG, whereas all patients in the control group who had a QTc of less than 500 msec. Factors associated with QT prolongation include:

- A higher methadone total daily dose

- Hypokalemia

- Low prothrombin level (suggestive of reduced liver function)

- Coadministration of a medication that inhibits the CYP3A4 enzyme system, which may increase methadone serum levels

It is also important to be mindful of other medications that can prolong the QTc interval. A comprehensive review of drug-related QT interval prolongation by Crouch and colleagues describes

Converting to Methadone from Other Opioids (e.g., Opioid-Tolerant Patients)

The majority of patients probably come to methadone as a second-line therapy, having converted from a different opioid such as morphine, oxycodone, hydromorphone, or hydrocodone. The $64,000 question is—how can we best convert a patient from a different opioid to methadone, achieve pain relief as quickly as possible, while not increasing the risk of immediate or delayed toxicity? If you walk outside on a clear night, and look up, you will probably see a lot of stars—count them, because that's how many proposed conversion charts we have for methadone!

One thing is very, very, VERY clear—the conversion from other opioids such as morphine to methadone is **NOT** a linear conversion. What do we mean by this? If you look at the equianalgesic conversion chart we've been using in previous chapters, you see recommendations such as: oxycodone 20 mg oral ~ morphine 30 mg oral. We can quibble and say the oral oxycodone:morphine ratio is 15:30, or 30:30, and we can argue whether or not this is a bidirectional equivalency, but one clear implication is that it's *linear*. In other words, if you buy the fact that oxycodone 20 mg oral ~ morphine 30 mg oral, then you also accept that oxycodone 200 mg oral ~ morphine 300 mg oral. In other words—it's *linear*. This is ***absolutely not*** the case when converting to methadone. The *higher* the dose of the original opioid, the more *potent* the methadone is. We have many methadone conversion charts, and the recommended morphine:methadone conversion ranges from 3:1 to 20:1 or more! Remember, "more potent" doesn't mean "more effective"—potency refers to an equivalent dose to achieve equivalent pain control.

Why is this? Why does methadone become more powerful with increasing prior exposure to other opioids? Bruera suggests three possible reasons for this observation.[23] First, the molecular structure and chemical characteristics of methadone may alter binding to the opioid receptors, possibly resulting in less cross-tolerance to methadone (making the patient more sensitive to the effects of methadone than you would have suspected). Second, we discussed earlier in this chapter how methadone has additional mechanisms of action. Antagonism at the NMDA receptor may significantly reverse opioid tolerance, which can dramatically enhance the patient's response to methadone. Third, Bruera hypothesizes that more traditional opioids such as morphine and hydromorphone are metabolized to pharmacologically active products that may have a **"proalgesic"** effect (refers to a "pain producing effect" such as seen with metabolites including morphine-3-glucuronide, normorphine, etc.). Whether or not it is due to one or more of these reasons, or other reasons, clearly the morphine to methadone conversion is not linear.

So what are the steps in converting from other opioids to methadone? Of course you follow all the steps discussed earlier in this text, as follows:

- **Step 1**—Globally assess the patient (e.g., PQRSTU) to determine if the uncontrolled pain is secondary to worsening of existing pain or development of a new type of pain.

- **Step 2**—Determine the total daily dose of the current opioid. This should include all long-acting and breakthrough opioid doses.

- **Step 3**—In this case, we have already decided we are going to switch to methadone. If the patient was not already on oral morphine, the first part of Step 3 is to convert the patient's current opioid regimen to an equivalent dose of oral morphine. Then, using one of the many methadone conversion tables, calculate the total daily dose of methadone.

- **Step 4**—Individualize the dosage based on assessment information gathered in Step 1 and ensure adequate access to breakthrough medication. It is important to determine if the patient is taking any other medications that may induce or inhibit the metabolism of methadone (this may affect your decision about the total daily methadone dose). In this step you will also have to decide which opioid to use to treat breakthrough pain (methadone or another opioid), the dose, and dosing frequency. The last decision in step four is whether or not to do a "rapid switch" (also known as a "stop-start") or a gradual titration from the patient's current opioid regimen to methadone.

- **Step 5**—Last, it is critical that you exercise very close patient follow-up and continued reassessment. Encourage the patient to use his or her rescue opioid while the methadone accumulates, and monitor the patient to make sure the accumulating methadone dose is too much for the patient.

Let's look at a case to illustrate the process of switching to methadone!

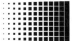 **CASE 6.4**
. . . .
Switching to Oral Methadone

AO is a 64 year old man with chronic low back pain. He is taking Kadian 80 mg po q12h with MSIR 20 mg q2h prn breakthrough pain (he uses on average two doses per day). He is not a surgical candidate, and his physician would like to switch him to methadone in hopes of achieving better pain control. AO is not taking any medications known to interact with methadone.

Step 1—Globally Assess the Patient (e.g., PQRSTU)

Of course we always start with complete analysis of the pain complaint. For patients with pain of mixed pathogenesis (e.g., nociceptive and neuropathic), methadone may be a preferred opioid. AO describes pain in his sacral area, with an occasional shooting pain down his leg and numbness in that extremity after standing a while. The physician hopes that switching to methadone will eliminate the need to add an adjuvant agent to the regimen, keeping things simpler for the patient.

Step 2—Determine Total Daily Dose of Opioid

Calculate the total daily dose of the patient's current opioid including long-acting tablets or capsules, and an average of their rescue opioid, particularly that used for spontaneous and nonvolitional incident pain. AO is taking Kadian 80 mg po q12h (160 mg TDD oral morphine) plus MSIR 20 mg for rescue (using about two doses a day for a total of 40 mg). His TDD of oral morphine is 200 mg.

Step 3—Convert to Daily Oral Morphine Equivalent Dose, then Convert to Methadone

If the patient is already taking oral morphine, your work is already almost done. If not, you need to do the mathematical calculations we discussed earlier in this text to determine the daily oral morphine equivalent dose. Be sure to consider both long-acting and short-acting opioids the patient is receiving (average the use of rescue opioid the patient takes). The patient may be taking more than one opioid—convert all opioids to the total daily oral morphine equivalent dose. Importantly, as we discussed with fentanyl you *do not* reduce the total daily oral morphine equivalent dose for lack of complete cross-tolerance. This is taken into consideration when we convert the daily oral morphine to methadone. In the case of AO, he is already taking oral morphine so we don't need to do any calculation.

As we discussed earlier, while there are many proposed ratios from morphine to methadone, there is one common theme—the higher the daily oral morphine equivalent dose, the more potent methadone is. This is *not* a linear relationship; the more morphine equivalent the patient was on, the lower the percentage of methadone needed to give an equianalgesic effect.

So, what is the magic number? First, it's a moving target—it depends on the daily oral morphine dose (or equivalent). The ratio tends to range from 4:1 to 40:1 (oral morphine:oral methadone). Let's look at some of the commonly used ratio conversion charts.

Ripamonti, 1998[24]

Morphine dose (mg/day)	30–90	90–300	Greater than 300		
Morphine: methadone EDR	4:1	6:1	8:1		

Mercadente, 2001[25]

Morphine dose (mg/day)	30–90	90–300	> 300		
Morphine: methadone EDR	4:1	8:1	12:1		

Ayonrinde, 2000[26]

Morphine dose (mg/day)	Less than 100	101–300	301–600	601–800	801–1000	1001 or more
Morphine: methadone EDR	3:1	5:1	10:1	12:1	15:1	20:1

EDR, equianalgesic dose ratio.

How do you use these charts? Let's look at applying each of these methods to the case of AO.

- Using the Ripamonti method, when the daily oral morphine dose is between 90 and 300 mg, you apply a 6:1 ratio (morphine:methadone). Therefore, applying a 6:1 (morphine:methadone) ratio to 200 mg a day of oral morphine would be approximately 200/6, or <u>33.3 mg oral methadone per day</u>.

- Using the Mercadente method, in the same dosage range, you apply an 8:1 ratio (200/8), giving you <u>25 mg oral methadone per day</u>.

- With the Ayonrinde method, it's a 5:1 ratio (200/5), or <u>40 mg per day of oral methadone</u>.

- The Fast Facts published by End-of-Life Physician Education Resource Center (EPERC) uses the Ayonrinde method, however after calculating the total daily dose of oral methadone they recommend reducing this dose by 50–75% (making this a fourth method!).[27] In this case, we would take our 40 mg oral methadone per day and reduce it by 50–75% to <u>10 or 20 mg oral methadone per day</u>.

- What does the manufacturer of Dolophine Hydrochloride (methadone hydrochloride) recommend as a conversion, as recently updated in their prescribing information and approved by the FDA (yes, this would be the fifth method!)?[29] Their recommended oral morphine to oral methadone conversion for chronic administration is as follows:

Total daily baseline ORAL morphine dose	Estimated daily ORAL methadone requirement as percent of total daily morphine dose
Less than 100 mg	20% to 30%
100 to 300 mg	10% to 20%
300 to 600 mg	8% to 12%
600 mg to 1000 mg	5% to 10%
Greater than 1000 mg	Less than 5%

Using the case of AO, receiving 200 mg of oral morphine per day, the estimated daily oral methadone requirement would be 10–20% of the total daily morphine dose, or <u>20 to 40 mg per day</u>. So, looking at these very popular methods, this gives us a range from 10 to 40 mg of oral methadone per day—nothing like a four fold difference to make you scratch your head! Just to make you crazy, let me lay one more "simplified methadone conversion on you!" Dr. William Plonk combined the above and other methods to derive a linear regression equation for dosing conversion (yes, by golly, this makes six, and I promise I'm going easy on you!).[28] His final equation is as follows:

$$\text{estimated oral methadone per day (mg)} = \frac{[\text{oral morphine equivalents per day (mg)}]}{15} + 15$$

Using AO, above, 200 mg oral morphine per day calculates to [(200/15) + 15] = <u>28.33 mg per day oral methadone</u>. This is in the ballpark of the answers we calculated using the other methods.

OK, OK, I know what you're thinking. Actually I know what you're saying—"I can't believe I bought this book. You would think the answer to methadone conversion calculations would be in the book—but no, she gives us 18 possible ways to do it. I might as well pick up a dart and throw it!" I share your pain. But it's not just me—I promise! Weschules and Bain conducted an exhaustive—exhaustive AND exhausting (I had to take a nap after reading it)—review of opioid conversion ratios used with methadone for treatment of pain.[29] They reviewed 22 clinical studies (none of which was deemed to be of high quality) and 19 case reports or series, which included 730 patients. Ratios used to convert patients from morphine to methadone ranged from 4:1 to 37.5:1. And after this mind-boggling review, what was their bottom line? And I quote "There was no evidence to support the superiority of one method of rotation to methadone over another. Patients may be successfully rotated to methadone despite discrepancies between rotation ratios initially used and those associated with stabilization. Further research is needed to identify patient-level factors that may explain the wide variance in successful methadone rotations."[29] I was particularly impressed with a passage in their discussion, as follows:

"One important distinction that needs to be made is between methadone rotations as a *care process* as opposed to a *dose calculation*. It may be less important to determine an exact opioid ratio when performing a methadone conversion than it is to assure that the patient is an appropriate candidate for methadone conversion, the switch is carried out over a time period consistent with the therapeutic goals, and that the patient is monitored closely by medical staff throughout the process."[29] Kinda brings a tear to your eye, doesn't it? This is *exactly* what we've been saying throughout this book—do the math based on the very best the literature has to offer, tempered with common sense clinical judgment, and monitor your patient like nobody's business!

However, to keep you from looking for your receipt for this book, I will share with you the method I use every day in my practice to convert patients to methadone. I learned of this method from Dr. Loren I. Friedman, therefore I refer to it as the "Friedman Method" (yes, this makes seven methods, but this is "lucky seven!").[30] This method is actually a modification of the widely-adopted "Morley-Makin United Kingdom model" (yes, an 8th method!)[31] which recommends the following strategy:

- Previous opioid is discontinued and replaced with a fixed dose of methadone. The methadone dose is 10% of oral morphine daily equivalent (this is a 10:1 morphine:methadone ratio), not to exceed 30 mg. The methadone dose is offered every 3 hours as needed. For example, with AO (receiving 200 mg per day of oral morphine) this model would result in an order of: "methadone 20 mg po every 3 hours as needed for pain." If a patient receiving 800 mg oral morphine per day, the order would be "methadone 30 mg po every 3 hours as needed for pain" because the maximum methadone dose is 30 mg.

- On day 6, the amount of methadone given over the previous 2 days is averaged, then converted to a twice-daily schedule.

- Ten to 15% of the total daily methadone dose should remain available for breakthrough pain, offered every 3 hours as needed.

Friedman and colleagues use an adaptation of this model, with a couple important differences. First, they have scheduled methadone doses, and don't rely solely on "prn dosing." Second, they use a more conservative conversion ratio for older adults, and patients on higher doses of opioid: for patients over 65 years of age, and/or receiving more than 1,000 mg/day of oral morphine they use a 20:1 ratio (morphine:methadone) instead of a 10:1 ratio.

Using this "Modified Morley-Makin Model" by Friedman and colleagues, we would use as 10:1 (oral morphine:oral methadone) conversion for AO because he is less than 65 years old and on less than 1,000 mg of oral morphine per day. This means we would convert his 200 mg oral morphine per day to 20 mg per day of oral methadone. If you want to work it out the long way you could set it up as a ratio, as follows:

$$\frac{\text{"X" mg TDD oral methadone}}{200 \text{ mg TDD oral morphine}} = \frac{1 \text{ mg oral methadone}}{10 \text{ mg oral morphine}}$$

$(10)(X) = (1)(200)$

$10X = 200$

Divide both sides by 10: $\dfrac{10X}{10} = \dfrac{200}{10}$

$X = 20$ mg TDD oral methadone

We would recommend methadone <u>10 mg po every 12 hour</u>. We'll discuss the rescue dose in the next step. In my practice, I generally do not use methadone for breakthrough pain; instead use 10–15% of the total daily morphine dose (or equivalent amount of another opioid). Figure 6-2 depicts this model graphically.

Step 4—Individualize the Dosage Regimen

With methadone one of the most important steps is individualizing the dose based on interacting medications in the patient's medication regimen. As discussed earlier, we

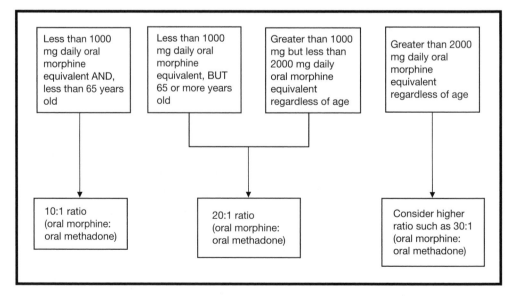

Figure 6-2. Graphic depiction of "Modified Morley-Makin Model" (aka "Friedman Model").[28] *Source*: reference 30.

would reduce our calculated dose by 25% or more if the patient is taking an enzyme-inhibiting drug. Again, the prospective 25% decrease in oral methadone dose secondary to the anticipated drug interaction is only an estimate; the actual level of inhibition varies from drug to drug. If the patient is taking an enzyme-inducing medication, go with your calculated dose, but be liberal with the rescue medication. AO is not taking any medications that inhibit methadone metabolism so we have no need to reduce our calculated TDD of oral methadone.

Many methadone conversion models advocate using methadone not only for continuous pain control, but for rescue as well. Some pain experts prefer *not* to use methadone for breakthrough pain in addition to the standing dose of methadone.[32] If the patient takes rescue doses of methadone as needed, it may be more difficult to predict when you are finally at steady-state. The more serious issue is the disparity in time to pain relief vs. time to steady state—if a patient keeps taking rescue doses of methadone for unrelieved pain, by the time it reaches steady state, it may be a potentially fatal dose.

Although there is not a shred of evidence to support this statement, most end-of-life practitioners will tell you that methadone doesn't seem to work as well as morphine in treating **dyspnea** (shortness of breath or an uncomfortable awareness of breathing). Therefore, if you are treating a patient with end-stage COPD, lung cancer, or any other disease associated with dyspnea, it may be more prudent to use short-acting morphine for breakthrough pain OR dyspnea.

If you chose to use morphine or another short-acting opioid for breakthrough pain, follow the 10–15% of the total daily dose guideline we've discussed throughout the book. You would base the breakthrough dose on the total daily morphine equivalent you calculated back in step one. In the case of AO, his total daily oral morphine dose was 200 mg, therefore you could suggest MSIR 20 mg po q2h prn breakthrough pain. It somehow seems a bit cleaner to use an opioid other than methadone if you have other variables influencing the situation such as converting from transdermal fentanyl in a cachectic patient where you're not sure how much benefit they were getting from the patch, or a patient with multiple co-morbid conditions such as renal and/or hepatic impairment, or a patient on multiple interacting medications. Using a short-acting opioid such as morphine, oxycodone, oxymorphone, or hydromorphone for breakthrough introduces one less variable you have to worry about.

On the other hand, if you are switching to methadone because the patient had a poor outcome with morphine or another short-acting opioid (e.g., allergic reaction) if would certainly be acceptable to use methadone for breakthrough pain. While on the way to steady-state, you could offer 50% of the regularly scheduled methadone dose (dose not to exceed 30 mg of oral methadone) for rescue every 3–4 hours. Because it takes days to get to steady-state with methadone therapy, in this case the rescue methadone is part of the initial titration; once at steady-state, apply the 10–15% of the total daily dose rule. For example, with AO, we could suggest an order such as methadone 10 mg po every 12 hours, plus an additional 5 mg every 3 hours as needed for additional pain. Of course we would ask AO to keep a pain diary and document use of rescue methadone, and we would expect to see less and less use of the rescue opioid as the days went by and he approached steady-state. If on Day 7 of therapy we found that AO was taking his regularly scheduled methadone 10 mg po q12h, plus 2 extra doses of methadone 5 mg per day, we could change his regimen to methadone 15 mg po q12h, plus 5 every 3 hours for breakthrough pain. In this case, the rescue dose is slightly more than 15% of his TDD oral methadone (TDD is 30 mg oral methadone; 10% = 3 mg, 15% = 4.5 mg).

The last burning question in this step is whether we should switch to methadone suddenly (known as a "rapid switch" or "stop-start" method) or sneak in the door one foot at a time. Of the 21 clinical trials Weschules and Bain reviewed in their article, only 9 involved a "rapid conversion."[29] A rapid switch refers to stopping the previous opioid, and with the next scheduled dose, begin the methadone. The Morley-Makin and Friedman models are examples of a rapid switch.

Other practitioners prefer a gradual conversion to methadone (although this method is falling out of favor due to the risk of respiratory depression). The "Edmonton Model" is a classic example of a "slow transition."[33] The rules of play with the Edmonton Model are as follows:

- Calculate the total daily oral morphine equivalent. On Day 1, decrease the morphine dose by 30% and replace with oral or rectal methadone every 8 hours using a 10:1 ratio for morphine:methadone.

- On day 2, if pain control is adequate, further reduce the original dose of morphine by 30%. The methadone dose should remain stable unless the patient experiences moderate to severe pain (in which case you may need to increase the methadone dose). Breakthrough pain should be treated with a short-acting opioid.

- On day 3, discontinue the morphine entirely, and keep the patient on their scheduled methadone every 8 hours. Also, offer 10% of the total daily methadone dose for breakthrough pain.

In my practice, I generally do the rapid switch, unless one of the following situations exist:

- The patient is on a high dose of morphine (e.g., greater than 400–600 mg total daily oral morphine dose)

- It's a complicated conversion calculation (e.g., converting from multiple opioids simultaneously

- The patient is very cachectic, and we're converting from transdermal fentanyl

- We need to build trust with the patient/family

In very complicated cases we will frequently admit the patient to an inpatient hospice unit to facilitate the conversion to methadone, where we can provide closer patient monitoring and better rescue for breakthrough pain crises. With the case of AO, I would stop the Kadian, begin the methadone 12 hours later, and continue the MSIR 20 mg q2h prn breakthrough pain.

Step 5—Patient Monitoring

Your work is not over yet—not by a long shot! The *most* critical step is to monitor your patient very closely! We're even dragging AO's wife into the fray! We will ask AO's wife to observe AO several times a day for changes in his respirations (depth, rhythm, and rate), difficulty in waking him up, snoring, and other signs of opioid overdose. We will either see or speak to AO daily over the next week.

Titrating the Methadone Regimen

As we discussed previously, the patient probably will not achieve steady state before four or more days. You can increase the methadone regimen by an absolute milligram amount, or you can calculate how much opioid they are using for breakthrough pain (methadone or another opioid), and adjust the standing methadone regimen accordingly. Well, we've talked methadone conversion calculations to death—let's get our hands dirty and try a few more cases, shall we?

CASE 6.5
Switching to Oral Methadone: Comparing Different Methods

SM is a 63 year old woman with significant osteoarthritis pain in both knees, both hips and the sacral area of her spine. She has been referred to your pharmacotherapy service for evaluation and possible conversion to methadone, because she describes occasional electric shooting pains down both legs. Her prescriber would like to keep her analgesic regimen as simple as possible. At present, SM is taking MS Contin 45 mg po q8h, plus MSIR 20 mg every 4 hours as needed (she generally takes 3 times a day).

You have done your history and physical, and agree that converting to methadone is a good idea. Next step, calculate your total daily oral morphine dose—we don't need to calculate the daily oral morphine equivalent because the patient is already *on* morphine. She's getting MS Contin 45 mg po q8h (totals 135 mg oral morphine) plus three doses of the MSIR 20 mg (60 mg) for a total daily dose of 195 mg oral morphine.

SM lives with her husband, who is very interested in her care; therefore you are comfortable doing a rapid switch. Just for kicks, let's use some of the methods we described above to calculate an equivalent dose of methadone.

- Ripamonti—90–300 mg oral morphine is a 6:1 conversion; 195/6 = 32.5 mg oral methadone per day
- Mercadente—90–300 mg oral morphine is an 8:1 conversion; 195/8 = 24.4 mg oral methadone per day
- Ayonrinde—101–300 mg oral morphine is a 5:1 conversion; 195/5 = 39 mg oral methadone per day
- Fast Facts and Concepts—Ayonrinde method and reduce by 50–75%; 39 mg × 0.25 (75% reduction) or 0.50 (50% reduction) = 9.8–19.5 mg oral methadone per day
- Friedman—Less than 1000 mg per day oral morphine and patient less than 65 years old is a 10:1 conversion; 195/10 = 19.5 mg oral methadone per day

So our range is between 9.8 and 39 mg per day, and the Friedman method is right in the middle. Let's go with methadone 10 mg po q12h. We're comfortable doing this as a rapid switch, so we advise the patient to begin the methadone 8–12 hours after her last MS Contin dose, starting at a time that sets her up for a convenient every 12-hour dosing schedule.

We would like to continue the morphine for breakthrough pain; ten percent of her total daily dose of oral morphine would be 19.5 mg, 15% would be 29.25 mg. The patient stated that the 20 mg dose of MSIR was barely effective; therefore we will go with MSIR 30 mg po q2h prn breakthrough pain.

It is important to educate SM and her husband that achieving good pain control with methadone is like climbing a set of stairs—it takes 4 or more days to "get to the top"—achieving steady state. She should be encouraged to use her rescue opioid as needed, and *document* use of the MSIR. Mr. M needs to be directed to systematically, explicitly assess (and document would be nice) SM's level of arousal. As described in the FDA Public Health Advisory, twice a day the husband should stop and purposefully take notice of any trouble or difficulty breathing by SM (slowed breathing, periods of apnea, possibly faster breathing, or shallow breathing), excessive tiredness or sleepiness, or snoring (unless SM routinely sucks the curtains off the wall while asleep!). He should question SM about changes in mentation (e.g., confusion), observe for gait imbalance, or signs of confusion. If Mr. M suspects anything is amiss, he should contact you immediately.

CASE 6.6

· ·

Switching to Oral Methadone: What a Difference a Day Makes!

Let's look at the case of QG, a 67 year old man with low back pain. He has been taking half of a Percocet tablet (5 mg oxycodone/325 mg acetaminophen) about 4 times a day with good success, but he complains about having to carry the Percocet tablets around with him, and it's am inconvenience having to cut them in half. He asks about a longer-lasting opioid. You think of OxyContin, but the lowest dosing regimen would be 10 mg po q12h, or 20 mg oxycodone per day. He is only using 10 mg oxycodone per day. Your assessment of his pain does not indicate an adjuvant medication would be of particular help. Then you think of methadone—this can be dosed twice daily as well. How do we come up with an equivalent dose of methadone to maintain pain control?

Next we have to determine the total daily oral morphine equivalents QG is receiving. He is taking 10 mg oxycodone per day. Using our 20 mg oral oxycodone ~ 30 mg oral morphine, we see this is approximately 15 mg of oral morphine per day. Remember—we do *not* reduce this amount for lack of cross-tolerance; this is already taken into account when we convert to methadone.

Let's use the Friedman model because I want to emphasize a particular point with this case. Even though the patient is getting a low dose of morphine equivalents, the model directs us to a 20:1 ratio because he is over 65 years old. Using this ratio, 15 mg oral morphine per day is approximately equivalent to 0.75 mg oral methadone per day (15 mg/20). That's equivalent to licking the label on the bottle once a day! Seriously, the Friedman model tends to be overly conservative with patients who are over 65 years of age, and on a low oral morphine equivalent dose per day. As a matter of fact, it calculates a dose lower than what we would start for this patient if he were opioid-naïve!

We have all seen patients over 65 years old who look and act ten or more years younger, just as we have seen patients 60 years old who could pass for 80 physiologically. We know that when a patient goes to bed 64 years old and wakes up 65 years old the next day he did not suffer a huge physiologic decline. We have to use common sense about this. I frequently ask nurses about patients whose age is *close* to 65 years old "Is he a *young* 67 or an *old* 67?"

Also, it wouldn't make sense to recommend a methadone dose *lower* than what you would use in an opioid-naïve patient. So, for QG, he's only 67, you learn that he's in great shape other than the low back pain (he still works full time and exercises daily). Minimally I would recommend methadone 2.5 mg po once daily (perhaps in the a.m.), but it's very likely he'll do just fine on methadone 2.5 mg po q12h. You can still keep the Percocet tablets (1/2 tablet every 4 hours as needed) for breakthrough pain (although QG wasn't too happy with the Percocet tablets to begin with; hopefully he won't need a rescue opioid once he's at steady-state on methadone). And of course you would closely monitor your patient for therapeutic effectiveness and potential toxicity.

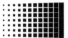

CASE 6.7
• •
Switching to Oral Methadone from Multiple Opioids

JK is a 54 year old man referred to hospice care with a diagnosis of end-stage lung cancer. On admission to hospice he is taking the following analgesics:

- Transdermal fentanyl 75 mcg/h every 3 days
- OxyContin 20 mg po q12h
- Morphine 10 mg every 2 hours as needed (taking about 5 doses per day)

Despite this regimen, he rates his worst pain as an 8, his best as a 4 and his daily average as 5. Plus, it makes little sense clinically to have a patient take two long-acting opioid formulations (transdermal fentanyl and OxyContin). After a careful symptom analysis you decide that switching him to methadone is a good option. He is not receiving any medications known to interact with methadone. How would you convert him to methadone?

Next we have to calculate the total daily morphine equivalent dose. Transdermal fentanyl 75 mcg/h is approximately equivalent to 150 mg oral morphine (JK is not cachectic). OxyContin 20 mg po q12h equals 40 mg oxycodone per day which is approximately equivalent 60 mg oral morphine per day. Plus he's taking 5 doses of morphine solution 10 mg per dose which totals 50 mg. Altogether he is receiving 260 mg oral morphine equivalent per day.

Using the Friedman method, the patient is under 65 years of age, and he is receiving less than 1000 mg oral morphine equivalent per day, so we can use the 10:1 ratio, which is 26 mg methadone per day (260/10). Because he is still in pain, we can increase to 30 mg per day and order methadone 10 mg po q8h. Because the patient has lung cancer and he experiences occasional shortness of breath, we will keep the morphine for breakthrough pain, but we will increase the dose to 30 mg, offered every 2 hours. Encourage use of a pain diary, monitor the patient and adjust the methadone therapy as appropriate.

PITFALL •••
Adjusting Oral Methadone Regimens

Because methadone has a long terminal half-life, it takes 4 or more days to achieve steady state (range 4–14 days). Unless the patient is experiencing magnificent pain, do *not* increase the scheduled doses of methadone *before* 5–7 days; instead use rescue opioids to treat additional pain. If you increase the scheduled methadone dose one or more times *before* the patient achieves steady-state (e.g., a stable blood concentration of methadone), by the time the *last* dosage increase achieves steady-state, it may be a toxic dose for the patient!

•••

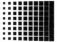 # CASE 6.8
•••
Titrating Oral Methadone at Steady-State

AZ is a 48 year old man with end-stage AIDS, referred to hospice. He was started on morphine around the clock, but it caused extreme itching and he was switched to an equivalent dose of methadone, 5 mg po q12h. His physician also ordered the 5 mg methadone dose for breakthrough pain every three hours as needed. Let's take a look at AZ's pain diary:

Day	Scheduled Methadone Dose	# of Rescue Doses Methadone Taken for Spontaneous Pain	Average Pain Rating
1	Methadone 5 mg po q12h	4 doses	7
2	Methadone 5 mg po q12h	4 doses	5
3	Methadone 5 mg po q12h	3 doses	4
4	Methadone 5 mg po q12h	2 doses	3
5	Methadone 5 mg po q12h	2 doses	2–3
6	Methadone 5 mg po q12h	2 doses	2–3

You see AZ in your clinic on Day 7. He is very content with his level of pain control. You have assessed his complaint of pain and feel that switching to methadone was still a good choice. Do you leave his regimen as is, or make a change?

You could make a good argument either way. Personally, I would increase his standing dose of methadone to 10 mg po q12h and keep the 5 mg dose for breakthrough pain. Even though the two extra doses he's been using is not an unspeakable burden, I think it's worth a shot to maximize the standing dose, and hopefully alleviate the need for breakthrough doses at this time. If however, you feel the patient is emotionally attached to regular use of the rescue opioid doses, you might be better off leaving well enough alone. Also, remember to review the other medications concomitantly prescribed and the adherence to taking them—antiretroviral therapy and antimicrobials commonly used in the management of opportunistic infections can significantly interact with methadone. The sudden withdrawal of an enzyme inducer such as rifabutin can result in potentially toxic levels of methadone.

CASE 6.9

Switching to Oral Methadone: Taking the Slow Road

TH is a 28 year old woman admitted to hospice with cervical cancer. She comes to you on an intravenous basal hydromorphone infusion at 10 mg/hour with a 5 mg bolus every 15 minutes as needed (taking about 6 doses per day). She is a very angry young woman; she has twin daughters who are turning 3 years old soon and she has several things she wants to accomplish before she dies. She wants to finish potty training the girls, and transition them to a regular bed. She finds the hydromorphone infusion cumbersome as it limits her ability to accomplish her remaining goals. After assessing her pain complaint you mention that you'd like to switch to oral methadone she snaps at you "My doctor tried that methadone stuff before. I was so loopy I was seeing two sets of twins. No way!" On closer questioning you find that TH's physician started her on methadone 10 mg q6h as her first opioid regimen, causing her to have an altered mental status, and extreme tiredness and weakness. You explain that this was probably too high of a dose at the time, which caused adverse effects. You explain that you you'd like to revisit methadone as a therapeutic option, and you will carefully calculate the appropriate dose, with a slow and careful conversion process!

TH reluctantly agrees, but she wants to do it cautiously and carefully over a period of time, not as a rapid switch. She has a love/hate relationship with her hydromorphone infusion—it's a pain in the neck, but it does give her good pain control. You agree to do this slowly over a several-week period.

Next, let's determine the total daily oral morphine equivalent based on her current analgesic regimen. She's getting hydromorphone 10 mg/hour, which is 240 mg parenteral hydromorphone per day) plus 6 doses of 5 mg breakthrough (an additional 30 mg parenteral hydromorphone per day) for a total of 270 mg parenteral hydromorphone per day. Looking at our equianalgesic opioid dosing table, we see that 1.5 mg parenteral hydromorphone (HM) is equivalent to 30 mg oral morphine. Let's set up our ratio and see where we stand:

$$\frac{\text{"X" mg TDD oral morphine}}{\text{270 mg TDD parenteral HM}} = \frac{\text{30 mg equianalgesic factor of oral morphine}}{\text{1.5 mg equianalgesic factor of parenteral HM}}$$

Cross multiply:

$(1.5) \times (X) = (270) \times (30)$

$1.5X = 8,100$

$X = 5,400$

Wow—that's a lot of oral morphine—5,400 mg per day! You saw in the Friedman model for patients on more than 2,000 mg oral morphine a day to consider using a higher ratio such as 30:1. Using this ratio, the dose comes out to 180 mg oral methadone per day. Even though the Friedman model generally uses a "rapid switch," in this case it makes more sense to make this transition slowly. Knowing that this may be my eventual dose, I would like to do this inpatient, or very slowly if she insists on remaining at home (which of course she does). Also, I would make sure I had a baseline ECG showing a normal QTc interval, and that she is not receiving other medications that prolong the QTc interval, or inhibit the metabolism of methadone.

OK, here's the plan. On Day 1 of Week 1, we reduce the hydromorphone infusion to 7 mg/hour, and keep the bolus at 5 mg. Simultaneously we start methadone 20 mg po q8h. So how did we come up with those numbers? We have empirically picked a 3 mg/hour reduction in the hydromorphone infusion (from 10 mg/hour to 7 mg/hour); this is about a one-third reduction in the patient's total daily IV hydromorphone dose. Therefore it would be reasonable to replace this with about 1/3 of the calculated total oral methadone dose (180 mg oral methadone per day), or 60 mg oral methadone. We will encourage TH to use the breakthrough dose liberally as needed. On Day 1 of Week 2, if TH continues to have good pain control (now we're at steady-state), we will reduce the hydromorphone infusion to 3 mg/hour (another 1/3 reduction), reduce the breakthrough dose of hydromorphone to 3 mg, and increase the methadone to 40 mg po every 8 hours (another 1/3 increase from 60 mg oral methadone a day to 120 mg oral methadone a day). Assuming all goes well, on Day 1 of Week 3, we will discontinue the hydromorphone infusion but keep the bolus option, and increase the methadone to 60 mg po q8h (the total daily dose of methadone initially calculated). In this case we decided to use methadone for breakthrough pain as well due to the sheer amount of opioid she was taking. We recommended methadone 20 mg po q3h prn breakthrough pain and encourage TH to use the oral methadone breakthrough dose instead of the IV hydromorphone. In this case we have chosen to use methadone for breakthrough pain, because we would need a very large dose of morphine or oxycodone if we chose to use one of those opioids for breakthrough pain. If, after a week TH is still comfortable and not using the IV hydromorphone at all, we can discontinue it entirely.

Yes, this was a fairly long process, but TH was very fearful of giving up the hydromorphone pump, and she was leery of methadone. This slow process over several weeks allowed us to successfully transition her while allowing her to stay home with her family. Of course if we had admitted her to out inpatient hospice unit, we could have done the transition more quickly. Of note, TH accomplished all her goals prior to her death.

Titrating/Converting OFF Methadone

Cue the orchestra—"To Dream the Impossible Dream." OK, it's not that bad, but I am reminded of a line from a Stephen King book, "You can't get there from here!" There is only a very small amount of literature (mostly case reports) that evaluate the methadone to morphine conversion. Between this scanty literature, and personal correspondence with other pain practitioners, it seems a 3:1 conversion (oral morphine : oral methadone, going TO oral morphine) is probably a safe bet, although it could very well be a higher ratio (e.g., 5 or 6:1).[29, 34]

Walker and colleagues evaluated the conversion ratio from methadone (oral and IV) to different opioids.[35] Data from 29 patients was evaluated; the mean dose ratio for oral methadone to oral morphine equivalent daily dose (MEDD) was 1:4.7, and for IV methadone to MEDD was 1:13.5 (a surprising finding given methadone's high oral bioavailability). The authors acknowledged a number of limitations to this study, such as its retrospective nature, low number of subjects, homogeneity in the study population, lack of control for a host of potentially confounding factors, and limited data available related to pain scores. Their final conclusion was that pending additional study, it would be judicious to rotate patients off methadone using a more conservative ratio than what they found in this study, and rely on rescue opioid to maintain pain control.

Obviously frequent monitoring for opioid withdrawal symptoms, pain ratings and oversedation is critically important. Also, as the methadone serum concentration falls, additional morphine may be required. In some cases it may not be possible to completely titrate a patient off methadone and switch them to another opioid completely. However, in such patients a dosage reduction of methadone and titration of the newly substituted opioid may resolve methadone-related adverse events (if this was the reason for the switch) and still provide adequate pain relief.

 CASE 6.10
. . . .
Switching Off Oral Methadone

GW is a 62 year old woman with history of osteoarthritis in both knees and hips. Her pain was not adequately controlled with non-opioids, and her prescriber started her on methadone 2.5 mg po twice daily. Over several weeks GW was titrated up to 7.5 mg methadone po twice daily. She does not have any opioids available for breakthrough pain. Her pain is improved, but GW continues to complain of a "hung-over" feeling that she has experienced the entire time she's been taking methadone. Today in clinic she tells you that she wants to stop taking the methadone. You do not want her to stop opioid therapy cold turkey, and she reluctantly agrees to switch to oral morphine. What dose, and how do we go about this?

GW's total daily dose of oral methadone is 15 mg. If we use the conversion ratio described by Walker et al., above, it would be 15 × 4.7, or 70.5 mg oral morphine per day. However, based on the researcher's own advice, it would probably be more prudent to use a lower conversion, such as 3:1, which would be 45 mg of oral morphine per day. A reasonable plan would be to advice GW to stop the methadone once she got her prescription filled for morphine, and 12 hours after her last methadone dose, begin morphine sulfate 7.5 mg every 4 hours. Also, you can suggest she take morphine 5 mg by mouth every 2 hours as needed for additional pain. I would anticipate that she will probably not need the rescue opioid in the first few days after stopping the methadone (because it takes days for the methadone concentration to fall), but she may need these extra morphine doses to achieve pain control. In about a week you can make a better assessment of how much morphine GW actually needs per day to keep her comfortable and you may choose to switch to a long-acting oral morphine product at that time.

Parenteral Methadone

Required reading for any practitioner even *thinking* about working with parenteral methadone is the consensus guideline document on parenteral methadone by Shaiova and colleagues.[36] Parenteral methadone may be given by IV or SQ patient-controlled analgesia, continuous and/or intermittent bolus infusion. Subcutaneous administration is a bit more challenging because it may cause local erythema and induration in some patients. Strategies to limit this include rotating the infusion site every 1–2 days, limiting the volume (less than 2–3 mL/hour), adding dexamethasone 1–2 mg/day to the infusate, or if irritation occurs, injecting hyaluronidase into the infusion site.[36]

Converting from Oral to Parenteral Methadone

The consensus guidelines recommend if the patient is not already on oral methadone, convert the patient's current opioid regimen to oral methadone using one of the methods described in this chapter. The total daily dose (TDD) of parenteral methadone is then calculated as 50% of the total daily oral methadone dose (actual or as calculated from a different opioid regimen). The TDD parenteral methadone can then be divided by 24 to determine an hourly infusion rate, or divided into intermittent doses to be administered every 6–8 hours.

Patient-controlled analgesia is recommended as the preferred method for the administration of parenteral methadone in the consensus guidelines.[36] Some specific recommendations include the following:

- Calculate a conservative initial basal rate based on current opioid use. Do not increase the basal rate for the first 12 hours after starting IV PCA therapy because both analgesic and sedative properties increase at the 12-hour mark (with infusion initiation or dose increase).

- A patient demand bolus dose should be available, equivalent to the hourly infusion rate during the titration phase, offered every 15 to 30 minutes.

- Clinician-activated boluses should be available (a dose given by the health care provider), usually at twice the hourly infusion rate, and may be given hourly.

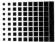 **CASE 6.11**
....
Switching from Oral to IV Methadone

BL is a 42 year old man with end-stage HIV disease. He has been admitted to the hospital with esophagitis leaving him unable to swallow his MS Contin tablets. Also, he has significant neuropathic pain which is only partially controlled with his current oral morphine regimen. The prescriber has asked for your assistance in transitioning BL to an IV PCA infusion of methadone. Let's take a look at our 5 step process as we make this switch.

First step, assess of the patient's pain. You review the physicians admission note, and talk briefly with BL who confirms that he has considerable pain in his throat, leaving him unable to swallow anything, and he has complaints of wide-spread pain that indeed have a neuropathic component. He is rating his pain as an 8 or 9 (on a 0–10 scale). Our second step is to determine BL's TDD of opioid use. At present he is taking MS Contin 120 mg po q12h plus MSIR 30 mg every 4 hours as needed (using about 4 doses per day for spontaneous pain). This gives us a grand total of 240 mg plus 120 mg, or 360 mg TDD oral morphine. Step 3 is to convert this TDD oral morphine to TDD oral methadone. The patient is less than 65 years of age, and on less than 1,000 mg of oral morphine a day, so using our Friedman model of 10:1 (morphine:methadone) we calculate a TDD oral methadone of 36 mg (360/10). The last part of this step is to convert the TDD oral methadone to a TDD parenteral methadone. Using the 2:1 guideline described above, 36 mg TDD oral methadone would be 18 mg TDD parenteral methadone (36/2).

Step 4 is to individualize the dose for this patient. He is not taking any medications that are known or suspected to interact with methadone, and this is very important given his past medical history (HIV medications and anti-infectives frequently interact with methadone). The other aspect of individualization is to understand that BL is in significant pain right now, therefore it would be appropriate to increase his dose a bit. Eighteen milligrams of parenteral methadone calculates to 0.75 mg/hour of IV methadone. Given his current pain complaint, it would be reasonable to increase the PCA continuous infusion to 1 mg/hour. We will also set the PCA demand dose at 1 mg every 15 minutes, and the clinician-activated bolus as 2 mg, available hourly. BL will likely require a 2 mg bolus as soon as we switch him to the PCA methadone infusion. We should stay with the continuous infusion at 1 mg/hour for at least 12 hours; at that time we may adjust the dose up as indicated clinically. Step 5—the most important step of all—is to monitor BL closely for both pain relief and methadone overdose. The clinician should be prepared to administer the clinician-activated bolus hourly as needed, and BL should be monitored for oversedation, respiratory difficulties, confusion, or other methadone-related toxicities; should such occur the PCA dose may need to be reduced.

Converting from Parenteral to Oral Methadone

The ratio for converting methadone from the oral to parenteral route has been cited as 2:1 by the guidelines described above as well as others.[36-39] Conversely, the recommended ratio for converting from parenteral to oral methadone is 1:2.[39] However, this is inconsistent with our knowledge of the oral bioavailability of methadone, which is 70–80% on average (range of 36–100%).[2] A 1:2 (parenteral:oral methadone) conversion implies an oral methadone bioavailability of 50%; if in fact this is a low estimate and the oral bioavailability is *higher*, we may be causing neurocognitive adverse effects such as sedation and confusion when switching from parenteral to oral methadone. González-Barboteo and colleagues evaluated conversions from parenteral to oral methadone in eight cancer patients with good pain control (patients were being switched to oral methadone for each of administration).[40] Their results showed the most accurate conversion ratio to maintain pain control and minimize adverse effects was a oral:parenteral methadone ratio of 1:0.7. Practically, one would multiply the TDD parenteral methadone by 1.3 to determine the TDD of oral methadone. Mathematically this is consistent with the average bioavailability of methadone 70–80%). The researchers acknowledged the limitation of the small number of patients they reported on, but darn it, their results just *make sense*! González-Barboteo and colleagues use a "stop and go" approach in their parenteral to oral conversion: the first dose of oral methadone is given at the discontinuation of the continuous IV or SQ infusion. Let's look at a case using the conversion ratio suggested by this research.

 CASE 6.11 CONTINUES
• •
Switching from IV to Oral Methadone

One week after admission, BL's pain is very well controlled on a IV PCA methadone infusion at 3 mg/hour with a 3 mg bolus, which he has only used twice in the past 12 hours. He is able to swallow oral solutions and soft foods, and would very much like to be discharged home on oral methadone solution. Let's work out the math for this switch-a-roo.

BL is getting 3 mg/hour of IV methadone; this makes his TDD of parenteral methadone 72 mg. Using the guideline proposed by González-Barboteo and colleagues, we multiply the TDD parenteral methadone by 1.3, which gives us 93.6 mg TDD oral methadone. When we stop BL's PCA infusion we can immediately begin methadone 30 mg po q8h, administering the first dose when we discontinue the infusion. We can also offer methadone 15 mg po q4h as needed for additional pain, and of course we will monitor our patient carefully during this transition.

The parenteral methadone consensus guidelines offer additional guidance in converting from other IV opioid to IV methadone with patient-controlled analgesia, which are shown in Table 6-3.

Table 6-3

Suggested Safe and Effective Starting Doses when Rotating Patients from Other IV Opioids to IV Methadone with Patient-Controlled Analgesia

		Methadone		
	Basal[a]	Basal[a]	Demand[b]	CAB[c]
Morphine	10 mg	1 mg	1 mg	5 mg
Hydromorphine	1.5 mg	0.3 mg	0.3 mg	5 mg
Fentanyl	250 mcg	1.25 mg	1.25 mg	5 mg

Source: Reprinted with permission from reference 36.

[a]Continuous hourly infusion. Decrease the initial dose of methadone by 25–50% for high previous opiate doses (e.g., 50 mg/h of morphine) and increase the dose by 25–50% for low doses (e.g., 5 mg/h of morphine).

[b]Dose available every 15 min by the patient pressing the demand button on the infusion pump.

[c]Clinician-activated bolus: dose administered by nurse upon request if pain persists despite the self-administration of demand doses.

The consensus guidelines are clear in pointing out that the risk of methadone-induced QT prolongation is significantly greater with parenteral methadone than with oral methadone. This increased risk in QT prolongation association with parenteral methadone is thought to be due to the preservative chlorobutanol in the IV preparation, therefore preservative-free methadone may be more appropriate for patients at high risk (although this formulation is considerably more expensive and difficult to obtain). They recommend close monitoring in patients with risk factors such as unexplained syncope (in the patient or a family member), seizures or congenital deafness, history of abnormal serum potassium or magnesium levels, renal impairment, advanced age, female gender, cardiovascular disease, bradycardia, heart failure, hypotension, myocardial ischemia, hypothermia and pituitary insufficiency.[36] These are in addition to the recommendation for close monitoring when there is concurrent administration with a medication known to inhibit methadone metabolism. The consensus guidelines recommend a screening ECG prior to starting parenteral methadone, after 24 hours of therapy, after 4 days of therapy, when methadone dose is significantly increased, and with any change in patient's condition that increases risk for QT prolongation. They also recommend monitoring electrolytes in patients receiving parenteral methadone.

In this amazing chapter we have talked about everything worth discussing regarding the incredibly versatile yet demanding opioid, methadone. As with the chapters that preceded this one, the important things with conversion calculations involving methadone are to understand the pharmacokinetics of the drug, use evidence-based medicine as best we can, and above all be guided by common sense and close monitoring of our patients.

PRACTICE PROBLEMS

P6.1: Starting Oral Methadone in an Opioid-Naïve Patient

KG is a 72 year old woman with a 1-year history of postherpetic neuralgia. She has tried several adjuvant analgesics with minimal success, therefore you decide to start methadone. She is not taking any other opioids. Her medications at this time include:

- Lisinopril 20 mg po once daily
- Hydrochlorothiazide 25 mg po once daily
- Zoloft 50 mg po once daily
- Multivitamin with iron one tablet po daily

What is your recommendation for starting methadone in this patient?

P6.2: Starting and Titrating Oral Methadone in an Opioid-Naïve Patient

BM is 50 year old man with a history of low back pain. The patient has had recent imaging studies and no surgical intervention is indicated at this time. He describes it as an achy-type feeling, which worsens with bending, stooping, or lifting more than 20 pounds. He rates the constant pain as 6 out of 10, increasing to an 8 or 9 with exacerbating activities. He states that when he stands for more than 15 minutes his left leg goes numb, and he frequently experiences shooting pain down his left leg as well. BM's physician has him on pregabalin 100 mg q8h; he had tried duloxetine 60 mg po qd, but the patient complained of nausea and discontinued therapy. BM's physician would like to begin methadone therapy. BM is receiving no drugs known to interact with methadone. What starting dose of methadone would you recommend? BM's physician does *not* want to give BM an opioid for breakthrough pain due to suspected abuse of Percocet (oxycodone/acetaminophen) years earlier. If BM's pain is not entirely controlled on the methadone dose you recommend, when would you increase the dose, and to what dose? What should you monitor while titrating BM for potential methadone-induced side effects?

P6.3: Switching to Oral Methadone; What to Do with an Interacting Drug?

GH is a 42 year old man who suffered an accident while working at a construction site. There was a cave-in and he was crushed under an I-beam, requiring reconstruction of his left hip. This has left him with residual pain for which he takes MS Contin 60 mg po q12h plus MSIR 20 mg every 4 hours as needed (and he takes about 6 doses per day). This regimen, in addition to the pregabalin (Lyrica) he is already taken, has not successfully controlled his pain. GH is also taking sertraline (Zoloft) 100 mg a day for depression. You decide to switch him to methadone. Perform the calculation using all the methods described. Once you decide on a total daily dose of methadone, recommend a dosing strategy for both the "rapid-switch" method and the "slow conversion" method. That should keep you off the streets for a while!

P6.4: Switching from Transdermal Fentanyl to Oral Methadone

JR is a 64 year old man admitted to hospice with a terminal diagnosis of pancreatic cancer. His analgesic regimen on admission is transdermal fentanyl 200 mcg/h and oxycodone 20 mg q4h prn breakthrough pain (taking about 6 doses per day). Convert to methadone using the Friedman method as a rapid switch. Patient is not receiving any medications known to interact with methadone. JR's pain is fairly well controlled on this regimen but transdermal fentanyl is not on your formulary. He is slim, but not cachectic.

P6.5: Switching off Oral Methadone to Another Oral Opioid

AH is a 34 year old woman with HIV-related neuropathy, receiving pregabalin 100 mg three times daily. Oral hydromorphone was eventually added to her regimen after her pain progressed and the patient did not tolerate antidepressant agents known to reduce neuropathic pain. AH's pain never responded 100% to the hydromorphone so her prescriber transitioned her to methadone, currently at 15 mg three times daily. Unfortunately, AH's prescriber suspects that the methodone is responsible for the edema AH has been experiencing, and in fact worsening as the methadone dose has been increased. The prescriber asks your advise on transitioning AH to morphine. What do you suggest? AH is taking no other medications that are likely to interact with methadone.

P6.6: Switching from Oral to IV Methadone

PV is a 68 year old man with end-stage lung cancer, receiving hospice care at home. He is receiving oral methadone 20 mg every 12 hours, with methadone 5 mg ever 3 hours for breakthrough pain. His pain has been increasing in intensity over the past week, with PV using six doses per day of his breakthrough methadone in addition to the two scheduled doses. The physician suspected bone metastases and naproxen 500 mg po q12h was added, with marginal success. PV is now requesting euthanasia; since you are unable to honor this request, you counter with an offer to move PV to an inpatient facility, switch him to parenteral methadone and titrate to relief. You are unwilling to do this switch in the home environment because PV is very debilitated and he has an unreliable caregiver situation. You further agree that if you are successful at managing PV's pain you will transition him back to oral methadone so he can return to his home. PV agrees with this plan and is admitted to a hospice bed in your local hospital. How do you transition PV to a PCA methadone infusion?

P6.7: Switching from IV to Oral Methadone

One week later, PV, our patient from case 6.6 has been stabilized for several days now on a methadone IV PCA infusion at 2.5 mg/hour with a demand bolus of 2.5 mg, which he uses about once per 8 hour shift. He is very happy with his level of pain control, no longer requesting euthanasia, and would like to return home on oral methadone therapy. A repeat ECG shows you are still on firm ground (his QTc is still below 450 msec); what dose of oral methadone do you recommend for discharge?

REFERENCES

1. Sandoval JA, Furlan AD, Mailis-Gagnon A. Oral methadone for chronic noncancer pain. A systematic literature review of reasons for administration, prescription patterns, effectiveness and side effects. *Clin J Pain*. 2005;21:503–512.

2. Lugo RA, Satterfield KL, Kern SE. Pharmacokinetics of methadone. *J Pain Palliat Care Pharmacother*. 2005;19:13–24.

3. Eap CB, Buclin T, Baumann P. Interindividual variability of the clinical pharmacokinetics of methadone. Implications for the treatment of opioid dependence. *Clin Pharmacokinet*. 2002;41:1153–1193.

4. Dale O, Sheffels P, Kharasch ED. Bioavailability of rectal and oral methadone in healthy subjects. *Br J Clin Pharmacol*. 2004;58(2):156–162.

5. Baselt RC, Casarett LJ. Urinary excretion of methadone in man. *Clin Pharmacol Ther.* 1972;13:64–70.

6. Weschules DJ, Bain KT, Richeimer S. Actual and potential drug interactions associated with methadone. *Pain Med.* 2008;9:315–344.

7. Ferrari A, Coccia CP, Bertolini A, et al. Methadone: metabolism, pharmacokinetics and interactions. *Pharmacol Res.* 2004;50:551–559.

8. Drug Interactions. Indiana University School of Medicine. http://medicine.iupui.edu/flockhart/index.htm, Accessed August 4, 2008.

9. Dolophine® Hydrochloride (Roxane Laboratories) Prescribing Information. http://www.fda.gov/cder/foi/label/2006/006134s028lbl.pdf, Accessed August 5, 2008.

10. Evidence-based recommendations for medical management of chronic non-malignant pain: reference guide for physicians. The College of Physicians and Surgeons of Ontario. November 2000. Accessed August 5, 2008, at: http://www.cpso.on.ca/Publications/pain.htm.

11. Mercadente S, Sapio M, Serretta R, et al. Patient-controlled analgesia with oral methadone in cancer pain: preliminary report. *Ann Oncol.* 1996;7:613–617.

12. Caplehorn JR, Drummer OH, Cyrne A, et al. Fatal methadone toxicity: signs and circumstances, and the role of benzodiazepines. *Austr New Zealand J Public Health.* 2002;26:358–363.

13. Webster LR, Choi Y, Desai H, et al. Sleep-disordered breathing and chronic opioid therapy. Pain Medicine 2008;9:425–432.

14. Toombs JD, Kral LA. Methadone treatment for pain states. *Am Family Physic.* 2005;71:1353–1358.

15. VA/DoD (Veterans Administration/Department of Defense). Clinical Practice Guideline for the Management of Opioid Therapy for Chronic Pain. 2003. Accessed August 8, 2008 at http://www.oqp.med.va.gov/cpg/cot/ot_base.htm.

16. Shir Y, Rosen G, Zeldin A, et al. Methadone is safe for treating hospitalized patients with severe pain. *Can J Anesth.* 2001;48:1109–1113.

17. FDA Public Health Advisory: Methadone use for pain control may result in death and life-threatening changes in breathing and heart beat. Created November 27, 2006, updated July 2007. Accessed August 8, 2008 online at: http://www.fda.gov/CDER/drug/advisory/methadone.htm.

18. Ehret GB, Voide C, Gex-Fabry M, et al. Drug-induced long QT syndrome in injection drug users receiving methadone. *Arch Intern Med.* 2006;166:1280–1287.

19. U.S. Food and Drug Administration. Guidance for Industry: E14 Clinical Evaluation of QT/QTc Interval Prolongation and Proarrhythmic Potential for Non-Antiarrhythmic Drugs. Rockville, MD: Center for Drug Evaluation and Research; 2005.

20. Bednar MM, Harrigan EP, Ruskin JN. Torsades de pointes associated with nonantiarrhythmic drugs and observations on gender and QTc. *Am J Cardiol.* 2002;89:1316–1319.

21. Crouch MA, Limon L, Cassano AT. Clinical relevance and management of drug-related QT interval prolongation. *Pharmacotherapy.* 2003;23:881–908. Also can be accessed online at: http://www.medscape.com/viewarticle/458868_print.

22. Krantz MJ, Martin J, Stimmel B, et al. QTc interval screening in methadone treatment. *Ann Intern Med.* 2009;150:387–395.

23. Bruera E, Sweeney C. Methadone use in cancer patients in pain: a review. *J Palliat Med.* 2002;5:127–138.

24. Ripamonti C, Groff L, Brunelli C, et al. Switching from morphine to oral methadone in treating cancer pain: what is the equianalgesic dose ratio? *J Clin Oncol.* 1998;16:3216–3221.

25. Mercadente S, Casuccia A, Fulfaro F, et al. Switching from morphine to methadone to improve analgesia and tolerability in cancer patients: a prospective study. *J Clin Oncol.* 2001;19:2898–2904.

26. Ayonrinde OT, Bridge DT. The rediscovery of methadone for cancer pain management. *Med J Aust.* 2000;173:536–540.

27. Gazelle G, Fine PG. Fast Facts and Concepts #75: Methadone for the treatment of pain, 2nd Edition. July 2006. End-of-Life Physician Resource Center: http://www.eperc.mcw.edu.

28. Plonk WM. Simplified methadone conversion. *J Palliat Med.* 2005;8:478–479.

29. Weschules DJ, Bain KT. A systematic review of opioid conversion ratios used with methadone for the treatment of pain. *Pain Med.* 2008;9:595–612.

30. Friedman LL, Rodgers PE. Pain management in palliative care. *Clin Fam Prac.* 2004;6:371–393.

31. Morley J, Makin M. The use of methadone in cancer pain poorly responsive to other opiates. *Pain Rev.* 1998;5:51–58.

32. Lipman AG. Methadone: A double-edged sword. *J Pain Palliat Care Pharmacother.* 2005;19:3–4.

33. Bruera E. Pereira J, Watanabe S, et al. Opioid rotation in patients with cancer pain. A retrospective comparison of dose ratios between methadone, hydromorphone, and morphine. *Cancer.* 1996;78:852–857.

34. Peng PWH, Tumber PS, Gourlay D. Review article: perioperative pain management of patients on methadone therapy. *Can J Anesth.* 2005;52:513–523.

35. Walker PW, Palla S, Pei, B, et al. Switching from methadone to a different opioid: what is the equianalgesic dose ratio? *J Palliat Med.* 2008;11:1103–1108.

36. Shaiova L, Berger A, Blinderman C, et al. Consensus guidelines on parenteral methadone use in pain and palliative care. *Palliat Support Care.* 2008;6:165–176.

37. Davis MP, Walsh D. Methadone for relief of cancer pain: a review of pharmacokinetics, pharmacodynamics, drug interactions, and protocols of administration. *Support Care Cancer.* 2001;9:73–83.

38. Gagnon C. The use of methadone in the care of the dying. *Eur J Pallit Care.* 1997;4:152–158.

39. Inturrisi CE. Clinical pharmacology of opioids for pain. *Clin J Pain.* 2002;18:S3–S13.

40. González-Barboteo J, Porta-Sales J, Sanchez D, et al. Conversion from parenteral to oral methadone. *J Pain Palliat Care Pharmacother.* 2008;22:200–205.

SOLUTIONS TO PRACTICE PROBLEMS

P6.1: Starting Oral Methadone in an Opioid-Naïve Patient

KG is opioid naïve, therefore 2.5 mg by mouth one to three times daily is the dosage range we're considering. KG is also taking Zoloft (sertraline), a selective serotonin reuptake inhibitor, which is known to inhibit the metabolism of methadone. Based on this, it would be prudent to start KG on methadone 2.5 mg po qhs, and use an alternate opioid for rescue as needed such as morphine or oxycodone 2.5 mg q4h prn. Once KG achieves steady state (e.g., a week to 10 days) we can safely increase the methadone if necessary. An alternate strategy would be to order methadone 2.5 mg po at bedtime and methadone 2.5 mg po q3h prn pain. This will allow for good pain control through self-titration while not risking an overdose due to the drug interaction with sertraline.

P6.2: Starting and Titrating Oral Methadone in an Opioid-Naïve Patient

Because BM is a relatively young patient with no co-morbid conditions, we can start methadone at 2.5 mg po q8h. We would educate the patient and his wife to look for feelings of faintness, dizziness, confusion, trouble breathing or shallow breathing, loud snoring, extreme tiredness or sleepiness, blurred vision, and difficulty thinking, walking or talking.

BM should also maintain a diary tracking his pain ratings per day, including the best (0-10), the worst, and the average. He should comment on his ability to perform activities, and the presence or absence of symptoms such as numbness, radiating or shooting pain. If his pain is not controlled after a week, you could recommend increasing to 5 mg po q8h. One week later if necessary, increase to 7.5 mg po q8h, 1 week later to 10 mg po q8h. If an additional increase is needed beyond this, consider changing the dosing interval to every 12 hours (e.g., 20 mg po q12h). And during all this, don't forget the bowels!

P6.3: Switching to Oral Methadone; What to Do with an Interacting Drug?

You have assessed GH's pain and feel that switching to methadone is preferable to adding another adjuvant analgesic at this time. The next step is to calculate the total daily morphine dose GH is receiving. Between his MS Contin (120 mg per day) and MSIR (120 mg per day) he is receiving 240 mg oral morphine per day. Step 3 is to convert the TDD oral morphine to a TDD oral methadone. Looking at our different methods, we get the following potential methadone doses:

- Ripamonti: 90–300 mg per day oral morphine is a 6:1 conversion: calculated total daily oral methadone dose is 40 mg

- Mercadente: 90–300 mg per day oral morphine is 8:1 conversion: calculated total daily oral methadone dose is 30 mg

- Ayonrinde: 101–300 mg per day oral morphine is 5:1 conversion: calculated total daily oral methadone dose is 48 mg

- Fast Facts: Ayonrinde reduced by 50–75%: calculated total daily oral methadone dose is 12–24 mg

- Friedman: Patient less than 65 years old and on less than 1000 mg oral morphine per day is a 10:1 conversion: calculated total daily oral methadone dose is 24 mg

So our calculated range is 12-48 mg oral methadone per day. Step 4—Let's remember two things—this patient is receiving sertraline (Zoloft) a known enzyme inhibitor and his pain isn't well controlled either. Let's take the 24 mg oral methadone total daily dose we calculated with the Friedman method and reduce it to 20 mg per day to allow for the influence of the sertraline. Our dose therefore, would be methadone 10 mg po q12h. This isn't a full 25% decrease to allow for enzyme inhibition because the patient is also in pain. To keep things simpler, let's keep the morphine for breakthrough pain; 10–15% of 240 mg total daily oral morphine is 24–36 mg, therefore let's go with MSIR 30 mg po q2h prn breakthrough pain.

The second part of your mission was to recommend a "rapid switch" and a "slow conversion" plan. For the "rapid switch" you would discontinue the MS Contin, and begin oral methadone 10 mg 12 hours later after the last dose (methadone 10 mg po q12h). Increase the MSIR from 20 to 30 mg immediately and advise patient he can take it as frequently as every 2 hours as needed. Step 5 is to monitor your patient like a maniacal stalker!

If you want to slow things down, smell the roses, enjoy the experience, you can do it over 3 days. On Day 1 reduce the MS Contin to 30 mg po q12h (you have to choose between MS Contin 45 mg po q12h and MS Contin 30 mg po q12h because that's the way the tablets come) and start methadone 10 mg po q12h. Also, I would increase the MSIR to 30 mg q2h prn breakthrough pain at this point. On Day 2 reduce the MS Contin to 15 mg po q12h (of course this means you'll have to get the 15 mg tablet) and keep methadone dose at 10 mg po q12h. Continue using MSIR 30 mg po q2h prn pain. On Day 3 discontinue the MS Contin, and either continue the MSIR 30 mg po q2h prn pain or switch to methadone 2.5 mg po q3h prn breakthrough pain. Most practitioner would prefer to do this type of "slow switch" in an acute care facility due to the increased risk for respiratory depression.

P6.4: Switching from Transdermal Fentanyl to Oral Methadone

You have assessed JR's pain and have no reason to suspect neuropathic or bone pain, therefore no adjuvant analgesics are necessary at this time. The first step is to calculate the total daily oral morphine equivalent for JR. He is on transdermal fentanyl 200 mcg/h, which is approximately equivalent to 400 mg oral morphine. He is taking 6 doses per day of oxycodone 20 mg, which is 120 mg oral oxycodone. Using our oxycodone:morphine ratio of 20:30, 120 mg oral oxycodone is equivalent to 180 mg oral morphine. This gives us a grand total of 580 mg oral morphine total daily equivalent for JR.

The patient is less than 65 years old, and receiving less than 1,000 mg oral morphine equivalent per day, therefore the recommended ratio is 10:1, or 58 mg per day of oral methadone. Using a rapid switch transition, after we're sure the methadone has been delivered to JR's home (this is an important logistical point!), we instruct him to remove the transdermal fentanyl (TDF) patch, and begin methadone 20 mg po q8h approximately 12 hours after the TDF was removed. We have increased the oxycodone oral solution to 40 mg, and have instructed the patient to use his rescue opioid every 2 hours as needed for breakthrough pain. But before we sign off on this case, how did we get that dose of oxycodone for breakthrough? The patient was on the equivalent of 600 mg TDD oral morphine, which is about a TDD of 400 mg oral oxycodone. Using our 10–15% rescue analgesia guideline, oxycodone 40 mg oral solution every 2 hours seems reasonable.

P6.5: Switching off Oral Methadone to Another Oral Opioid

You agree with the prescriber's assessment of AH; her total daily dose of methadone is 45 mg (15 mg po q8h). Using the 1:3 (oral methadone:oral morphine) conversion, you calculate an oral morphine TDD of 135 mg. You suggest using the immediate-release morphine for the time being, at 20 mg oral morphine every 4 hours, starting 12 hours after the last methadone dose. You also recommend an additional 10 mg of oral morphine every 2 hours as needed for additional pain. After 5–7 days on this regimen, the prescriber can evaluate AH's response to therapy, increase or decrease the TDD oral morphine, and switch to long-acting oral morphine if appropriate.

P6.6: Switching from Oral to IV Methadone

You agree with the prescriber's plan and meet with PV to assess his pain. Just to be safe, you recommend getting an ECG to make sure PV's QTc interval is not excessively long. Remember, parenteral methadone is even more likely to prolong the QTc than oral methadone. You get the ECG and all is well (430 msec). What a relief!

Your next step is to calculate PV's TDD of oral methadone. He is taking 20 mg every 12 hours scheduled (40 mg a day) plus six doses per day according to his diary of the 5-mg rescue methadone (5×6 doses = 30 mg per day) for a TDD of 70 mg oral methadone. According to the parenteral methadone consensus guidelines, we give 50% of this as parenteral methadone, or 35 mg (70/2). We divide this by 24 to determine our hourly infusion rate, which calculates to 1.46 mg/hour (35/24)—you recommend beginning IV methadone at 1.5 mg/hour, with a 1.5 mg bolus every 15 minutes and a 3 mg clinician-activated bolus. You would wait 12 hours before adjusting the infusion rate so as to avoid dose-stacking and potential toxicity, and of course you recommend a fairly aggressive monitoring plan.

P6.7: Switching from IV to Oral Methadone

Congratulations on doing such a terrific job controlling PV's pain on the IV methadone PCA infusion! Let's get busy switching him to oral methadone! He is receiving 2.5 mg/

hour by continuous infusion, and approximately 3 extra doses of 2.5 mg per day for breakthrough pain. This gives us a TDD of 67.5 mg parenteral methadone. Using our guideline to multiple the TDD IV methadone by 1.3, we get a TDD of oral methadone of 87.75 mg. For ease of administration you recommend methadone 30 mg po every 8 hours. You can also offer methadone 10 mg po every 3 hours for additional pain. Ask PV to continue his pain diary, and pay close attention to his response to therapy during this transition. Good job!

CHAPTER 7

Patient-Controlled Analgesia and Neuraxial Opioid Therapy

OBJECTIVES

After reading this chapter and completing all practice problems, the participant will be able to:

1. Calculate, monitor and adjust patient-controlled analgesia opioid therapy for acute and chronic pain management, with and without a continuous opioid infusion.

2. Convert a patient between parenteral PCA therapy and an oral opioid regimen.

3. Using the limited evidence available, recommend a conservative strategy to convert a patient between epidural or intrathecal opioid therapy and other opioid regimens.

INTRODUCTION

In this chapter we will explore more advanced methods of treating pain—specifically, patient-controlled analgesia (PCA) and neuraxial (epidural, intrathecal) opioid administration. Much of neuraxial opioid administration comes under the purview of a specialist such as an anesthesiologist, but practitioners "in the trenches" often inherit patients receiving these therapies and need an understanding of them.

Patient-Controlled Analgesia (PCA)

Patient-controlled analgesia (PCA) is a precise and convenient method of providing opioid therapy to patients with moderate to severe acute or chronic pain. The convenience aspect is the patient's ability to decide when they need a dose of opioid, without having to rely on the nurse to administer it. A PCA system uses a computerized pump that has a syringe, cartridge, or infusion bag that contains the opioid locked inside the pump. The PCA pump can be configured in different ways (with or without a continuous infusion of opioid), but it generally has the capability for a patient to self-administer a small dose of opioid fairly frequently. When we say a "small dose" this means relative to an "every 4 hours" dose.

There are several features that you need to be familiar with regarding PCA pumps. First, the pump needs to be programmed for the drug concentration in the cartridge, syringe, or infusion bag.

In other words, we tell the pump what volume is available for infusion or bolus dosing, and the concentration of the opioid solution (e.g., mg/mL). We must also program the rate of the continuous opioid infusion, if applicable; the PCA bolus dose (the amount of drug the patient receives when they push the bolus button), the delay interval, known as the lockout period (the period of time during which no additional bolus doses will be administered despite the patient pushing the demand bolus dose button); and the 1- or 4-hour limit (the total amount of opioid the patient can receive in one or four hour(s) by PCA bolus plus basal infusion). We can also retrieve historical information from the PCA pump which includes the number of PCA bolus attempts the patient has made, the number of PCA bolus doses given, the volume given and the volume remaining in the syringe, cartridge, or infusion bag. Wow—that sounds complicated! While it's not rocket science, it can get confusing, and PCA pump therapy is an error-prone, high-risk source of medication errors.

PCA therapy is usually administered intravenously but can be administered subcutaneously, or epidurally, as well. Let's first consider the use of PCA therapy post-operatively using the SQ or IV route of administration.

Patient-Controlled Analgesia Post-Operatively

Most patients who receive PCA therapy post-operatively are opioid-naïve. In opioid-naïve persons, generally practitioners use standardized dosing unless there is a compelling clinical reason to use a different dosing strategy. For example, standard orders are typically for 1 mg of morphine or its equivalent (0.2 mg hydromorphone or 20 mcg fentanyl) every 8 minutes (6 minutes for fentanyl) (see Table 7-1).[1-3] These doses should be

Table 7-1

Starting IV PCA Prescription Ranges for Opioid-Naïve Adults

Drug	Typical Concentration	Loading Dose[1]	Starting PCA Dose[2]	Usual Lockout	Range Lockout	Approx. Time to Onset of Action	Approx. Time to Peak Effect	Approx. Duration of Effect
Morphine	1 mg/mL	2.5 mg	1.0 mg	8 min	5–10 min	2–4 min	15–20 min	~2 hr
Hydromorphone	0.2 mg/mL	0.4 mg	0.2 mg	8 min	5–10 min	2–3 min	10–15 min	~2 hr
Fentanyl	50 mcg/mL	25 mcg	20 mcg	6 min	5–8 min	1–2 min	5 min	1–2 hr

[1]Repeat prn; administered and response monitored by clinician. May be repeated every 10 minutes up to 3–5 times or until pain controlled (e.g., a 50% reduction in pain).

[2]Reduce usual starting PCA dose by 50% for frail or elderly patients.

Source: Adapted from the following references:

- *Principles of Analgesic Use in the Treatment of Acute Pain and Cancer Pain.* 6th ed. American Pain Society: Glenview, IL; 2008.
- McCaffery M, Pasero C. *Pain Clinical Manual.* 2nd ed. Mosby: Baltimore, MD; 1999.
- Strassels SA, McNicol E, Ruleman R. Postoperative pain management: A practice review, part 1. *Am J Health-Syst Pharm.* 2005;62:1904–16.

reduced for frail or elderly patients, or for patients with less than severe pain. When beginning PCA therapy in the immediate post-operative period, the patient will likely be in pain. In this case, the clinician (e.g., recovery room nurse, or anesthesiologist) would administer one or more loading doses (referred to as "clinician loading dose") of the opioid to get the patient comfortable. This may be given every 10 minutes until the pain is reduced by at least 50%, or up to 3-5 times as indicated by hospital policy. Strassels and colleagues recommend that the loading dose can be increased by 50% if the patient has not achieved pain relief within an hour. If pain relief has not been achieved in another hour, consider reducing the dosing interval to 6 minutes.[3]

Let's consider a variety of scenarios regarding level of pain control, and the development of adverse effects with IV or SQ PCA therapy (see Table 7-2).

Table 7-2

Improvement of Pain Control and Reduction of Adverse Effects Associated with IV or SQ PCA Analgesia

Clinical Situation	Proposed Interventions
Patient has insufficient or no pain relief, and no adverse effects	Verify infusion system is patient and functional; verify pump is assembled, loaded and programmed correctly
	Confirm lockout interval is appropriate
	Administer a clinician loading dose
	Increase PCA bolus dose by 25–100%
Patient has insufficient or no pain relief, but experiences adverse effects	Treat adverse effects
	Add or increase non-opioid or adjuvant analgesic (be careful of bleeding risk with NSAIDs on post-operative patients)
	Decrease opioid dose cautiously by 25%
	Rotate to a different opioid
Pain relief, but patient experiencing adverse effects	Treat adverse effects
	Reduce opioid dose by 25–50%, possibly more with excessive sedation and/or respiratory depression
	Rotate to a different opioid
Pain relief with adverse effects immediately after PCA bolus dose administration (such as excessive sedation)	Treat adverse effects
	Give smaller doses more often (e.g., decrease the PCA bolus dose by 25–50% and shorten the lockout interval)
	Rotate to a different opioid
Pain relief except during periods of activity	Remind patient to use PCA bolus prior to activity (2–5 minutes beforehand) and continue to self-administer during activity

Table 7-2 (contd.)

Improvement of Pain Control and Reduction of Adverse Effects Associated with IV or SQ PCA Analgesia

Clinical Situation	Proposed Interventions
Maximum programmed amount of opioid used (in 1- or 4-hour block)	In patient still in pain, administer clinician loading dose
	Verify hourly or 4-hourly limit was calculated correctly, and PCA pump is programmed correctly and functional and IV line is patent
	Determine amount of pain relief obtained; if < 50%, increase programmed 4-hourly limit by 100%. If pain relief > 50% but less than optimal, increase programmed 4-hourly limit by 50%
Patient somnolent and difficult to arouse, or experiencing respiratory depression	In opioid-naïve patient, discontinue opioid. If patient opioid-tolerant, reduce opioid dose by 75% (do not stop opioid: may precipitate opioid withdrawal)
	Consider use of naloxone if necessary (titrate to respiratory rate of 10 breaths/min and recovery of cognition; do not titrate to reversal of analgesia)
	Add non-sedating non-opioid analgesic
	When adverse effects resolve, resume opioid at 50% of previous dose
Disproportionate number of injections and attempts (injection/attempt ratio)	Determine if someone other than patient is pressing the demand button (proxy dosing); this practice is not allowed
	Determine if patient fully understands use of the demand button; re-educate if appropriate
	If patient gets less than one injection for every 2–3 attempts and is not in pain, do nothing
	If patient gets less than one injection for every 2–3 attempts and patient has pain, administer clinical loading dose(s) and increase PCA bolus dose by 25–100%
	If patient gets more than one injection to 3 attempts and has no pain relief administer supplemental clinical loading dose(s) and remind patient to use PCA bolus dose (remind them to self-dose before pain gets away from them, and redose *after* evaluating response to initial dose)

Source: Adapted with permission from reference 2.

Let's do a case or two!

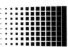

CASE 7.1

Your Mama Told You Not to Get a Motorcycle!

BT is a 32 year old man who was involved in a motor vehicle accident. He was riding his motorcycle and an unexpected pile-up accident caused him to flip off the back of the car in front of him. He flew 50 feet in the air, landed hard on his ankle, and skidded for about

30 more feet. He has broken several bones and peeled off a considerable amount of skin. He was brought to Shock Trauma at your institution, and he is now in the PACU post-operatively from having several rods placed in his ankle. The surgical team has asked that you write the orders for BT's IV PCA with morphine. What order do you write?

You consult your IV PCA dosing chart, and order morphine at 1 mg/mL, with a PCA dose of 1 mg every 8 minutes as needed. You also write for a "clinician bolus" (loading dose) of 2.5 mg every 10 minutes up to 5 doses, until pain is reduced by 50%. The PACU nurse hunts you down about 40 minutes later to say she's given four doses of 2.5 mg and the patient is still complaining of pain that is 10 out of 10 (0 = no pain, 10 = worst imaginable). You and the nurse together verify the infusion system is patent and functional, and the PCA pump is programmed correctly. The patient is moaning in significant pain. What do you do now?

At this point you increase the clinician loading dose to 4 mg, and increase the PCA bolus dose to 2 mg. After 2 additional clinician loading doses (another 8 mg), the patient reports his pain is now a 6 and tolerable. You educate him about using the PCA bolus button as often as he needs it. The nurse in the PACU will continue to follow the patient for another hour or so, at which point he'll be transferred to the floor.

 ## CASE 7.2
. . . .
The Perils of Proxy!

VP is a 58 year old woman who was recently diagnosed with colon cancer. She was admitted for tumor resection, and is receiving hydromorphone by IV PCA pump. Her prescription order is 0.2 mg every 8 minutes, and a clinician loading dose of 0.4 mg every 30 minutes for uncontrolled pain to be administered by the nurse. She is in her hospital room, 8 hours after surgery. When the nurse checks on VP she sees that the patient is asleep, is snoring loudly and has a respiratory rate of 6 breaths/minute, and breathing is irregular and erratic. With vigorous shaking the RN is able to awaken her, but she falls right back asleep. Her oxygen saturation (O_2) is 88%, which increases to 96% with oxygen at 2 L per nasal cannula. Mr. P is visiting his wife; the nurse asks if VP has been hitting her PCA bolus button, and he admits that VP has been asleep so he has continued to hit the button so VP won't awaken in pain. What do you do now?

This is known as PCA by proxy, meaning the PCA demand bolus button has been activated by someone other than the patient such as a family member, a friend, or even a clinician, more times than not at times when the patient is *not* in need! This practice is obviously strongly discouraged! The beauty of *patient*-controlled analgesia is that the *patient* takes a dose, and if pain-free, frequently falls asleep. While sleeping, the patient is unable to hit the demand button, preventing further doses from being administered. Obviously Mr. P needs to be educated about how he has put Mrs. P's very life in jeopardy. Your action at this time is to hold the hydromorphone, and consider the use of naloxone, particularly if the clinical situation worsens.

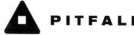

PITFALL •••

PCAs Are Error-Prone

PCA pumps are frequently involved in medication errors, which may result in severe adverse effects. The United States Pharmacopeia (USP) has an alert to practitioners about the high rate of medication errors associated with PCA pump use. The most common errors include: improper dose/quantity (38.9%), unauthorized drug (18.4%), omission error (17.6%), prescribing error (9.2%), and a variety of other types of errors comprising the remainder.[5] Education of prescribers, dispensers, and nursing staff is critical with PCA therapy.

•••

Adding a Continuous Infusion to the PCA in Opioid-Naïve Patients

A continuous infusion of opioid is generally not used in opioid-naïve patients. Most practitioners prefer the patient rely on the bolus dose option to avoid inadvertently overdosing the patient. If you choose to give a continuous infusion, it is especially important not to start it until at least 8 hours after surgery to allow for resolution of the residual effects from anesthesia.[3] If, however, the patient is free of adverse effects, and is consistently using the PCA bolus such that sleeping would be difficult, some practitioners would consider giving a portion of the opioid requirement by continuous infusion. For examples, Strassels recommends averaging the analgesic dose administered during the previous two 8-hour shifts and providing half that amount by continuous infusion; of course the bolus option would remain in place in addition to that.[3]

Other practitioners take exception to the concept of continuous infusion, because it has been noted that continuous infusion PCA does not necessarily improve pain control, may increase the risk of adverse effects including respiratory depression, and patients may end up receiving more opioid than they otherwise would have.[4] Let's look at an example of incorporating a continuous infusion into PCA.

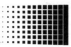 **CASE 7.3**

•••

Adding Continuous Infusion to the PCA in an Opioid-Naïve Patient

CG is a 32 year old woman status-post C-section at 6 a.m. this morning. She had been in hard labor for 14 hours prior to the surgical intervention, and she has been quite vocal about the pain and suffering she's been through. CG has been on a PCA pump since surgery, receiving morphine 1 mg every 8 minutes, and ringing the call button ceaselessly, crying "I can't stand the pain, and I'm exhausted. How am I going to get any rest when I have to keep hitting this button! Can't you DO something?" The nurse taking care of CG threatens to hurt you if you don't address this situation. So you decide to start a continuous infusion during the night so CG can get a little rest (not to mention the nurse!).

Over the first 8 hours she used 30 mg IV morphine, over the second 8 hours she used 22 mg IV morphine. You could average these, or just go with the amount used during the second 8-hour shift. The amount used in the second 8 hours is probably more reflective of steady-state blood levels of the opioid, and her pain may already be lessening. Twenty-two milligrams of IV morphine over 8 hours is 2.75 mg/hour; half of this is 1.375 mg/hour. You could round up to 1.5 mg/hour of IV morphine as a continuous infusion, and leave the 1 mg every 8 hour order on top of that. Don't forget to leave explicit instructions for exemplary nursing care and close observation of CG during the night so she will not experience a serious adverse drug reaction (especially respiratory depression) secondary to adding the continuous infusion. So much for the nurse getting some well-deserved R & R!

Switching from Parenteral to Oral Opioid Therapy

As acute pain begins to subside, the pain stabilizes and the patient is able to tolerate oral medications, it is appropriate to consider calculating an oral opioid regimen to transition from the PCA pump (with or without the continuous infusion). Since most acute pain patients receiving IV PCA therapy do not receive a continuous infusion, let's look at a more typical case.

 CASE 7.4
. . . .
Switching from Parenteral to Oral Opioid Therapy

FO is a 71 year old man who had a below the knee amputation several days ago. He has been on an IV PCA morphine pump since surgery. His current regimen is 2 mg every 8 minutes. Over the past 24 hours he has used on average one or two boluses per hour (a total of 32 boluses, or 64 mg, in 24 hours). His physician anticipates FO will continue to experience moderate pain after discharge, so he would like to transition FO to oral long-acting oxycodone. What would be an equivalent dose to what FO has received via IV PCA over the past 24 hours?

FO has received 32 boluses of 2 mg morphine over the past 24 hours, for a total daily dose of 64 mg IV morphine. Let's set up an equation to convert this to oral oxycodone.

$$\frac{\text{"X" mg TDD oral oxycodone}}{\text{64 mg TDD parenteral morphine}} = \frac{\text{20 mg equianalgesic factor of oral oxycodone}}{\text{10 mg equianalgesic factor of parenteral morphine}}$$

$(10) \times (X) = (64) \times (20)$

$10X = 1280$

$X = 128$ mg oral oxycodone

Because we are switching from one opioid to another, let's reduce this by 25–50% (because of incomplete cross-tolerance), which would be 64–96 mg total daily dose oral oxycodone. OxyContin is available as a 30 mg tablet; therefore an appropriate around-the-clock order would be OxyContin 30 mg po q12h. Next you need to determine what dose of immediate-release oxycodone to order for breakthrough pain. On one hand, FO tells us a 2 mg dose of IV morphine did a very fine job relieving his pain. Two mg of IV morphine is equivalent to 4 mg of oral oxycodone (which rounds up well to 5 mg). On the other hand, ten to fifteen percent of our total daily dose of scheduled oxycodone (TDD is 80 mg) is 6–9 mg (which rounds nicely to 5 or 10 mg). Therefore, you could initially recommend OxyIR 5 mg po q2h prn breakthrough pain, and increase to 10 mg if needed. You can leave the IV PCA bolus option in place for several hours after beginning oral opioid therapy (OxyContin peaks at about 3 hours), but should encourage FO to use the OxyIR for breakthrough pain instead.[6]

Patient-Controlled Analgesia in Patients with Advanced Illness

Patient-controlled analgesia can be used very successfully by opioid-naïve and -tolerant patients with advanced illness. We frequently turn to parenteral opioid therapy for patients with rapidly escalating pain, for patients who can't swallow or who don't have a feeding tube, when transdermal fentanyl is not an option, or when the patient has a bowel obstruction. The same or similar PCA pumps are used for patients with advanced illness whether they are at home, in a facility, or in the hospital. The prescriber will still have to determine the PCA bolus dose, possibly a clinician loading dose, a continuous infusion if appropriate, and sometimes an hourly (or 4 hourly) limit. The 1-hour limit, if set, is usually 3–5 times the estimated required hourly dose, although frequently this is omitted in palliative care due to the need for frequent dosage adjustments based on patient status (which may be rapidly changing). Just as with acute or post-operative pain, PCA therapy in this setting may be used to deliver morphine, hydromorphone, or fentanyl. Parenteral methadone is now also being used more often for patients with advanced illness (see Chapter 6). Intravenous and subcutaneous PCA remain the primary routes of PCA therapy, although it can also may be used for epidural, intrathecal or intracerebral ventricular administration.[7]

A word about subcutaneous opioid infusions—morphine, hydromorphone, and fentanyl are commonly given by this route. Methadone has also been given, but may cause skin irritation (see Chapter 6). As discussed in earlier chapters, we consider SQ and IV doses to be equivalent (1 mg IV = 1 mg SQ). The big issue with a subcutaneous infusion is the volume limitation—it is generally recommended that we not exceed 3 mL/hour because the subcutaneous tissue cannot absorb much more volume than that. Some practitioners actually prefer to limit SQ volume to less than 2 mL/hour; to exceed 3 mL/hour imperils your site of administration. When patients have high opioid requirements that result in larger volumes of drug that need to be administered, you might want to consider switching from morphine to hydromorphone because it is more potent and results in a smaller infusion volume. When administering PCA by the SQ route, it is recommended that the 25- or 27-gauge butterfly SQ needle be placed on the upper arm, shoulder, abdomen or thigh. The American Academy of Hospice and Palliative Medicine (AAHPM) recommends avoiding needle placement in the chest wall to prevent iatrogenic pneumothorax during needle insertion.[8] Generally speaking a SQ site will last about a week unless a high volume is infused, or local skin irritation, itching, site bleeding or infection occurs.

PCA Infusions in Opioid-Naïve Patients with Advanced Illness

When beginning PCA therapy in an opioid-naïve patient with advanced illness, you can choose to either begin solely with demand dosing, or start a low dose opioid infusion. It is probably preferable to start with demand dosing (and clinician loading dose if needed), using dosages shown in Table 7-1. For very frail or elderly patients, consider halving these doses. For example, you might want to start morphine PCA demand dosing in an older frail patient at 0.5 mg every 8 minutes (and possibly a clinician loading dose of 1 mg every 10 minutes, as discussed previously). One technique that has been published for determining the appropriate dose for your continuous infusion is to calculate the amount of opioid that was needed over the first 4 hours to achieve patient comfort.[7] For example, if the patient received 9.2 mg over the first 4 hours, you can calculate an infusion rate of 9.2/4 = 2.3 mg/hour, and therefore start your continuous infusion at 2 mg/hour. Because the patient is not yet at steady-state, this may be an over-estimation of what the patient continuously, therefore you may chose to reduce this to 1 or 1.5 mg/hour, and use a demand PCA dose to titrate to effect.

Another strategy for dose-finding a PCA infusion for an opioid-naïve patient with advanced illness is to use clinician bolus doses until the pain achieves pain relief. One recommended dosing guideline is IV morphine 0.03 mg/kg (or the equivalent dose of a different opioid), administered every 10 minutes until pain is reduced by 50% and the patient achieves satisfactory pain relief. At that point the maintenance opioid infusion dose can be approximated based on our knowledge of the opioid elimination half-life (2–4 hours for morphine or hydromorphone). Every 2 hours, up to half of the administered dose is eliminated and must be replaced to maintain steady state blood levels, therefore the hourly maintenance dose would be approximately equal to ¼ the loading dose. For example, if a patient received three clinician bolus doses of 2 mg over a 30-minute period, and achieved a 50% reduction in pain, ¼ of 6 mg could be ordered as the hourly maintenance dose (1.5 mg). This calculation is based on a 2-hour half life for morphine; most literature estimates put the half-life as closer to 4 hours, therefore it might be prudent to reduce the hourly maintenance dose to 1.0 mg morphine.

It is important to note that there is a difference between the role of the PCA demand bolus dose and the continuous infusion in patients with *acute pain* (e.g., post-operative pain) and *chronic pain*. The purpose of the continuous infusion with *acute pain* (if used at all) is to give the patient a "leg up" so they can get a little sleep and not have to activate the PCA bolus button every 8 minutes or so. You do *not* use the continuous infusion in this case to eliminate the need for the PCA bolus. In *chronic pain* patients however, the purpose of the continuous infusion (assuming the patient has persistent pain) is to minimize the need for the PCA bolus dose, but it is still there if the patient needs it. This is the same principle as using an oral long-acting opioid with an oral short-acting opioid for breakthrough pain.

Back to the discussion at hand—an opioid-naïve patient with an advanced illness—we've established a continuous infusion rate that we anticipate will meet the majority of the patient's opioid needs, but of course we also have the PCA bolus dose available. How do we calculate that dose? A good starting point is 50% of the hourly infusion.[7] This dose can of course be increased or decreased based on patient response; one reference suggests the bolus be 50–150% of the hourly infusion rate.[9] As we discussed in Chapter 4, occasionally a patient will experience incident pain that is significantly more painful than we anticipate; in this case you may need a higher dose for the PCA bolus. For IV PCA you can offer the PCA bolus dose every 10–15 minutes; for SQ PCA you may want to consider every 15–30 minutes. These lockout periods should also be tailored to meet patient needs. For example, with stable pain control the "prn" dosing interval could be extended to every 1 or 2 hours.

Titrating the PCA Infusion

An important safety point is when in doubt, be conservative with the continuous infusion, and more liberal with the PCA bolus dose. You can adjust the continuous infusion rate every 20–24 hours (once the patient has achieved steady-state serum concentrations) based on PCA bolus dose use and patient response, and you can adjust the PCA bolus dose amount itself every 30–60 minutes. When adjusting the continuous infusion rate, you would never increase more than 100%.

In an AAHPM Fast Facts, Dr. David Weissman offers the following example of a typical opioid infusion titration order: "Morphine 2–10 mg/hour, titrate to pain relief."[10] What's wrong with this order? First, an order of this type leaves the hard work to the nurse—there is no guidance on how fast to titrate or how the dose should be incrementally increased (1 mg at a time, 2 mg at a time?). Dr. Weissman suggests a better order would be: "Morphine 2 mg/hour and morphine 2 mg every 15 minutes for breakthrough pain (or 2 mg via PCA bolus). Nurse may dose escalate the prn dose to a maximum of 4 mg within 30 minutes for poorly controlled pain." I would suggest that we can even tighten this up a bit more by giving parameters for the bolus dose increase, such as "…nurse may dose escalate the prn dose to a maximum of 4 mg within 30 minutes for pain rated as 6 or higher (0 = no pain, 10 = worst pain imaginable)."

CASE 7.5

PCA Continuous Infusion Dosing

SW is a 60 year old man residing in a long-term care facility admitted to hospice with a diagnosis of end-stage esophageal cancer. He has an order for Darvocet-N-100, 1–2 tablets every 6 hours as needed for pain. He has tried a few in the past, but now refuses to take them because they "didn't do any darn good!" (Well there's a surprise!) The Darvocet has also become a moot point because the patient can't swallow tablets or capsules. He is complaining of significant pain, which he rates as high as a 9 or 10 on average. He has a central line that is still patent. You decide to begin him on a PCA morphine pump, and would like to start with just demand dosing. Your original order is for 0.5 mg every 8 minutes as needed. An hour into therapy he has taken seven doses and his pain is only down to a 7 out of 10. You increase the demand bolus to 1 mg, and order a clinician loading dose of 2 mg. Approximately six hours later he has received two clinician loading doses, and is averaging about 4 doses per hour of the PCA demand dose and he is fairly comfortable (he rates pain as a 4 on a 0–10 scale). After 18 hours, you review his opioid use—you see that he has taken on average three demand PCA doses per hour over the past few hours. You would like to begin him on a morphine infusion—what rate do you write for?

SW is at, or close to steady-state on his morphine PCA therapy. He has been getting about 3 mg/hour of IV morphine to achieve his current level of pain control, therefore you could begin SW on an infusion at 3 mg/hour with a bolus of 1.5 mg every 10 minutes. You would continue to evaluate his pain control hourly for the next few hours (to determine if you need to adjust his PCA continuous infusion or bolus dose).

Converting to PCA Infusions in Opioid-Tolerant Patients

Patients already receiving opioids also frequently need to be converted to parenteral therapy, as discussed above. The only thing different from the entire discussion above is the need to calculate the appropriate starting dose, based on the patient's current opioid regimen. Weinstein and colleagues offer the following step-wise process (which thankfully coincides with everything we've already discussed in this book!) as follows[9]:

Step 1—Determine the patient's current opioid regimen and calculate a conversion to the parenteral opioid you will be using. For example, if the patient is taking extended-release morphine 30 mg po q12h with immediate-release morphine 10 mg po q4h prn (taking 4 doses per day), this is a total of 100 mg oral morphine per day. Converting to parenteral morphine is a 3:1 (oral:parenteral) ratio, therefore 100 mg per day of oral morphine represents 33 mg per day of parenteral morphine. If we use this as the basis for our continuous infusion, we would divide 33 mg/day by 24, to get 1.375 mg/hour of parenteral morphine. Ok, that's a weird, unlikely number, but wait…

Step 2—If the patient's current opioid regimen is effective, go with the dose you calculated in Step 1. If not, and opioid therapy remains the appropriate therapy for the patient, increase the dose by 25–100% (see Chapter 4 on titration). For example, if this patient's pain never got below a 4–5, it would be appropriate to increase by 25–50%, which calculates to be 1.7–2.1 mg/hour. You could choose 1.7 or 2.0 mg/hour as your continuous infusion (or a number in between!).

Step 3—If the continuous infusion you will be starting represents a dosage increase from the patent's previous opioid regimen, you will want to provide a clinician loading dose at the start of the infusion (e.g., twice the hourly infusion rate). This will boost their blood level of the opioid, so they patient won't have to wait several hours to achieve pain relief.

Step 4—Bolus calculation time! We discussed earlier selecting a bolus dose anywhere from 50–150% of the hourly infusion rate. You may have decided to be a bit more conservative with the continuous infusion above (e.g., 1.7 mg/hour), therefore you might want to be a bit more aggressive with the bolus (e.g., 2 mg).

Step 5—Select a dosing interval for the PCA bolus dose. As you can see from Table 7-2, the onset of IV opioids range from 1–4 minutes, with a peak effect of 15 to 20 minutes. Table 7-1 recommends a lockout of 5–10 minutes, but that is for opioid-naïve adults. We are discussing converting an opioid-tolerant patient to a PCA infusion, therefore a bolus every 30 minutes is likely sufficient.

Step 6—Assess, assess, assess your patient. Assess for therapeutic effectiveness and potential adverse events every 10–15 minutes until the patient is stable. As discussed above, you can adjust your PCA bolus dose every 30–60 minutes.

Step 7—And you thought you were done assessing—you silly goose! You need to reassess the need to alter the continuous infusion rate every 6–8 hours, using the number of PCA bolus doses and patient response as a guide to increase or potentially decrease the continuous infusion. However, it is important not to increase the continuous infusion rate more than 100% at any one time. When you increase the continuous infusion, you should give a clinician loading dose to more rapidly achieve steady-state blood levels of the opioid.

Of course everything discussed above should be customized for your patient, with consideration given to their functional status, organ function, and response to therapy.

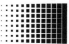

CASE 7.6

● ●

Converting from Multiple Opioids to PCA Therapy

HY is a 34 year old woman with end-stage breast cancer, with widespread metastases including the bones and brain. She is admitted to hospice on the following medications: Transdermal fentanyl 50 mcg/h, MS Contin 60 mg po q12h, and hydromorphone 2 mg po q2h (taking about 4 times per day). She is also taking dexamethasone 8 mg po q12h. Despite this regimen, she rates her pain as 8 to 10 constantly, and off the chart with movement. HY is 5'3" and weighs 120 pounds. You decide to convert her to IV PCA morphine (she has a PICC line in place). How do you convert HY to IV PCA morphine? First things first—this is a complicated conversion, and is best done in a monitored environment. Just so you know, HY is just starting Day 2 of her current 50 mcg/h TDF patch, and her last MS Contin dose was about 6 hours ago. To keep me out of jail, we'll be doing HY's conversion in our inpatient palliative care unit!

Step 1—Determine the patient's current opioid regimen and calculate a conversion to IV morphine. Let's do this one opioid at a time:

1. Transdermal fentanyl 50 mcg/h ~ 100 mg oral morphine total daily dose ~ 33 mg IV morphine total daily dose (using guideline 1 mcg/h TDF ~ 2 mg po morphine)
2. MS Contin 60 mg po q12h = 120 mg oral morphine total daily dose ~ 40 mg IV morphine total daily dose (used equivalency of 1:3; 1 mg parenteral morphine ~ 3 mg oral morphine)
3. Hydromorphone 2 mg × 4 doses = 8 mg oral hydromorphone (HM) total daily dose. This one is a bit harder to do in our head—let's set up a ratio:

$$\frac{\text{"X" mg TDD parenteral morphine}}{8 \text{ mg TDD oral HM}} = \frac{10 \text{ mg equianalgesic factor of parenteral morphine}}{7.5 \text{ mg equianalgesic factor of oral HM}}$$

(7.5) × (X) = (10) × (8)
7.5X = 80
X = 10.7 mg TDD parenteral morphine

Now we need to combine all the parenteral morphine amounts we've calculated:

33 mg IV morphine TDD (from transdermal fentanyl)
40 mg IV morphine TDD (from MS Contin)
10.7 mg IV morphine TDD (from hydromorphone)

Add these all together and we get 83.7 mg IV morphine as her equianalgesic total daily dose. Wow, that's a lotta morphine! I sure hope she's on a bowel protocol such as senna plus docusate!

Step 2—What do we do with the number we've just calculated? We generally don't apply the 25–50% reduction rule with conversions involving transdermal fentanyl (see Chapter 5), and the MS Contin does not require dosage reduction (going from morphine to morphine), but maybe we should consider a slight reduction for the hydromorphone. On the other hand, she's complaining of pain that she rates from 8 to "off the chart." Therefore, let's take our number and run with it or even increase a bit. When we divide 83.7 by 24 (hours) we get 3.5 mg/hour. Because the patient is experiencing severe pain, let's increase by 25%, which calculates out to 4.4 mg/hour of morphine. It would be reasonable to start her IV morphine at 4 mg/hour as the continuous infusion.

Step 3—If we're increasing her opioid, we need to give her a clinician loading dose. Previously when we discussed this seven step process published by Weinstein and colleagues[9] we discussed giving a clinician loading dose of twice the hourly infusion rate. But, remember, we're just taking the transdermal fentanyl patch off now and we have that depot effect to worry about. But recall, the patch only represents about a third of our calculated IV morphine dose, and, the patient is in a lot of pain *now*. I think I need a Tylenol, how about you? Think like a Boy Scout—safety first. I vote we give her a 4 mg IV morphine bolus now, take off the transdermal fentanyl patch, begin the infusion at 2 mg/hour for the first six hours, and then kick it up to the calculated 4 mg/hour rate. We will also make a PCA bolus option available to her (see Step 4).

Step 4—Speaking of the bolus calculation—the bolus is anywhere from 50–150% of the hourly infusion rate. Let's be conservative and go with a 2-mg bolus.

Step 5—Now we get to pick a dosing interval for the PCA bolus. Because we're giving it IV, and because she's in pain, let's go with every 15 minutes.

Step 6—Now we're going to assess HY like nobody's business. We have given the 4 mg IV morphine clinician loading dose, we removed the transdermal fentanyl patch, we've started the continuous infusion at 2 mg/hour (for the first 6 hours), and HY has the PCA bolus option of 2 mg every 15 minutes. One hour later HY is still telling you her pain is a 10 out of 10. Be bold men—let's repeat the clinician bolus of 4 mg, and increase her bolus dose to 4 mg every 10 minutes. We will continue to evaluate the effectiveness of the bolus dose, and adjust every 30–60 minutes.

Step 7—It has now been 18 hours since HY was admitted to the palliative care unit and she was switched to IV PCA morphine. Her continuous infusion was increased from 2 to 4 mg/hour about 12 hours ago; over the past 12 hours she has received 2 clinician boluses at 4 mg, 5 PCA bolus doses at 2 mg, and 20 PCA bolus doses at 4 mg. However, over the past 2 hours she has only used two PCA bolus doses and she tells you she is comfortable. You could increase the continuous infusion at this time, but with the wearing off of the transdermal fentanyl and the MS Contin, and her apparently stability over the past 2 hours, I would probably hold the course at 4 mg/hour continuous IV infusion with 4 mg every 30 minutes for breakthrough pain. You should plan on re-evaluating both the continuous infusion and PCA bolus dose in about 2–4 hours, and every shift thereafter. Importantly, you should only change one parameter at a time: the PCA demand dose, the PCA demand dose lockout interval, or the continuous infusion dose.

Converting from a PCA Infusion to Oral or Transdermal Opioid Therapy

There are many occasions where we need to convert a patient from a continuous infusion PCA to oral or transdermal therapy. We simply use the reverse process we used in converting from oral to the PCA infusion. There are of course some timing considerations (e.g., when to start the oral long-acting or transdermal fentanyl relative to discontinuing the infusion), and the calculation of breakthrough doses.

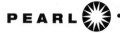

PEARL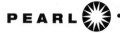

Switching from PCA to Oral Long-Acting Opioid Therapy

When converting to an oral long-acting opioid from a PCA or continuous infusion, you must consider the lead time necessary for the new opioid to achieve adequate serum levels before stopping the parenteral infusion. For example, in Chapter 5 we discussed one protocol when switching to a transdermal fentanyl patch from parenteral fentanyl. In that protocol, six hours after application of the TDF patch, the continuous infusion was reduced 50%, then discontinued 12 hours after TDF patch application. When switching to an oral long-acting opioid, it would be appropriate to administer the first dose 3–6 hours before discontinuing the parenteral opioid infusion.

PEARL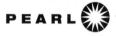

Incident Pain is Not Incidental!

We talked in Chapter 4 about not including opioid rescue doses that were administered for incident *pain when doing conversion calculations. This is because* incident *pain, particularly those under the patient's control, varies significantly depending on the frequency of the precipitating events.*

PEARL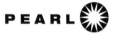

Timing is Everything when Switching Off PCA Therapy

When converting a patient from PCA therapy (continuous plus demand) it is important not to convert the patient until pain is controlled. For example, it is important to achieve the correct continuous infusion rate, such that the patient requires only occasional PCA demand doses, otherwise we end up chasing the person's pain and having to start over.

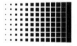 **CASE 7.7**

Converting from Parenteral PCA Therapy to Oral or Transdermal Opioid Therapy

NA is a 62 year old woman with cancer who had been admitted to the hospital for pain which is out of control. She now has good pain control and would like to go home. She is taking naproxen 500 mg po q12h, gabapentin 300 mg po q8h, and SQ PCA morphine running at 1.5 mg/hour, plus a 2-mg bolus she takes before her physical therapy. You have been asked to convert her to a long-acting opioid regimen.

First we calculate her total daily dose of opioid—she's getting 1.5 mg/hour × 24 hours = 36 mg SQ morphine total daily dose. Multiplying by three gives us the total daily oral morphine dose, or 108 mg. For long-acting morphine our choices are Avinza 100 mg po qd, Kadian 50 mg po q12h, MS Contin 45 mg po q12h, or OraMorph 30 mg po q8h.

Whichever you choose the tablet or capsule should be administered about 3 hours prior to discontinuing the PCA infusion. You could give the tablet or capsule 3 hours before discontinuing the PCA infusion, but keep the PCA bolus dose in place for an additional period of time to assure the patient doesn't experience additional pain. Of course, you would also have available (preferable even to the PCA bolus dose) a dose of oral rescue morphine, such as MSIR 15 mg po q2h prn.

If you were going to switch NA to a transdermal fentanyl patch, 108 mg per day of oral morphine is approximately equivalent to a 50 mcg/h TDF patch. You would apply the patch; 6 hours later reduce the continuous infusion to 0.7 mg/hour, and then discontinue the continuous infusion 12 hours after patch application. You can still have the immediate-release morphine 15 mg po q2h prn available from the time of patch application.

So why didn't we include the 2 mg PCA bolus the patient takes before therapy when we calculated our total daily dose of morphine? Because physical therapy is *volitional incident* pain! If she doesn't participate in therapy, there is no need to include that dose. If she does participate in therapy, she can use the immediate-release morphine 15 mg 30–60 minutes before her scheduled appointment time.

Neuraxial Opioid Therapy

Neuraxial, or intraspinal, opioid therapy refers to administering opioids into the spaces or potential spaces surrounding the spinal cord. This generally refers to epidural and intrathecal (sometimes referred to as "spinal") opioid administration. The spinal cord is protected by the bony vertebral column and three connective tissue layers known as the meninges. The meninges are known as the dura mater (the outermost layer closest to the skin), the arachnoid mater (the middle of the three layers), and the pia mater (the membrane closest to the spinal cord and brain).

The epidural space (also known as the extra dural space) is outside the dura mater, and contains blood vessels, nerve roots, fat and connective tissue. There is a potential cavity between the dura and the arachnoid mater, referred to as the subdural space. The space between the arachnoic mater and the pia mater is the subarachnoid space, or the intrathecal or spinal space. The subarachnoid space contains the cerebrospinal fluid (CSF) that bathes the spinal cord. Therefore, we can provide opioid therapy either by the intraspinal route (inserting a needle into the subarachnoid space) or by the epidural route (injecting the opioid or threading a catheter into the space outside the dura mater—see Figure 7-1). Medications can be administered into the epidural or intrathecal space as an injection or infusion, or by patient-controlled analgesia.

When medications are administered intraspinally, it is important to use only preservative-free solutions. Also, it is critical to recognize the extreme potency of medications administered by these routes. You can appreciate the difference in dosing depending on the opioid, and the site of administration (see Table 7-3).

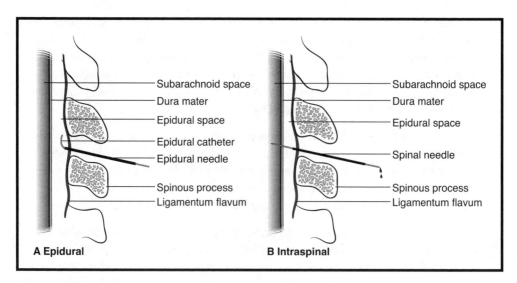

Figure 7-1 (A and B). Neuraxial opioid administration sites. (A) Epidural. (B) Intraspinal.

Table 7-3

Intraspinal Analgesic Dosing Guidelines for Acute Pain in Adults[1]

Drug	Single Dose (mg)[2]	Infusion Rate (mg/h)[3]	Onset (minutes)	Duration of Single Dose (hours)
Epidural				
Morphine	1.0–6.0	0.10–1.0	30	6–24
Fentanyl	0.025–0.100	0.025–0.100	5	4–8
Clonidine[4]	–	0.30	–	–
Hydromorphone	0.8–1.5	0.15–0.3	5–8	4–6
Intrathecal				
Morphine	0.1–0.3	[5]	1.5	8–34
Fentanyl	0.005–0.025	[5]	5	3–6

[1]Infusions injected into the epidural and intrathecal space must be preservative free.

[2]Doses must be adjusted for age, injection site, and patient's medical condition and degree of tolerance to opioids by a clinician experienced in using intraspinal drugs.

[3]If a local anesthetic is used in conjunction with an infusion, 0.06% bupivacaine is recommended.

[4]Recently approved by FDA for severe pain in cancer patients in combination with opioids. Available as a preservative-free preparation (100 mcg/mL) in 10-mL vials.

[5]Continuous subarachnoid infusions are not recommended in acute pain management as the risk of accumulation of drug in the CSF is excessive. For chronic cancer pain, infusion of very small doses may be practical.

Source: Reprinted with permission from the American Pain Society, *Principles of Analgesic Use in the Treatment of Acute Pain and Cancer Pain.* 6th ed. 2008.

Converting Between Routes of Administration (Including Intraspinal) with the Same Opioid

Now we come to the tricky part—the discussions about conversion calculations that involve neuraxial opioid therapy (this won't take long!). A couple fairly common examples which would necessitate conversion from epidural to IV opioid, include a case where the epidural catheter is accidently pulled out or the patient is not achieving satisfactory pain relief, and epidural catheter placement is questioned. In these cases, it would be appropriate to switch from the epidural to IV opioid, and possibly on to the oral opioid. There is very little data that provides guidance on switching between routes of administration (including epidural and intrathecal) for any one opioid. One commonly referenced guide is the following[11]:

- 300 mg oral morphine, equals
- 100 mg parenteral morphine, equals
- 10 mg epidural morphine, equals
- 1 mg intrathecal morphine

Even though this conversion is seen *everywhere* in the neuraxial literature, it is not evidence-based (it was based on modeling), and in personal discussion with anesthesiologists, a recurring theme is "don't believe everything you read." One anesthesiologist comments that it's probably safe (e.g., conservative, and won't get you in trouble, but won't necessarily be 100% equivalent in terms of effective pain relief) to use this equivalency when going in the direction of oral to intrathecal, but not the other way. As an example, in the late 1980s and early 1990s a survey of experts showed a range of intravenous to epidural conversion ratios ranging from 10:1 to 10:2 to 10:5, but none have been validated in clinical trials or even garnered consensus.[12] DuPen reported that his experience converting from IV morphine to epidural morphine indicated that the ratio was approximately 3:1 (this is an unpublished observation).[12] Unfortunately we don't know if this information is bidirectional, or just applicable when going from IV to epidural. Kalso and colleagues also described the conversion of 10 cancer patients from epidural to subcutaneous morphine.[13] The authors concluded the median epidural:subcutaneous ratio was 1:3, but ranged from 1:1 to 1:10, and recommended individualization of conversion ratios. Many clinicians use a ratio of 1:5 for switching from epidural hydromorphone to IV hydromorphone, and a ratio of 1:3 for switching patients from epidural fentanyl to IV fentanyl.[2]

DuPen further states that he has found 90 mg oral morphine to be approximately equivalent to 1 mg of intrathecal morphine.[12] He further advises that after doing the mathematical conversion, to reduce the oral opioid administered by "no more than 50%," then titrate the dose down by about 1/3 of the dose per week while at the same time increasing the intrathecal dose by 10–15%.[12] How do we deal with all these differences of opinion? At least everyone agrees that we begin at a low dose, titrate slowly, and always have rescue medication available.

Let's look at an epidural to IV conversion and see if we go completely blind.

CASE 7.8

● ●

Uh-oh! The Epidural Catheter Got Pulled Out. What Do I Do Now?

LK is a 62 year old woman who has had severe chronic pain for years. She had an above-the-knee amputation 3 days ago. Her pain was well controlled on an epidural PCA infusion with a continuous infusion of 0.4 mg/hour of morphine with a 0.2 mg PCA bolus every 15 minutes. While in therapy today, LK's epidural catheter was accidently pulled out. LK cannot swallow solid dosage formulations, so you've been called to calculate an appropriate IV PCA prescription.

If we go with the 10 mg IV morphine ~ 1 mg epidural morphine (10:1 ratio), then an appropriate basal infusion rate would be 4 mg IV morphine/hour. If we go with the 3 mg IV morphine ~ 1 mg epidural morphine (3:1 ratio), the basal infusion rate would be 1.2 mg/hour IV morphine. The answer is probably somewhere between 1.2 and 4 mg/h IV morphine. I would err on the conservative side, and go with 1.5 mg/hour, being generous with the IV PCA bolus dose. Using the 10:1 rule, an equivalent IV PCA bolus dose would be 2 mg; using the 3:1 it would be 0.6 mg, therefore our bolus dose range is 0.6–2.0. We could compromise and start LK on IV PCA with the continuous infusion running at 1.5 mg/h, and the IV PCA bolus at 1.5 mg every 10 minutes. This allows us to be conservative, particularly since we don't know the exact conversion. Additionally, it will probably take hours for the epidural morphine to wear off. Meanwhile, we've given the patient a generous IV PCA bolus dose, which we can increase up or down every 30–60 minutes.

Converting Between Neuraxial Opioids

So, how's life treating you WAY out there on the limb? If you thought we were on thin ice calculating conversions to and from an intraspinal route of administration and another route using one opioid, we are completely without ice when we think about converting from one opioid to another by the same intraspinal route. According to the "Polyanalgesic Consensus Conference 2007: Recommendations for the Management of Pain by Intrathecal (Intraspinal) Drug Delivery: Report of an Interdisciplinary Expert Panel" there is no definitive evidence of a true conversion factor for calculating dose changes when switching from one intrathecal opioid to another.[14] Panelists did comment that switching from a more lipophilic drug (sufentanil, fentanyl) to a less lipophilic drug (morphine, hydromorphone) carried a high risk for respiratory depression when using conventional equianalgesic dosing charts. The conclusion was to start a very low dose of the new opioid, titrating slowly while tapering down on the initial opioid.

Do you remember this case way back at the beginning of the book:

WE is a 54 year old man with an end-stage malignancy referred to hospice with an implanted intrathecal pump, which is delivering 1 mg of morphine per day. The hospice nurse calls you and wants to know what would be an appropriate dose of oral morphine to give the patient for breakthrough pain?

Believe it or not, this was the impetus for me to write this book. This was a real case and I had no clue how to answer the question (that sure burst my bubble!). I went home, pulled as much literature as I could find, and basically ended up with the conversion recommendations from that modeling study (1 mg intrathecal morphine = 10 mg epidural morphine = 100 mg IV morphine = 300 mg oral morphine). Based on this, I advised the nurse to request an order for immediate release morphine 40 mg every 2 hours as needed for breakthrough pain—my rationale was that 1 mg intrathecal ~ 300 mg oral morphine, and 20% of that was 60 mg. The nurse asked the physician for an order for immediate release morphine 20 mg with a 20 mg repeat in an hour, every 4 hours as needed for breakthrough pain, and the 20 mg dose was more than enough. Was I wrong? (Never—I think everyone is entitled to my opinion!). This just points out the variability in doing this kind of calculation. Now that I'm older and wiser (and much better looking!), I probably would have gone with the 20 mg dose—safety first!

Well, we've done some wild and crazy conversion calculations in this chapter! We started this book with a discussion of "safety first" and that principle is still extremely important with the calculations we describe in this chapter. Consideration of patient-related variables, and exemplary patient monitoring are the keys to success with difficult opioid conversion

PRACTICE PROBLEMS

P7.1: Determining an Initial PCA Dose

JB is a 62 year old woman status-post total abdominal hysterectomy. She has just been moved to the recovery room and has been started on a morphine PCA pump. You have been asked to write the orders including a clinician loading dose for the recovery room nurse to give at her discretion. What parameters should the recovery room nurse, and surgical floor nurse case manager follow to manage JB's pain?

P7.2: Adjusting PCA Doses

GK is a 68 year old man status-post total hip replacement. He was started on a hydromorphone PCA pump at 0.2 mg every 8 minutes, with a clinician bolus (loading dose) of 0.4 mg as needed. GK was transferred to the floor about 6 hours ago, and the nurse case manager has called you to assess GK. He is complaining of pain that he rates as 10 out of 10. "This stuff doesn't work," he huffs, indicating the hydromorphone PCA pump. "I want the good stuff—I have the best health insurance money can buy!" And here you were holding out on GK giving him the mediocre stuff! When you check historical data on the PCA pump you see that GK has made three bolus attempts over the last 6 hours, and received 2 doses. How will you handle the case of GK and the second-rate hydromorphone PCA order?

P7.3: Calculating a PCA Continuous Infusion Dose

LD is a 42 year old man who has been admitted to the ICU after an automobile accident and emergency abdominal surgery. He was started on a fentanyl PCA pump, 20 mcg every 6 minutes, which was increased to 30 mcg every 6 minutes. Over the past 16 hours he has received a total of thirty 20 mcg doses and eighty 30 mcg doses. His pain is about a 4–5 at this time which he finds to be acceptable. LD insists that he wants to get this medication automatically overnight so he can sleep and not have to push the button. LD's physician asks that you calculate the dose of a continuous infusion that provides 50% of what he has been getting on average, but keep the hourly limit the same as if he were only getting the bolus option. What do you recommend?

P7.4: Converting from IV PCA to Oral Morphine

MJ is a 75 year old woman status-post Whipple procedure 4 days ago. She has been receiving IV PCA morphine for the pain, initially with a continuous infusion (2 mg/hour IV) plus a bolus (1 mg IV q8h morphine). For the past 24 hours she has only been getting the bolus, and she has received 34 doses. What would be an equivalent oral morphine regimen to send her home on?

P7.5: Converting from Oral to SQ PLA Morphine

DT is a 60 year old man with a history of widespread metastatic cancer, with no identified primary site. His pain has been controlled on Avinza 60 mg po once per day with MSIR 10 mg po q2h prn breakthrough pain until recently. Co-analgesics have been added with no success. A decision has been made to admit DT to the inpatient palliative care unit and convert him to a SQ PCA infusion. DT is admitted at 6 p.m.; he took his last dose of Avinza at 8 a.m. that morning. He has been averaging 6 doses per day of the MSIR, and he has taken 3 doses since 8 am this morning. DT rates his pain as a 6 on average, but it can increase to 8 or more without provocation. What prescription will you write for DT's SQ PCA morphine?

P7.6: Converting from IV PCA Hydromorphone to Oral Oxycodone

GJ is a 62 year old man who has a history of pancreatic cancer. He was admitted for a Whipple procedure, and his current oral opioid regimen was converted to a parenteral PCA regimen for ease of administering post-operative analgesia. It is now several days post-op and GJ's pain is stable and he would like to go home. He is receiving hydromorphone 0.5 mg/hour by IV PCA, with a PCA bolus dose of 0.3 mg, which he uses about 4 times in a 12-hour period. He would like to resume taking OxyContin and OxyIR. What dosage regimen do you recommend and how do you make this conversion?

REFERENCES

1. *Principles of Analgesic Use in the Treatment of Acute Pain and Cancer Pain.* 5th ed. Glenview, IL: American Pain Society; 2003.

2. McCaffery M, Pasero C. *Pain Clinical Manual.* 2nd ed. Baltimore, MD: Mosby; 1999.

3. Strassels SA, McNicol E, Ruleman R. Post-operative pain management: A practice review, part 1. *Am J Health-Syst Pharm.* 2005;62:1904–1916.

4. Hagle ME, Lehr VT, Brubakken K et al. Respiratory depression in adult patients with intravenous patient-controlled analgesia. *Orthop Nurs.* 2004;23:18–27.

5. U.S. Pharmacopeia. http://www.usp.org/hqi/practitionerPrograms/newsletters/qualityReview/qr812004-09-01a.html Accessed August 13, 2008.

6. OxyContin Prescribing Information. http://www.purduepharma.com/PI/Prescription/Oxycontin.pdf Accessed August 13, 2008.

7. Prommer E. "Fast Fact and Concept #92. Patient Controlled Analgesia in Palliative Care." 2nd ed. November 2007. End-of-Life/Palliative Education Resource Center, www.eperc.mcw.edu.

8. Weissman DE. "Subcutaneous opioid infusions Fast Fact and Concept #28." 2nd ed. July 2005. End-of-Life Palliative Education Resource Center, www.eperc.mcw.edu.

9. Weinstein R, Arnold R, Weissman DE. "Fast Facts and Concepts #54." September 2006. End-of-Life Physician Education Resource Center, www.eperc.mcw.edu.

10. Weissman DE. "Fast Facts and Concepts #72: Opioid infusion titration orders." 2nd ed, July 2006. End-of-Life Physician Education Resource Center, www.eperc.mcw. edu.

11. Krames ES. Intraspinal opioid therapy for chronic nonmalignant pain: current practice and clinical guidelines. *J Pain Symptom Manage*. 1996;11:333–352.

12. DuPen SP, DuPen AR. Neuraxial analgesia by intrathecal drug delivery for chronic noncancer pain. Medscape. http://www. medscape.com/viewprogram/2872_pnt, Accessed August 18, 2008.

13. Kalso E, Heiskanen T, Rantio M, et al. Epidural and subcutaneous morphine in the management of cancer pain: a double-blind cross-over study. *Pain*. 1996;67:443–449.

14. Deer T, Krames ES, Hassenbusch SJ, et al. Polyanalgesic consensus conference 2007: recommendations for the management of pain by intrathecal (intraspinal) drug delivery: report of an interdisciplinary expert panel. *Neuromodulation*. 2007;10:300–327.

SOLUTIONS TO PRACTICE PROBLEMS

P7.1: A reasonable order would be a 1.0 mg morphine PCA bolus dose every 8 minutes, and a loading dose (clinician bolus) of 2.5 mg as needed every 10 minutes, up to 5 doses, until the patient experiences a 50% reduction in pain. The recovery room and floor nursing staff should monitor JB's pain rating and her ability to perform activities such as moving about in bed, transferring, ambulating, going to the bathroom, and providing personal care. For toxicity, the nursing staff should monitor JB's respiratory rate, pupil size, level of arousal (difficulty arousing patient), snoring, excessive sleepiness, bowel habits (constipation), itching, nausea and vomiting.

P7.2: Clearly GK missed a memo! He isn't hitting the PCA bolus button enough. As discussed in Table 7-2, if the patient has received more than one injection to 3 attempts and has no pain relief, the patient should be re-instructed on the idea and use of the PCA pump. GK should be given a clinician loading dose bolus now (0.4 mg) and taught to hit the PCA button *before* the pain gets ahead of him, and frequently to keep the pain at bay. And reassure GK—hydromorphone is *quality* stuff!

P7.3: Over the past 16 hours, LD has received 30 × 20 mcg (600 mcg) plus 80 × 30 mcg (2400 mcg) of fentanyl for a total of 3000 mcg. This averages 187.5 mcg/hour. Half of this would be 93.8 mcg/hour. Therefore you recommend a continuous infusion of 90 mcg/hour, keep the bolus of 30 mcg every 6 minutes, but with an hourly limit of 300 mcg (which would be if he took all ten boluses of 30 mcg during an hour).

P7.4: MJ received 34 doses × 1 mg/dose of IV morphine over the past 24 hours, for a total daily dose of IV morphine of 34 mg. Since the oral:parenteral morphine ratio is 3:1, this is equivalent to 102 mg of oral morphine per day. Since we're converting from morphine to morphine we do not have to reduce for lack of cross-tolerance, however her pain is improving each day. You could start MJ on short-acting oral morphine 15 mg po q4h (total daily dose of 90 mg), or extended-release morphine 45 mg po q12h with MSIR 10 mg po q2h prn. You can overlap either regimen with the IV PCA morphine since she is just receiving demand boluses.

P7.5:

Step 1—The first step in calculating DT's SQ PCA morphine is to determine the patient's total daily opioid regimen. He is taking Avinza (once daily oral morphine) 60 mg plus six doses per day of MSIR (10 mg each), for another 60 mg, or 120 mg total daily dose oral morphine. One hundred twenty milligrams of oral morphine per day is equivalent to 40 mg parenteral morphine per day.

Step 2—Next we have to decide whether to increase, decrease, or go with this number. DT's pain is not well controlled, and we don't have to worry about reducing for lack of complete cross tolerance. If we go with the 40 mg parenteral morphine per day, this works out to 1.6 mg/hour. A 25% increase would be just over 2 mg/hour, therefore that seems to be a reasonable starting dose for the continuous infusion. Because DT is about half way through the dosing interval from the Avinza dose he took this morning, we will begin with 50% of the infusion rate for now (1 mg/hour) and increase it in 6 hours to 2 mg/hour.

Step 3—Do we want to give DT a clinician dose? Since he's in pain right now, it would be reasonable to give him a dose of twice the anticipated infusion rate, or 4 mg.

Step 4—We calculate the bolus dose (50–150% of the hourly rate), therefore we will go with 2 mg (since he's in pain and we're not sure how much he's going to need).

Step 5—Dosing interval for the bolus dose; let's go with every 20 minutes since its being administered subcutaneously.

Step 6—Assess the efficacy of the PCA bolus dose; if the patient is consistently demanding a bolus dose, increase this by 50–100%.

Step 7—Do the same process with the continuous infusion rate.

P7.6: First let's calculate GJ's total daily dose of IV hydromorphone. He's getting 0.5 mg/hour, which is 12 mg/day, plus 2.4 mg from his bolus doses. This gives us a total daily dose of 14.4 mg parenteral hydromorphone. Let's set up a conversion between parenteral hydromorphone (HM) and oral oxycodone:

$$\frac{\text{"X" mg TDD oral oxycodone}}{\text{14.4 mg parenteral HM}} = \frac{\text{20 mg equianalgesic factor of oral oxycodone}}{\text{1.5 mg equianalgesic factor of parenteral HM}}$$

$(20) \times (14.4) = (1.5) \times (X)$
$288 = 1.5X$
$X = 192$ mg oral oxycodone total daily dose

Because we are switching from one opioid to another and the patient's pain is well controlled, we will need to reduce this amount by 25–50%, to 96–144 mg of oral oxycodone per day. Because GJ was still using 8 doses a day of her rescue opioid, let's err on the side of being a bit more aggressive with her standing opioid dose, and recommend OxyContin 60 mg po q12h with OxyIR 20 mg po q2h prn breakthrough pain. We can give the first dose of OxyContin about 3 hours before discontinuing the PCA opioid infusion.

CHAPTER 8

Calculating Doses from Oral Solutions and Suspensions

OBJECTIVES

After reading this chapter and completing all practice problems, the participant will be able to:

1. Define what is meant by a medication solution or suspension.

2. Explain why these dosage formulations are used in caring for patients with advanced illnesses, and how they should be administered.

3. Calculate the appropriate volume of a medication solution or suspension to administer a specific prescribed dose.

4. Verify the calculated volume of an oral solution or suspension intended to deliver a specific prescribed dose.

INTRODUCTION

Medications are available in a wide range of dosage formulations, suitable for various routes of administration (e.g., oral, rectal, parenteral, topical). Oral dosage forms may be solid (tablets or capsules), semi-solid (troches, lozenges) or liquid (solutions, suspensions or emulsions). This chapter is not about opioid *conversion* calculations specifically; rather it is to learn how to calculate an appropriate volume of an oral solution or suspension to give a specific prescribed dose. This may seem like a simple calculation, but done incorrectly, the results could be disastrous.

A **solution** is a homogeneous mixture (uniform in composition throughout) prepared by mixing two or more substances. The **solute** (the substance being added for dissolution, usually present in the smaller amount) may be a solid, liquid or gas. The **solvent** (volume to which the solute is added) is a liquid, hence the reference to "**oral solution**." Since one substance is completely dissolved in another, there is generally no need to shake the oral solution prior to administration, as there is with a **suspension**. A suspension is a mixture in which solid particles are suspended in a fluid; the particles are prone to settle on standing therefore the mixture must be shaken prior to administration.

Oral solutions are used to treat patients with advanced illnesses for several reasons, including:

■ The dose of medication may be individualized to a greater degree than that allowed by dividing tablets or taking multiple tablets or capsules. This is especially important in managing small dose increments in upward or downward titration.

- The administration of certain medications at higher dosages would not be feasible due to pill burden (e.g., taking 18 tablets at a time)

- Most commonly, patients with advanced illnesses are often unable to swallow solid oral dosage formulations, or may have a feeding tube in place. Also, some patients of all ages have an aversion or inability to swallowing pills or capsules

- Opioids may be administered as a concentrated oral solution in the sublingual or buccal cavity when the oral route is not available (e.g., bowel obstruction, difficulty swallowing, nausea or vomiting, reduced level of consciousness), or when parenteral or rectal routes of opioid administration are not desired or feasible.

Oral solutions may be administered by mouth to be swallowed or administered via a feeding tube. They may be administered by the **sublingual** (under the tongue) route or into the **buccal** cavity (cheek of the mouth) if the oral solution is sufficiently concentrated. Boehringer Ingelheim Roxane Laboratories makes a line of "**intensol**" drug products: these are highly, or "intensely," concentrated oral solutions of medication. Examples include alprazolam 1 mg/mL, dexamethasone 1 mg/mL, diazepam 5 mg/ mL, lorazepam 2 mg/mL, methadone 10 mg/ mL, and prednisone 5 mg/mL. Other pharmaceutical manufacturers offer morphine and oxycodone as a 20 mg/mL oral solution.

Some "oral solutions" are simply referred to as "liquids" while others are called "elixirs," "concentrates," "syrups," or "drops." Elixirs historically referred to oral solutions that contained alcohol, and syrups used to contain sugar. Today the terms do not hold these meanings. "Drops" generally refers to an oral solution in a dropper bottle, and "concentrates" are concentrated solutions as discussed in the preceding paragraph.

Principles

So, how do you go about calculating the appropriate volume of an oral solution to give a specific prescribed dose? Look at the following equation. On the left is the concentration of the oral solution in milligrams per milliliters. On the right is the desired dose in the numerator, and the "unknown" variable ("X"), the appropriate volume, in the denominator.

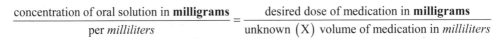

$$\frac{\text{concentration of oral solution in } \textbf{milligrams}}{\text{per } \textit{milliliters}} = \frac{\text{desired dose of medication in } \textbf{milligrams}}{\text{unknown } (\text{X}) \text{ volume of medication in } \textit{milliliters}}$$

Note in the above equation that **milligrams** are in the numerator on both sides of the equation, and *milliliters* are in the denominator on both sides of the equation.

To determine the appropriate volume of medication to administer, cross multiply and solve for the unknown ("X"), as shown in the following example.

Case Examples

CASE 8.1
· ·
Calculating the Volume of an Oral Solution

Patient is an 82 year old man with esophageal cancer. He had been receiving morphine extended-release tablets 15 mg po q12h with good pain control. His cancer has progressed and now he struggles to swallow the morphine tablets. His prescriber would like to discontinue the morphine extended-release tablets and instead switch to morphine 5 mg by mouth every 4 hours around the clock using a 10 mg/5 mL morphine oral solution. What volume should you administer?

Set up your ratio as described above.

$$\frac{10 \text{ mg}}{5 \text{ mL}} = \frac{5 \text{ mg}}{\text{"X" mL}}$$

Cross multiply: 10 mg × X mL = 5 mg × 5 mL

Solve for X by dividing both sides of the equation by 10 mg and canceling units that appear in both the numerator and denominator, as follows:

$$\frac{10 \text{ mg} \times X}{10 \text{ mg}} = \frac{5 \text{ mg} \times 5 \text{ mL}}{10 \text{ mg}}$$

$$\frac{\cancel{10 \text{ mg}} \times X}{\cancel{10 \text{ mg}}} = \frac{5 \cancel{\text{ mg}} \times 5 \text{ mL}}{10 \cancel{\text{ mg}}}$$

$$X = \frac{25 \text{ mL}}{10}$$

X = 2.5 mL

You would administer 2.5 mL of the 10 mg/5 mL oral morphine solution to the patient every 4 hours.

How can you check your math? First, **THINK** about it. You are giving 5 mg from a 10 mg/5 mL solution. Five milligrams is one-half of the 10 milligrams in the numerator, so the volume should be ½ the 5 milliliters in the denominator. So, this passes the "it makes sense" test. To be sure however, you know that multiplication is the reverse of division, so multiply the volume you plan to administer by the oral solution concentration, to make sure you end up with the intended dose, as follows:

$$2.5 \text{ mL} \times \frac{10 \text{ mg}}{5 \text{ mL}}$$

Solve by canceling units that appear in both the numerator and denominator as follows:

$$2.5 \; \cancel{mL} \times \frac{10 \; mg}{5 \; \cancel{mL}} = \frac{2.5 \; x \; 10 \; mg}{5} = \frac{25 \; mg}{5} = 5 \; mg$$

This leaves an answer of 5 milligrams, the correct, intended dose.

 FAST FACT ▶ **Accurately Measuring a Dose of an Oral Solution**

What's the best way to accurately measure a dose of a medication in an oral solution? Many people associate a "teaspoonful" with a volume of 5 mL, and a "tablespoonful" with 15 mL. However, the household teaspoon is insufficiently accurate to reliably deliver 5 milliliters, just as a household tablespoon is unreliable for administering 15 milliliters when dosing accuracy is important. Alternate methods include the use of medicine cups, dosing spoons, droppers and *oral* syringes. According to USP standards, an appropriate measuring device should deliver a dose with no more than a ± 10% dosing error. Calibrated droppers and *oral* syringes are the best bet for minimizing dosing errors.

This calculation works the same way when administering a dose of a combination analgesic oral solution. For example, Roxicet is available as an oral solution, containing 5 mg oxycodone plus 325 mg acetaminophen per 5 mL. Generally the calculation is based on the opioid component, not the non-opioid component. Therefore in this case the oxycodone dose is generally the more important component of the calculation. However, it is important to remember that patients with normal renal and hepatic function should not receive in excess of 4 grams of acetaminophen per day (less than 4 grams per day in patients with organ dysfunction or a history of alcoholism). Let's look at an example.

CASE 8.2
Calculating the Volume of a Combination Drug Solution

LS is a 62 year old woman with end-stage breast cancer. She has intermittent fevers, and abdominal pain. She has grown too weak to swallow her Percocet tablets (7.5 mg oxycodone/500 mg acetaminophen per tablet) so her prescriber would like to switch her to the oral solution. Generally LS takes one tablet every 4 hours; knowing that Roxicet is available as a 5 mg oxycodone plus 325 mg acetaminophen per 5 mL solution, what would be an equivalent volume of Roxicet oral solution?

The more important component of LS's analgesic regimen is the oxycodone. If LS is taking 7.5 mg oxycodone every 4 hours, how much of the Roxicet oral solution should be administered?

Set up your ratio as described above, focusing on the opioid component of the solution.

$$\frac{5 \; mg \; oxycodone}{5 \; mL \; Roxicet \; soln} = \frac{7.5 \; mg \; oxycodone}{"X" \; mL \; Roxicet \; soln}$$

Cross multiply: 5 mg × X mL = 7.5 mg × 5 mL

Solve for X by dividing both sides of the equation by 5 mg and canceling units that appear in both the numerator and denominator, as follows:

$$\frac{\cancel{5\ mg} \times X}{\cancel{5\ mg}} = \frac{7.5\ \cancel{mg} \times 5\ mL}{5\ \cancel{mg}}$$

$$X = \frac{37.5\ mL}{5}$$

X = 7.5 mL

You would administer 7.5 mL of the Roxicet solution, which contains 5 mg oxycodone and 325 mg acetaminophen per 5 mL. However you still have two tasks to perform before administering this dose.

First, check your math. Multiply the volume you intend to administer by the oral solution concentration, to make sure you end up with the correct oxycodone dose, as follows:

$$7.5\ mL \times \frac{5\ mg}{5\ mL}$$

Solve by canceling units that appear in both the numerator and denominator as follows:

$$7.5\ \cancel{mL} \times \frac{5\ mg}{5\ \cancel{mL}} = \frac{7.5 \times 5\ mg}{5} = \frac{37.5\ mg}{5} = 7.5\ mg$$

This leaves an answer of 7.5 mg, the correct prescribed dose.

But you're not done! Remember what we said about keeping an eye on the total daily acetaminophen dose. When you administer 7.5 mL of Roxicet solution, six times daily, what is the patient's total daily dose of acetaminophen, and is it less than 4 grams?

Let's check it out, as follows:

$$7.5\ mL \times \frac{325\ mg\ acetaminophen}{5\ mL} =$$

Solve by canceling units that appear in both the numerator and denominator as follows:

$$7.5\ \cancel{mL} \times \frac{325\ mg\ acetaminophen}{5\ \cancel{mL}} = 2437.5\ mg/5 = 487.5\ mg\ acetaminophen\ per\ dose$$

If you're administering 487.5 mg acetaminophen per dose, and the patient receives 6 doses per day, this is a total daily acetaminophen dose of 2,925 mg, which is safely below 4 grams per day. Remember that a lower total daily dose of acetaminophen may be appropriate for some patients.

As discussed earlier in this chapter, practitioners frequently use concentrated oral solutions to administer opioids to patients with advanced illnesses who have difficulty swallowing, or other reasons why swallowing the solution is not the best option by instilling the drug in the buccal or sublingual cavity. Although it was hoped that administering an opioid such as morphine or oxycodone by the sublingual or buccal route of administration would show a faster onset of action (as is seen with other medications such as nitroglycerin) this has not been seen. This is probably because morphine, oxycodone and hydromorphone are more water-soluble, which does not favor true oral transmucosal absorption. Highly lipid-soluble opioids, such as methadone or fentanyl are better absorbed (e.g., oral transmucosal fentanyl citrate lozenges and effervescent tablets are commercially available).

Having said all that, when morphine or oxycodone are administered in the sublingual or buccal cavity, the clinical effect is approximately equal to oral or rectal administration of the same dose. Most practitioners are comfortable administering up to 1 mL in the sublingual or buccal cavity with a few caveats. If the patient has copious oral secretions, the opioid may be washed away in the tide, and have little hope for absorption. Patients with diminished consciousness may be given oral concentrated solutions in the sublingual or buccal cavity, but it would be prudent to prop the patient's upper body up about 30 degrees, and administer no more than 1 mL at a time. Probably only a small portion of the dose is absorbed transmucosally; the majority of the oral solution trickles down the throat and is swallowed. The dose can be repeated when the initially administered volume has dissipated if necessary.

PEARL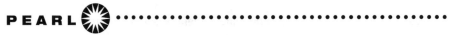

Administering Oral Concentrated Solutions

For patients with an impaired level of consciousness, it is important to prop the upper body up a bit (approximately a 30-degree elevation) to minimize the risk of aspiration before administering up to 1 mL of concentrated oral solution in the buccal cavity. And remember, higher volumes (> 1 mL), and ALL suspensions should be administered ONLY to patients who can swallow, or be administered via feeding tube if the patient has one in place; otherwise a different formulation and route must be chosen.

Calculating the volume of oral concentrated opioid solution to be administered transmucosally is the same process as we've been discussing throughout this chapter. Consider this example:

 CASE 8.3

Calculating the Volume of a Concentrated Oral Solution

GW is a 92 year old man with end-stage dementia. He was receiving oxycodone extended-release tablets, 15 mg every 12 hours, for generalized discomfort. He has become confused and intermittently somnolent, and is not reliably swallowing the oxycodone tablets. His provider wants to switch him to oxycodone oral solution, 5 mg every 4 hours, instilled in the buccal cavity. Using the commercially available oxycodone 20 mg/mL oral solution, what volume should you administer?

Set up your ratio as described earlier in this chapter:

$$\frac{20 \text{ mg}}{1 \text{ mL}} = \frac{5 \text{ mg}}{\text{"X" mL}}$$

Cross multiply: 20 mg × X mL = 5 mg × 1 mL

Solve for X by dividing both sides of the equation by 20 mg and canceling units that appear in both the numerator and denominator, as follows:

$$\frac{20\ mg \times X}{20\ mg} = \frac{5\ mg \times 1\ mL}{20\ mg}$$

X = 5 mL/20

X = 0.25 mL

You would administer 0.25 mL of oral oxycodone 20 mg/mL solution. You can accomplish this with an oral syringe, or a calibrated dropper. Most oral concentrated solutions come with a calibrated dropper, and this would be the preferred medication administration tool.

Check your math: first the "does this MAKE SENSE" approach. You're trying to administer 5 mg from a 20 mg/mL solution. Five milligrams is ¼ of 20 mg, so the appropriate volume should be ¼ of a mL, or 0.25 mL. But don't rely on this method! Do the second step to make SURE you are on firm ground. You really don't want to make a mistake with an oral concentrated opioid solution, so sharpen that pencil my friend!

$$0.25\ mL \times \frac{20\ mg}{1\ mL} = dose$$

Solve by canceling units that appear in both the numerator and denominator as follows:

$$0.25\ mL \times \frac{20\ mg}{1\ mL} = 0.25\ x\ 20\ mg = 5\ mg$$

This leaves an answer of 5 milligrams, the correct prescribed dose. If GW is obtunded, be sure to prop him up a bit, and gently place the 0.25 mL of 20 mg/mg oral oxycodone solution in the buccal cavity. After approximately 30 minutes, check to make sure the volume has dissipated, and you can return GW to a more supine position if desired.

 PITFALL •
"Intensol" is NOT a Drug Name!

Roxane Pharmaceuticals manufacturers several drug products as "Intensols" (see text). However, use of the term "Intensol" may lead to medication errors. One error reported to the USP Medication Error Reporting (MER) Program was an incident where a nursing supervisor didn't realize that the term "Intenol" could refer to several different medications, and the after-hours order for dexamethasone Intensol was inadvertently filled with chlorpromazine Intensol. The term "Intensol" refers to Roxane Pharmaceutical's "system of concentrated solutions of drugs with calibrated dropper." Be sure you have the right DRUG. *Always double check the actual drug name on the medication label.*

Source: http://www.usp.org/hqi/practitionerPrograms/newsletters/practitionerReporting-News/prn912001-08-08.html. Accessed September 3, 2007.

• •

What do you do when you need to give an opioid dose that requires administration of more than 1 mL of oral solution in the buccal or sublingual cavity? You have a couple of options – first, you could administer a smaller volume more often (e.g., 1 mL every 2 hours, in lieu of 2 mL every 4 hours), but this becomes a labor-intensive regimen, frequently unsuitable for family caregivers. Second, you could talk to your friendly neighborhood pharmacist who may be able to compound a more highly concentrated oral solution (e.g., morphine 50 mg/mL). Pharmacists who are able to draw on an evidence base of knowledge and prepare extemporaneous products to facilitate medication administration in patients with advanced illnesses are worth their weight in gold! Of course, this excludes this author (too much like cooking!).

 PITFALL •••
Writing the Right Prescription with Oral Solutions!

Oral solutions and suspensions should be prescribed using mg, not mL. When Elan Pharmaceuticals produced and marketed Roxanol Concentrated Oral Solution (20 mg/mL), the FDA mandated they send a "Dear Healthcare Professional" letter reporting serious adverse events and deaths that resulted from accidental overdose of this highly concentrated oral morphine solution when the order in milligrams (mg) was mistakenly interchanged for milliliters (mL). Elan recommended prescribers write a prescription as follows:

Roxanol 20 mg/mL

Sig: 15 mg (0.75 mL) every 4 hours as needed for pain

Dispense: 30 mL

Source: http://www.accessdata.fda.gov/scripts/cdrh/cfdosc/psn/printer.cfm?id=199. Accessed September 3, 2007.
•••

Frequently we administer co-analgesics in hospice and palliative care that are **suspensions**. A suspension is a liquid formulation of a medication where the drug itself is "suspended" in the liquid phase. Examples include phenytoin suspension and naproxen suspension. Suspensions must be shaken prior to administration to assure the medication is equally distributed in the preparation, and each dose is consistent. The calculations are exactly as you're been doing throughout this chapter. Just for kicks, let's do one more example, shall we?

 CASE 8.4
•••
Calculating the Volume of an Oral Suspension

DS is a 72 year old woman with breast cancer which has spread to the bone. She has become very debilitated, and struggles to swallow her Aleve tablet (220 mg naproxen sodium). Her prescriber would like to switch her to naproxen suspension, which is available in a concentration of 125 mg per 5 mL. The prescribed regimen is 250 mg po every

12 hours. How much volume should you administer?

Set up your ratio as described previously.

$$\frac{125 \text{ mg}}{5 \text{ mL}} = \frac{250 \text{ mg}}{\text{"X" mL}}$$

Cross multiply: 125 mg × X mL = 250 mg × 5 mL

Solve for X by dividing both sides of the equation by 125 mg and canceling units that appear in both the numerator and denominator, as follows:

$$\frac{\cancel{125 \text{ mg}} \times X}{\cancel{125 \text{ mg}}} = \frac{250 \ \cancel{\text{mg}} \times 5 \text{ mL}}{125 \ \cancel{\text{mg}}}$$

$$X = \frac{1250 \text{ mL}}{125} = 10 \text{ mL}$$

You would administer 10 mL of the 125 mg/5 mL naproxen suspension. Obviously the patient would need to be able to SWALLOW this volume; this could NOT be administered in the buccal or sublingual cavity.

Before you tell the patient "bottoms up" let's check that math. First, think it through. If 5 mL of the naproxen suspension gives you 125 mg, then double that volume would give you double the dose, or 250 mg. So, your mental math works out. No offense, but let's put pencil to paper just to make sure you're firing on all burners!

$$10 \text{ mL} \times \frac{125 \text{ mg}}{5 \text{ mL}}$$

Solve by canceling units that appear in both the numerator and denominator as follows:

$$10 \ \cancel{\text{mL}} \times \frac{125 \text{ mg}}{5 \ \cancel{\text{mL}}} = \frac{10 \times 125 \text{ mg}}{5} = \frac{1250 \text{ mg}}{5} = 250 \text{ mg}$$

This leaves 250 mg, the prescribed dose. Go ahead and give DS 10 mL of the naproxen suspension, you'll both feel much better!

 PITFALL •••

Don't Mix Your Metaphors!

In Chapter 6 you learned about methadone dosing, but it important to recognize the benefits and risks associated with using a concentrated solution such as methadone. Methadone is the ONLY opioid that is inherently long-acting (dosed two or three times daily) and available as an oral solution (and even a concentrated oral solution). Palliative care providers frequently use methadone concentrated oral solution (10 mg/mL) for baseline pain control, with morphine or oxycodone 20 mg/mL concentrated oral solution for breakthrough pain. When prescribed in this way these different oral solution concentrations can be confusing for patients and caregivers likely because different volumes of each will be required. Be very clear when providing instruction on how to use these products.

•••

PRACTICE PROBLEMS

• •

Here are a few practice problems for you to work on. The answers are shown in the Appendix. Be sure to check your math!

P8.1. Calculating the Volume of an Oral Solution

BJ is a 30 month old boy with a sprained ankle (you TOLD him not to ride his tricycle DOWN the hill). The pediatrician has recommended acetaminophen 5 mg/kg every 4 hours. BJ weighs 26.4 pounds. The parents have selected an acetaminophen elixir that is 80 mg/5 mL. What volume do you recommend the parents administer per dose?

P8.2. Calculating the Volume of a Concentrated Oral Solution

PZ is a 62 year old man with liver cancer. The hospice nurse would like to switch him to an oral solution because she anticipates he will not be able to swallow tablets for much longer. After consultation with the hospice medical director, they decide to switch from his previous dose of morphine sulfate extended release tablets, 60 mg po q12h, with morphine sulfate immediate release tablets 15 mg (using about 2 per day) to methadone solution, 10 mg/mL. You have calculated a recommended methadone dose of 5 mg po every 8 hours (yes, that was magical—refer to Chapter 6 to see how I came up with that conversion!). What volume of methadone 10 mg/mL solution should the nurse instruct the family to administer?

P8.3. Calculating the Volume of a Co-analgesic Oral Solution

HG is a 54 year old woman with end-stage HIV. She is complaining of very painful burning in her legs and feet, which you determine to be neuropathic pain. You would like to start nortriptyline therapy, starting with 25 mg po at bedtime, then increasing to 50 mg on day 3, and again to 75 mg on Day 6. Unfortunately, HG has significant esophagitis, and she finds it very difficult to swallow tablets. Fortunately, you knew that, and that's why you selected nortriptyline because you know it is available as an oral solution, 10 mg/5 mL. What volume should you administer for the 25 mg dose? The 50 mg dose? The 75 mg dose? You should have this down pat after all that math!

P8.4. Calculating the Volume of an Oral Solution

PA is an 82 year old woman with end-stage dementia, and several large sacral pressure ulcers. She becomes quite agitated with wound care, and you decide it would be a quality idea to pre-medicate her with oral morphine solution. She has a feeding tube in place. The prescriber gives you an order for morphine 2.5 mg 30 minutes before wound care, administered via feeding tube. Your pharmacy carries morphine solution in the 20 mg/5 mL strength. What volume of oral morphine solution should be you administer prior to PA's wound care? By the way, nice pick-up on using a pre-emptive opioid in this situation. PA is much appreciative!

Appendix

Oral Solution and Suspension Non-opioid, Opioids, and Co-Analgesics

Non-Opioid Analgesics

Medication	Dosage Formulations
Acetaminophen (Tylenol, various)	**Liquid:** 160 mg/5 mL, 500 mg/15 mL **Suspension:** 160 mg/5 mL **Elixir:** 160 mg/5 mL **Drops (Concentrate):** 100 mg/mL
Choline Magnesium Trisalicylate (various)	**Oral Solution:** 500 mg of salicylate (contains 293 mg of choline salicylate and 362 mg of magnesium salicylate) per 5 mL
Ibuprofen (Motrin, Advil, various)	**Oral Suspension:** 100 mg/5 mL **Oral Drops:** 40 mg/mL
Indomethacin (various)	**Oral Suspension:** 25 mg/5 mL
Meloxicam (Mobic)	**Oral Suspension:** 7.5 mg/5 mL
Naproxen (Naprosyn, various)	**Oral Suspension:** 125 mg/5 mL

Opioid Analgesics

Medication	Dosage Formulations
Codeine (various)	**Oral Solution:** 15 mg/5 mL
Hydromorphone (various)	**Oral Solution:** 1 mg/mL
Methadone	**Oral Solution:** 5 mg/5 mL, 10 mg/5 mL **Oral Concentrate:** 10 mg/mL
Morphine (MSIR, Roxanol, various)	**Oral Solution:** 10 mg/5 mL, 20 mg/5 mL **Oral Concentrate:** 20 mg/mL, 100 mg/5 mL
Oxycodone (OxyFast, Roxicodone, various)	**Oral Solution:** 5 mg/5 mL **Oral Concentrate:** 20 mg/mL

Combination Opioid Analgesics

Medication	Dosage Formulations
Codeine with Acet-aminophen (Tylenol, various)	**Oral Elixir, Suspension, Solution:** 12 mg codeine plus 120 mg acet-aminophen/5 mL
Hydrocodone with Acetaminophen (Lortab, various)	**Oral Solution:** 2.5 mg hydrocodone plus 108 mg acetaminophen/5 mL **Oral Elixir:** 2.5 mg hydrocodone plus 167 mg acetaminophen/5 mL **Oral Solution:** 3.3 mg hydrocodone plus 108.3 mg acetaminophen/5 mL **Oral Solution:** 10 mg hydrocodone plus 500 mg acetaminophen/5 mL
Oxycodone with Acet-aminophen (Roxicet)	**Oral Solution:** 5 mg oxycodone plus 325 mg acetaminophen/5 mL

Selected Co-Analgesics

Medication	Dosage Formulations
Carbamazepine (Tegretol, various)	**Oral Suspension:** 100 mg/5 mL
Dexamethasone (various)	**Oral Solution:** 0.5 mg/5 mL **Oral Concentrate:** 1 mg/mL
Gabapentin (Neurontin)	**Oral Solution:** 250 mg/5 mL
Levetiracetam (Keppra)	**Oral Solution:** 100 mg/mL
Nortriptyline (various)	**Oral Solution:** 10 mg/5 mL
Phenytoin (various)	**Oral Suspension:** 125 mg/5 mL
Valproic acid (various)	**Oral Syrup:** 250 mg/5 mL

RECOMMENDED READING

American Academy of Pediatrics Committee on Drugs. Alternative routes of drug administration: advantages and disadvantages (subject review). *Pediatrics.* 1997;100:143–152.

Coluzzi PH. Sublingual morphine: efficacy reviewed. *J Pain Sympt Manage.* 1998;16:184–192.

Gilbar PJ. A guide to enteral drug administration in palliative care. *J Pain Sympt Manage.* 1999;17:197–207.

Lugo RA, Kern SE. Clinical pharmacokinetics of morphine. *J Pain Palliat Care Pharmacother.* 2002;16:5–18.

Reisfield GM, Wilson GR. Rational use of sublingual opioids in palliative medicine. *J Palliat Med.* 2007;10:465–475.

SOLUTIONS TO PRACTICE PROBLEMS

P8.1 BJ weighs 26.4 pounds, and you must first convert this to kilograms because the acetaminophen is dosed by weight in kilograms. There are approximately 2.2 pounds per kilogram; or to be precise, there are 2.20462262 pounds per kilogram for you purists out there!

$$26.4 \; \cancel{\text{pounds}} \times \frac{\text{kilogram}}{2.2 \; \cancel{\text{pounds}}} = 12 \text{ kilograms}$$

The dose is 5 mg/kg and he weighs 12 kilograms, so we must next figure out the dose:

$$\frac{5 \text{ mg}}{\cancel{\text{kilogram}}} \times 12 \; \cancel{\text{kilograms}} = 60 \text{ mg}$$

Using the 80 mg/5 solution we must now determine how much volume to advise the parents administer to little Evel Knievel.

$$\frac{80 \text{ mg}}{5 \text{ mL}} = \frac{60 \text{ mg}}{\text{"X" mL}}$$

Cross multiply: 80 mg × X = 60 mg × 5 mL

Solve for X by dividing both sides of the equation by 80 mg and canceling units that appear in both the numerator and denominator, as follows:

$$\frac{80 \; \cancel{\text{mg}} \times X}{80 \; \cancel{\text{mg}}} = \frac{60 \; \cancel{\text{mg}} \times 5 \text{ mL}}{80 \; \cancel{\text{mg}}}$$

$$X = \frac{300 \text{ mL}}{80}$$

X = 3.75 mL

You would instruct the parents to administer 3.75 mL of the 80 mg/5 mL oral acetaminophen solution, or round down to the closest easily administered dose.

Check your work before you turn them loose!
First, does this make sense? If 80 mg are delivered in 5 mL, 60 mg must be less than 5 mL. So, 3.75 mg sounds about right. Now, do the math:

$$3.75 \text{ mL} \times \frac{80 \text{ mg}}{5 \text{ mL}}$$

Solve by canceling units that appear in both the numerator and denominator, and solve for mg dose:

$$3.75 \; \cancel{\text{mL}} \times \frac{80 \text{ mg}}{5 \; \cancel{\text{mL}}} = 60 \text{ mg}$$

This leaves an answer of 60 mg, the correct, intended dose. And be sure to give little BJ a stern talking to about listening to his parents! And don't forget the helmet!

P8.2 You need to determine how much methadone oral solution to give a patient for a 5 mg dose, using the 10 mg/mL solution.

Set up your ratio:

$$\frac{10 \text{ mg}}{\text{mL}} = \frac{5 \text{ mg}}{\text{"X" mL}}$$

Cross multiply: $10 \text{ mg} \times X = 5 \text{ mg} \times 1 \text{ mL}$

Solve for X by dividing both sides of the equation by 10 mg and canceling units that appear in both the numerator and denominator, as follows:

$$\frac{\cancel{10 \text{ mg}} \times X}{\cancel{10 \text{ mg}}} = \frac{5 \cancel{\text{ mg}} \times 1 \text{ mL}}{10 \cancel{\text{ mg}}}$$

X = 5 mL/10
X = 0.5 mL

So, as Dr. Phil would say, "How's that working for ya?" If the methadone is 10 mg per milliliter, and you want to administer 5 mg, it would be HALF that, or 0.5 mL.

Check your math:

$$0.5 \cancel{\text{ mL}} \times \frac{10 \text{ mg}}{\cancel{\text{mL}}} = 5 \text{ mg}$$

This is the correct, intended dose. Don't forget: if PZ is becoming too weak to swallow tablets, keep a sharp eye out for when he has difficulty swallowing oral solutions as well. You can still use the methadone 10 mg/mL oral solution, but you will need to instill it in the buccal cavity, and make sure he is propped up about 30 degrees to minimize aspiration.

P8.3 We need to determine how much of the 10 mg/5 mL nortriptyline oral solution to administer to give a 25-, 50- and 75-mg dose. Let's do the 25-mg dose first:

$$\frac{10 \text{ mg}}{5 \text{ mL}} = \frac{25 \text{ mg}}{\text{"X" mL}}$$

Cross multiply: $10 \text{ mg} \times X = 25 \text{ mg} \times 5 \text{ mL}$

Divide both sides of the equation by 10 mg to solve for X:

$$\frac{\cancel{10\ mg} \times X}{\cancel{10\ mg}} = \frac{25\ \cancel{mg} \times 5\ mL}{10\ \cancel{mg}}$$

X = 125 mL/10
X = 12.5 mL

This makes sense. If every 5 mL gives you 10 mg, and you want two and a half times the 10 mg, you need two and a half times the 5 mL, or 12.5 mL

Checking your math also shows you are CORRECT!

$$12.5\ \cancel{mL} \times \frac{10\ mg}{5\ \cancel{mL}} = 125\ mg\ /\ 5 = 25\ mg$$

If you use this same process, you will find that the 50 mg dose requires 25 mL of the 10 mg/5 mL solution be administered, and the 75 mg dose requires 37.5 mL. Obviously for all THREE of the doses and volumes you calculated, you would have to make sure HG could **swallow** the oral solution; the volume is too high for buccal administration.

P8.4 You want to administer 2.5 mg of morphine prior to wound care for PA using a 20 mg/5 mL oral morphine solution.

$$\frac{20\ mg}{5\ mL} = \frac{2.5\ mg}{"X"\ mL}$$

Cross multiply: 20 mg × X = 2.5 mg × 5 mL
Solve for X:

$$\frac{\cancel{20\ mg} \times X}{\cancel{20\ mg}} = \frac{2.5\ \cancel{mg} \times 5\ mL}{20\ \cancel{mg}}$$

X = 12.5 mL/20 = 0.625 mL

Does this make sense? If 20 mg is in 5 mL, that's 4 mg per mL. We want to give a little more than half of 4 mg (2.5 mg), therefore our volume should be a little more than half of one mL, which it is (0.625 mL). Unfortunately, this is a tough dose to give EXACTLY. You actually might want to talk to the prescriber about reducing the dose to 2 mg, which would be precisely 0.5 mL, and much easier to accurately measure.

Glossary

Basal dose—Opioid administered around the clock; usually refers to a continuous parenteral infusion or regularly scheduled long-acting oral opioid.

Bioavailability—refers to the percentage of drug that is detected in the systemic circulation after its administration. Also defined as the rate and extent to which the active ingredient or active moiety (the active part of the drug molecule) is absorbed from a drug product and becomes available at the site of action.

Breakthrough pain—pain that "breaks through" controlled persistent pain.

Buccal—refers to the located in the cheek of the mouth (either side).

Cytochrome P450 system—an enzyme system involved in the biosynthesis of steroids, fatty acids and bile acids, and the metabolism of endogenous and exogenous substances including toxins and drugs.

Drug formulation—the active medication combined with other pharmaceutical ingredients in a form that is stable, efficacious, appealing, easy to administer and safe. Examples include tablets, capsules, lotions, ointments, transdermal patches, rectal suppositories and injectable formulations, among others.

Drug interaction—one drug alters the pharmacokinetic or pharmacodynamic properties of another drug, potentially changing the pharmacologic effect (therapeutic or toxic).

Drug moiety—the active part of a drug molecule.

Dysphagia—difficulty swallowing.

Dyspnea—shortness of breath or an uncomfortable awareness of breathing.

End-of-dose pain—pain that recurs before the next regularly scheduled dose of an analgesic.

Epidural space—also known as the extra dural space, refers to the area outside the dura mater.

Equianalgesic—two opioid regimens are said to be equianalgesic if they provide the same degree of pain relief.

Equipotent—having equivalent potency.

Excipient—ingredients in a drug formulation aside from the active drug, designed to solubilize, suspend, thicken, dilute, emulsify, stabilize, preserve, color, flavor, and fashion medications into useful drug products.

First pass effect—the metabolism of orally administered drugs by gastrointestinal and hepatic enzymes, resulting in a significant reduction in the amount of unmetabolized drug reaching the systemic circulation.

Immediate-release formulation—an unmodified tablet, capsule or other dosage formulation that begins to dissolve and be absorbed after administration.

Incident pain, nonvolitional—pain that occurs from an identifiable cause that is not under the patient's control.

Incident pain, volitional—pain that occurs from an identifiable cause that is under the patient's control.

Incomplete cross-tolerance—increased sensitivity to the new opioid when switching opioids.

Intensol—a highly, or "intensely" concentrated oral solution of medication.

Lipophilic—fat-soluble.

Neuraxial—refers to administering drugs (such as opioids) into the spaces or potential spaces surrounding the spinal cord; also referred to as intraspinal.

Odynophagia—pain with swallowing.

Opioid-naïve—refers to a patient who has not been regularly taking opioids; the opposite of an opioid-tolerant patient.

Opioid rotation—transitioning a patient from one opioid or route of administration to another opioid and/or route of administration.

Opioid switching—transitioning a patient from one opioid or route of administration to another opioid and/or route of administration.

Opioid substitution—transitioning a patient from one opioid or route of administration to another opioid and/or route of administration.

Opioid responsiveness—the degree of analgesia achieved as the dose is titrated to an endpoint defined either by intolerable side effects or the occurrence of acceptable analgesia.

Parenteral—situated or occurring outside the intestine; usually refers to administration of a drug by intravenous, intramuscular, or subcutaneous injection.

Patient-controlled analgesia—a system that allows self-administration of analgesics (usually parenteral) using a programmable infusion pump.

Persistent pain—continuous pain; pain that is always present, around the clock.

Pharmacodynamics—the pharmacologic effect of a drug, including both therapeutic and toxic effects.

Pharmacokinetics—describes what the body does to a drug: absorption, distribution, metabolism, excretion.

Physiochemistry—the physical and chemical processes of a drug binding to a receptor.

Potency—refers to the intensity of analgesic effect for a given dose, and is dependent on access to the opioid receptor and binding affinity at the receptor site.

Proalgesic effect—a pain-producing effect.

Sleep apnea—periods of breathing cessation during sleep.

Solute—Substance being added for dissolution in a solution; usually present in an amount smaller than the solvent.

Solution—a homogenous mixture (uniform in composition throughout) prepared by mixing two or more substances.

Solvent—volume to which a solute is added; usually a liquid.

Spontaneous pain—pain that requires no precipitating stimulus.

Sublingual—refers to the area under the tongue.

Subarachnoid space—space between the arachnoid mater and the pia mater.

Subdural space—cavity between the dura and the arachnoid mater.

Steady-state—a state of equilibrium where the rate of drug into the body is equal to the rate out of the body, resulting in a "steady" serum concentration of the drug in the blood.

Suspension—a mixture in which solid particles are suspended in a fluid; the particles are prone to settle on standing therefore the mixture must be shaken prior to administration.

Sustained-release formulation—a pharmaceutically modified tablet, capsule or other dosage formulation designed to provide sustained or repeated release of the drug, allowing a longer dosing interval.

Tolerance—a phenomenon where continued exposure to a drug reduces its effectiveness, occasionally necessitating a dosage increase.

Transcutaneous electrical nerve stimulation (TENS)—device that provides electrical stimulation to the skin to relieve pain; thought to act by interfering with neural transmission of pain.

Transdermal—absorption of a drug across the skin, usually intending a systemic effect. Most commonly refers to a drug-impregnated adhesive patch applied to the skin.

Transmucosal—administration of a drug through the mucous membrane.

Appendix: Opioid Formulations

Opioid Formulations

Medication	Dosage Formulations
Codeine	
Codeine sulfate (various)	Oral tablets: 15 mg, 30 mg, 60 mg
Codeine phosphate (Various)	Oral solution: 15 mg/5 mL
Codeine phosphate	Injection: 15 mg/mL, 30 mg/mL
Fentanyl	
Fentanyl (Fentora)	Buccal Tablets: 100 mcg, 200 mcg, 400 mcg, 600 mcg, 800 mcg
Fentanyl (Actiq, various)	Lozenge on a stick: 200 mcg, 400 mcg, 600 mcg, 800 mg, 1200 mccg, 1600 mcg
Fentanyl (Duragesic, various)	Transdermal patch: 12.5 mcg, 25 mcg, 50 mcg, 75 mcg, 100 mcg
Fentanyl (Sublimaze)	Injection: 50 mcg/m
Hydromorphone	
Hydromorphone hydrochloride (Dilaudid, various)	Oral tablets: 2 mg, 4 mg, 8 mg
Hydromorphone hydrochloride (various)	Oral solution: 1 mg/mL
Hydromorphone hydrochloride (Dilaudid, various)	Injection; 1 mg/mL, 2 mg/mL, 4 mg/mL, 10 mg/mL
Hydromorphone hydrochloride (Dilaudid, various)	Rectal suppository: 3 mg
Methadone	
Methadone (Dolophine, Methadose, various)	Oral tablets: 5 mg, 10 mg
Methadone (Methadose, various)	Dispersible tablet: 40 mg (only for use by substance abuse treatment centers)
	Oral solution: 5 mg/5 mL, 10 mg/5 mL
	Oral concentrate : 10 mg/mL
Methadone (various)	Injection : 10 mg/mL
Morphine	
Morphine sulfate (various)	Oral tablet : 15 mg, 30 mg
Morphine sulfate (MS Contin, Oramorph SR, various)	Controlled release tablet: 15 mg, 30 mg, 60 mg, 100 mg, 200 mg

Medication	Dosage Formulations
Morphine sulfate (various)	Extended release tablet: 15 mg, 30 mg, 60 mg, 100 mg, 200 mg
Morphine sulfate (various)	Tablets for solution (injection): 10 mg, 15 mg, 30 mg
Morphine sulfate (Avinza)	Extended-release pellets in capsule: 30 mg, 45 mg, 60 mg, 75 mg, 90 mg, 120 mg
Morphine sulfate (Kadian)	Extended-release pellets in capsule: 10 mg, 20 mg, 30 mg, 50 mg, 60 mg, 80 mg, 100 mg, 200 mg
Morphine sulfate (MSIR, various)	Oral solution: 10 mg/5 mL, 20 mg/5 mL
Morphine sulfate (MSIR, various)	Oral concentrate: 20 mg/mL, 100 mg/5 mL
Morphine sulfate (various)	Injection: 0.5 mg/mL, 1 mg/mL, 2 mg/mL, 4 mg/mL, 5 mg/mL, 8 mg/mL, 10 mg/mL, 15 mg/mL
Morphine sulfate (DepoDur)	Extended-release liposomal injection: 10 mg/mL
Morphine sulfate (Infumorph, various)	Solution for injection: 25 mg/mL, 50 mg/mL
Morphine sulfate in 5% Dextrose (various)	Injection: 1 mg/mL
Morphine sulfate (various)	Rectal suppository: 5 mg, 10 mg, 20 mg, 30 mg
Oxycodone	
Oxycodone hydrochloride (various)	Oral tablet: 5 mg, 10 mg, 15 mg, 20 mg, 30 mg
Oxycodone hydrochloride (OxyContin)	Controlled-release tablet: 10 mg, 15 mg, 20 mg, 30 mg, 40 mg, 60 mg, 80 mg
Oxycodone hydrochloride (OxyIR)	Oral capsule: 5 mg
Oxycodone hydrochloride (various)	Oral solution: 5 mg/5 mL
Oxycodone hydrochloride (OxyFast, Roxicodone Intensol, various)	Concentrate solution: 20 mg/mL
Oxymorphone	
Oxymorphone (Opana)	Oral tablet: 5 mg, 10 mg
Oxymorphone (Opana)	Extended-release tablet: 5 mg, 7.5 mg, 10 mg, 15 mg, 20 mg, 30 mg, 40 mg
Oxymorphone (Opana)	Injection: 1 mg/mL

Selected Opioid Analgesic Combination Products

Medication	Dosage Formulation	
Codeine Phosphate Products		
With acetaminophen (Tylenol w/Codeine, various)	Oral solution	12 mg codeine phosphate and 120 mg acetaminophen
	Oral suspension	
	Oral elixir	

Medication	Dosage Formulation	
With acetaminophen (Tylenol w/Codeine #2, various)	Oral tablet	15 mg codeine phosphate and 300 mg acetaminophen
With acetaminophen (Tylenol w/Codeine #3, various)	Oral tablet	30 mg codeine phosphate and 300 mg acetaminophen
With butalbital, acetaminophen, and caffeine (Fioricet, various)	Oral capsule	30 mg codeine phosphate, 325 mg acetaminophen, 40 mg caffeine and 50 mg butalbital
With acetaminophen (Vopac)	Oral tablet	30 mg codeine phosphate and 650 mg acetaminophen
With aspirin (various)	Oral tablet	15 mg codeine phosphate and 325 mg aspirin
With aspirin (aspirin w/ Codeine #3, various)	Oral tablet	30 mg codeine phosphate and 325 mg aspirin
With butalbital, aspirin, and caffeine (Fiorinal, various)	Oral capsule	30 mg codeine phosphate, 325 mg aspirin, 40 mg caffeine and 50 mg butalbital
With acetaminophen (Tylenol w/ codeine #4, various)	Oral tablet	60 mg codeine phosphate and 300 mg acetaminophen
With aspirin (aspirin w/ codeine #4, various)	Oral tablet	60 mg codeine phosphate and 325 mg aspirin
Hydrocodone Bitartrate Products		
With ibuprofen (Reprexain)	Oral tablet	2.5 mg hydrocodone bitartrate and 200 mg ibuprofen
With ibuprofen (various)	Oral tablet	5 mg hydrocodone bitartrate and 200 mg ibuprofen
With ibuprofen (Vicoprofen, various)	Oral tablet	7.5 mg hydrocodone bitartrate and 200 mg ibuprofen
With ibuprofen (various)	Oral tablet	10 mg hydrocodone bitartrate and 200 mg ibuprofen
With acetaminophen (various)	Oral solution	2.5 mg hydrocodone bitartrate and 108 mg acetaminophen
With acetaminophen (Lortab Elixir, various)	Oral elixir	2.5 mg hydrocodone bitartrate and 167 mg acetaminophen
With acetaminophen (Zamicet Oral Solution)	Oral solution	3.3 mg hydrocodone bitartrate and 108.3 mg acetaminophen
With acetaminophen (Lortab, various)	Oral tablet	2.5 mg hydrocodone bitartrate and 500 mg acetaminophen
With acetaminophen (various)	Oral tablet	5 mg hydrocodone bitartrate and 300 mg acetaminophen

Medication	Dosage Formulation	
With acetaminophen (Norco, various)	Oral tablet	5 mg hydrocodone bitartrate and 325 mg acetaminophen
With acetaminophen (Zydone)	Oral tablet	5 mg hydrocodone bitartrate and 400 mg acetaminophen
With acetaminophen (Lortab 5/500, Vicodin, various)	Oral tablet	5 mg hydrocodone bitartrate and 500 mg acetaminophen
With acetaminophen (Lorcet-HD, various)	Oral capsule	5 mg hydrocodone bitartrate and 500 mg acetaminophen
With acetaminophen (various)	Oral tablet	7.5 mg hydrocodone bitartrate and 300 mg acetaminophen
With acetaminophen (various)	Oral tablet	7.5 mg hydrocodone bitartrate and 325 mg acetaminophen
With acetaminophen (Zydone)	Oral tablet	7.5 mg hydrocodone bitartrate and 400 mg acetaminophen
With acetaminophen (Lortab 7.5/500, various)	Oral tablet	7.5 mg hydrocodone bitartrate and 500 mg acetaminophen
With acetaminophen (Lorcet Plus, various)	Oral tablet Oral caplet	7.5 mg hydrocodone bitartrate and 650 mg acetaminophen
With acetaminophen (Vicodin ES, various)	Oral tablet	7.5 mg hydrocodone bitartrate and 750 mg acetaminophen
With acetaminophen (various)	Oral tablet	10 mg hydrocodone bitartrate and 300 mg acetaminophen
With acetaminophen (Norco, various)	Oral tablet	10 mg hydrocodone bitartrate and 325 mg acetaminophen
With acetaminophen (Zydone)	Oral tablet	10 mg hydrocodone bitartrate and 400 mg acetaminophen
With acetaminophen (Lortab 10/500, various)	Oral tablet Oral solution	10 mg hydrocodone bitartrate and 500 mg acetaminophen
With acetaminophen (Lortab 10/650, various)	Oral tablet	10 mg hydrocodone bitartrate and 650 mg acetaminophen
With acetaminophen (Vicodin HP, various)	Oral tablet	10 mg hydrocodone bitartrate and 660 mg acetaminophen
With acetaminophen (various)	Oral tablet	10 mg hydrocodone bitartrate and 750 mg acetaminophen
With aspirin (Lortab ASA, various)	Oral tablet	5 mg hydrocodone bitartrate and 500 mg aspirin

Oxycodone Hydrochloride Products

With acetaminophen (various)	Oral tablet	2.5 mg oxycodone hydrochloride and 300 mg acetaminophen

Medication	Dosage Formulation	
With acetaminophen (Percocet)	Oral tablet	2.5 mg oxycodone hydrochloride and 325 mg acetaminophen
With acetaminophen (various)	Oral tablet	2.5 mg oxycodone hydrochloride and 400 mg acetaminophen
With acetaminophen (various)	Oral tablet	5 mg oxycodone hydrochloride and 300 mg acetaminophen
With acetaminophen (Percocet, Endocet, Roxicet, various)	Oral tablet Oral solution	5 mg oxycodone hydrochloride and 325 mg acetaminophen
With acetaminophen (various)	Oral tablet	5 mg oxycodone hydrochloride and 400 mg acetaminophen
With acetaminophen (Roxicet 5/500, Tylox, various)	Oral capsule Oral caplets	5 mg oxycodone hydrochloride and 500 mg acetaminophen
With acetaminophen (various)	Oral tablet ·	7.5 mg oxycodone hydrochloride and 300 mg acetaminophen
With acetaminophen (Endocet, Percocet, various)	Oral tablet	7.5 mg oxycodone hydrochloride and 325 mg acetaminophen
With acetaminophen (various)	Oral tablet	7.5 mg oxycodone hydrochloride and 400 mg acetaminophen
With acetaminophen (Endocet, Percocet, various)	Oral tablet	7.5 mg oxycodone hydrochloride and 500 mg acetaminophen
With acetaminophen (various)	Oral tablet	10 mg oxycodone hydrochloride and 300 mg acetaminophen
With acetaminophen (Endocet, Percocet, various)	Oral tablet	10 mg oxycodone hydrochloride and 325 mg acetaminophen
With acetaminophen (various)	Oral tablet	10 mg oxycodone hydrochloride and 400 mg acetaminophen
With acetaminophen (various)	Oral tablet	10 mg oxycodone hydrochloride and 500 mg acetaminophen
With acetaminophen (Endocet, Percocet, various)	Oral tablet	10 mg oxycodone hydrochloride and 650 mg acetaminophen
With ibuprofen (Combunox)	Oral tablet	5 mg oxycodone hydrochloride with 400 mg ibuprofen
With aspirin (Percodan, various)	Oral tablet	4.5 mg oxycodone hydrochloride, 0.38 mg oxycodone terephthalate and 325 mg aspirin

Pharmaceutical formulations are frequently added or withdrawn from the market; please consult a pharmacist for specific product availability.

Index

• • • • • • • • • • A

Acetaminophen, 2, 5, 6, 50, 65, 77, 113
  with codeine, 60, 62
  oral solution, 176, 179
  oral solutions and suspensions, 177
Acetaminophen/codeine, 60, 62
Actiq, 68, 71
Acute pain management, 153
  Opioid-naive patient, 59–60, 77, 80
Adverse effects, 41–42
  development of, 2–3
Advil, 177
Alcohol, 109, 115
Aleve, 174
Allergic reaction, 52
American Academy of Hospice and Palliative Medicine, 152, 154
  converting to/from transdermal fentanyl, 90
American Pain Society, 23–24
Amitriptyline, 111
Amprenavir, 111
Antidepressants, 109
"As needed" orders, 59
Avinza, 5, 19, 28, 35, 44, 61, 62, 74, 158, 164, 165
Ayonrinde method, 121, 122, 127, 141

• • • • • • • • • • B

Basal dose, 14
Baseline pain control, 57, 175
Beclomethasone cream, 87
Benzodiazepines, 109, 115
Bidirectional equivalencies, 9
Bioavailability, 4–5, 19–20, 21, 34, 42
Breakthrough pain, 57, 62–63, 97, 175
  assessing presence of, 65
  characterizing, 64
  determining rescue opioid dosage, 67–69
  fentanyl dosing, 70–71
  methadone-treated patients, 116
  opioid selection, 66
  therapeutic options, 65–66
  types of, 69, 71
Buccal cavity
  administration, 22, 168
  opioids, 172
Buccal fentanyl, 84
Buprenorphine
  equianalgesic doses, 5, 6
  routes of administration, 18

• • • • • • • • • • C

Cachectic patients, transdermal fentanyl and, 97–98
Cannabis, 115

Carbamazepine, 111, 178
Cardiac effects, methadone, 117, 118
Care process, 123
Case study
  acute pain management in opioid-naive patient, 59–60
  adding continuous infusion to PCA in opioid-naive patient, 150–51
  converting from multiple opioids to PCA therapy, 156–57
  dosage escalation, 75
  epidural catheter pulled out, 162
  methadone in opioid naive patient, 113
  opioid dose escalation, 75
  PCA, 148–49
  PCA by proxy, 148
  PCA continuous infusion dosing, 154
  Pre-empting volitional incident pain, 72
  same opioid, different formulation and route of administration, 29–30, 30–32, 33–35
  same opioid and route of administration, different formulation, 24–26, 26–27, 27–28
  switching immediate-release opioid to sustained-release opioid, 60, 62
  switching for multiple opioids to transdermal fentanyl patch, 92–95
  switching from oral acetaminophen/oxycodone to oral extended release morphine, 42–45
  switching for oral long-acting morphine to transdermal fentanyl patch, 91–92
  switching from oral meperidine to oral oxycodone, 49–51
  switching from oral morphine to parenteral hydromorphone, 48–49
  switching from oral opioid to IV fentanyl, 99
  switching from oral oxymorphone to oral oxycodone, 45–48
  switching from oral to IV methadone, 134–36
  switching from parenteral fentanyl to transdermal fentanyl, 101
  switching from parenteral to oral opioid therapy, 151
  switching from transdermal fentanyl to parenteral fentanyl, 100–101
  switching off methadone, 133
  switching off transdermal fentanyl, 96–97
  switching to oral methadone, 120, 128–29
  switching to oral methadone, different methods, 127–28
  switching to oral methadone from multiple opioids, 129
  switching to oral methadone slowly, 131–32
  titrating oral methadone at steady-state, 130
  total daily opioid dose determination, 115–16
  transdermal fentanyl and cachectic patients, 98
  transmucosal fentanyl dosing, 72–73
  volume of combination drug solution, 170–72

volume of concentrated oral solution, 172–73
   volume of oral solution, 169–70
   volume of oral suspension, 174–75
Celebrex, 75
Chlorpromazine Intensol, 173
Choline magnesium trisalicylate, 177
Chronic pain, 153
Ciprofloxacin, 111
Citalopram, 111
Clarithromycin, 111
Cleveland Clinic, 58, 74, 75
Clinical Opiate Withdrawal Scale, 76
Clonidine, intraspinal dosing guidelines, 160
Co-analgesics, 65, 178
Cocaine, 115
Cochrane review, 3–4
Codeine, 52, 60, 177
   with acetaminophen, 178
   equianalgesic doses, 5
   plus nonopioid, 18
   routes of administration, 18
College of Physicians and Surgeons of Ontario, 112, 113
Combination opioid analgesics, oral solutions and suspensions, 178
Continuous infusions, 73
Controlled pain, dose escalation, 74
Conversion calculator, 9
Corticosteroid fluticasone propionate, 87
Cross-tolerance, 94
Cymbalta, 113
Cytochrome P450 3A4 inhibitors, 86

●●●●●●●●●● D

Darvocet-N-100, 154
Demerol, 49
Desipramine, 36, 51, 52, 111
Dexamethasone, 30, 31, 156, 178
   Intensol, 173
Diltiazem, 86
Dolophine hydrochloride, 112, 122
Donner conversion, 89
Dosage
   calculations, 25, 123
   decrease, 75
   individualization, 13–14, 120, 124–26
   reduction, 75–76
Dose equivalencies, 42
Dose escalation strategies
   oral regimens, 73–74
   parenteral opioid, 78, 81
   parenteral regimens, 74–75
Dose reduction, 78, 81
Dosing intervals, double check, 45
Drug dosing, equianalgesic, 5–8
Drug formulation, 21
Duloxetine, 113
Duragesic, 61, 95
   package insert, 86, 87
   patch, 85
Dyspnea, 125

●●●●●●●●●● E

Edmonton Model, 126
Efavirenz, 111
Elan Pharmaceuticals, 174
End-of-dose failure pain, 63, 69
End-of-Life Physician Education Resource Center, 122
Epidural dosing, acute pain in adults, 160
Epidural space, 159
Epinephrine, 52
Equianalgesia, 4, 42
   data, source of, 8
   drug dosing, 5–8
Equianalgesic Opioid Dosing Table, 13
Equipotent, 4
Equivalent dosing
   converting oral morphine to methadone, 120, 121–24
   converting from transdermal fentanyl, 96
   converting to transdermal fentanyl, 87–90
Erythromycin, 86, 111
European Association for Palliative Care, 60
Excipient, 21
Existential pain, 8

●●●●●●●●●● F

Fast Facts and Concepts, 122, 127, 141
Fentanyl, 73, 83–84, 136, 152, 162, 172
   acute severe pain management, 58
   buccal administration, 22
   buccal tablet, 70, 72–73, 77, 80–81
   breakthrough pain, 65–66, 68, 70–71
   conversions, 102–3
   epidural to IV, 161
   equianalgesic doses, 5, 6–7
   intraspinal dosing guidelines, 160
   iontophoretic transdermal system, 84
   IV PCA ranges for opioid-naive adults, 146
   oral transmucosal dosing, 71
   patch, 1, 2, 12, 61
   PCA continuous infusion, 163, 165
   transmucosal administration, 61
   transmucosal, immediate-release properties, 66
Fentora, 68–69, 70, 71, 72–73
First pass effect, 20–21
Fluconazole, 111
Fluoxetine, 111
Fluvoxamine, 111
Food and Drug Administration, 86, 118
Friedman, Loren I., 123
Friedman method, 123–24, 126, 127, 131, 141
Furosemide, 73

●●●●●●●●●● G

Gabapentin, 36, 51, 52, 113, 158, 178
Global patient assessment, 10–11, 120
Grapefruit juice, 86

H

Haloperidol, 29
Healthcare Professional Advisory, transdermal
    fentanyl patch, 86
Hycodan, 5
Hydrochlorothiazide, 137
Hydrocodone bitartrate, 78
Hydrocodone, 119
    equianalgesic doses, 5, 7, 50
Hydrocodone with acetaminophen, 5, 41, 51, 61, 66,
    178
Hydrocodone-homatropine, 5
Hydromorphone, 1, 17, 33, 77, 78, 80, 81, 92, 93, 94,
    108, 116, 119, 136, 142, 152, 156, 162, 172
    acute severe pain management, 58
    breakthrough pain, 65–66
    converting IV PCA to oral oxycodone, 164, 166
    dose escalation, 73
    epidural to IV, 161
    equianalgesic doses, 5, 7, 8, 50
    immediate release, 61, 77
    infusion, 131
    injections, 36
    intraspinal dosing guidelines, 160
    IV PCA ranges for opioid-naive adults, 146
    oral, 34–35, 86
    oral, bioavailability of, 20, 34
    oral, immediate-release properties, 66
    oral solutions and suspensions, 177
    parenteral, 24, 33
    parenteral, switching from oral morphine, 48–49
    PCA, 163, 185
    rectal, 22, 35
    routes of administration, 18
    tablets, 36
Hydromorphone:morphine ratio, 9

I

Ibuprofen, 5, 177
Immediate-release opioid, 60–62
Implanted intrathecal pump, 1
Incident pain, 63, 69, 158
Incomplete cross-tolerance, 13
Indiana University School of Medicine, 111
Indomethacin, 177
Inhaled medications, 12
Injected medications, 12
Insulin, 12, 21
Intensol, 173
Intramuscular administration, 23–24
Intrathecal dosing, acute pain in adults, 160
Intravenous administration, 23
Itraconazole, 111
IV fentanyl, 99
    converting from transdermal fentanyl, 99–101,
      103
    switching to transdermal fentanyl, 103–4, 106
IV morphine, 150

K

Kadian, 5, 19, 28, 44–45, 53, 61, 62, 72, 80, 120, 158
Keppra, 178
Ketoconazole, 86, 111
King, Stephen, 132

L

Levetiracetam, 178
Levorphanol, 61
Lisinopril, 137
Long-acting opioid administration, timing of, 19
Lorazepam, 30, 31
Lortab, 78, 178
Lyrica, 42, 43, 137

M

Medication Error Reporting (MER) program, 173
Medication reconciliation, 11–12
Meloxicam, 177
Meperidine, equianalgesic doses, 5, 50
Mercadente method, 121, 122, 127, 141
Methadone, 12, 73, 107, 172
    absorption, 108
    breakthrough pain, 68, 116
    candidates for therapy, 112
    cardiac safety monitoring, 117
    concentrated oral solution, 175
    converting from other opioids, 119–20
    converting from parenteral to oral, 135
    Disket, 113
    distribution, 108
    drug interactions, 109–11
    elimination, 109
    enzyme inhibitors and inducers effect, 110
    equianalgesic doses, 6, 7
    hydrochloride, 122
    long-acting, 61
    metabolism, 108–9
    monitoring in opioid-naive patients, 114–15
    opioid-naive patients, 112–13
    oral dosage formulations, 113
    oral, immediate-release properties, 66
    oral solutions and suspensions, 177
    oral, terminal half-life of, 130
    oral, titrating at steady-state, 130
    overdose signs, 115
    pharmacodynamics, 108
    public health advisory, 118–19
    rapid conversion, 126
    rapid onset, 61
    routes of administration, 18
    serum concentration, 114
    solution, 176, 180
    switching from oral to IV, 134–36
    titrating, 127
    titrating/converting off, 132–33
    titrating in opioid-naive patients, 116–17
Milligrams, 168
Milliliters, 168

Mobic, 177
Moderate pain, dose escalation, 74
Modified Ramsey scale, 32
Moiety, 19
Morley-Makin United Kingdom model, 123, 124, 126
Morphine, 4, 12, 17, 22, 44, 77, 108, 116, 119, 136, 152, 162, 172
   acute severe pain management, 58
   and applesauce, 28
   around-the-clock, 60
   breakthrough pain, 65–66, 127–28
   capsule, extended-release, 35
   concentrated oral solution, 175
   dose escalation, 73
   equianalgesic doses, 5, 6, 8, 50
   extended release, 30–31, 32, 42, 44, 45, 176
   extended-release tablets to oral solution, 169–70
   immediate release, 30–31, 59, 60, 61, 176
   intraspinal dosing guidelines, 160
   intravenous, 31–32, 59
   IV PCA ranges for opioid-naive adults, 146
   Long-acting, 61
   to methadone conversion, 119–20
   oral, 1, 19, 27–28, 46–47, 61, 62, 86, 93, 94, 133
   oral, bioavailability of, 19–20
   oral, breakthrough pain dosage, 67, 68
   oral, buccal cavity, 35
   oral, conversion to Duragesic, 88–90, 91–92
   oral, immediate release, 66, 77, 80
   oral solutions and suspensions, 177
   oral, switching to parenteral hydromorphone, 48–49
   oral to intrathecal, 161
   oral to rectal, 29–30
   oral to SQ PCA, 164, 166
   oral vs. parenteral, 25
   parenteral, 24
   PCA, 164, 165
   Pre-empting volitional pain, 72
   rectal suppository, 22
   reduction, 78, 81
   role of, 2
   routes of administration, 18
   subcutaneous infusion, 2
   sustained release, 60
   tablets administered rectally, 22, 23
   tablets or capsules, 61
Morphine:hydromorphone ratio, 9
Morphine-6-glucuronide, 20
Motrin, 177
MS Contin, 1, 5, 30, 44, 61, 62, 67, 77, 78, 91, 127, 134, 137, 156, 157, 158
MSIR, 66, 74, 137, 141, 164, 165, 177
Multivitamin with iron, 137

• • • • • • • • • • N

Naloxone, 59, 149
Naprosyn, 177
Naproxen, 28, 48, 59, 158, 177
   sodium, 174
   suspension, 174–75

Narcan, 59
National Comprehensive Cancer Network Clinical Practice Guidelines on Oncology, 58
Nefazodone, 86
Nelfinavir, 111
Neuroaxial opioid therapy, 159
   administration sites, 160
   converting between opioids, 162–63
   converting between routes of administration, 161
   dosing guidelines for acute pain in adults, 160
Neuroleptics, 109
Neurontin, 51, 178
Nevirapine, 111
Nitroglycerin, 172
Nonsteroidal anti-inflammatory drug, 65, 100, 113
Nonvolitional pain, 63, 69
Nortriptyline, 176, 178, 180–81

• • • • • • • • • • O

Objective Opioid Withdrawal Scale, 76
Older adults, transdermal fentanyl and, 97–98
Opana ER, 27, 36, 45, 46, 61
Opana injection, 36
Opana IR, 26–27, 45
Opioid
   conversion calculations, process, 9–15
   reasons for changing, 2–3
   rescue dosage, 67–69
   responsiveness, 4
   rotation, 3
   substitution, 3
   switching, 3, 12–13
   switching, adverse effects, 41–42
   therapy, initiating, 57–59
   titration, 31–32, 57
Oral morphine
   solution, 176, 181
   switching to transdermal fentanyl, 103, 105
Oral rescue doses, 77, 80
Oral solution, 167–68
   accurately measuring dose of, 170
   administering concentrated, 172–73
   prescription writing, 174
   principles, 168
   volume of combination drug solution, 170–72
Oral solution and suspension
   non-opioid analgesics, 177
   opioid analgesics, 177
Oral transmucosal fentanyl citrate lozenge, 68, 77, 80–81
Oramorph, 76, 158
Oramorph SR, 5, 44
Oxycodone, 2, 3, 17, 22, 75, 77, 80, 108, 119, 137, 142, 172
   acute severe pain management, 58
   breakthrough pain, 65–66, 67
   concentrated oral solution, 175
   controlled release, 48
   converting IV PCA hydromorphone to oral, 164, 166
   dose escalation, 73

equianalgesic doses, 6, 7, 8, 50
immediate release, 61, 77
long-acting, 61
oral, 18, 86
oral, bioavailability, 20
oral, immediate-release properties, 66
oral solutions and suspensions, 1, 172–73, 177
oral, switch from oral oxymorphone, 45–48
plus nonopioid, routes of administration, 18
routes of administration, 18
switching to transdermal fentanyl, 103, 105
tablets administered rectally, 22, 23
tablets or capsules, 61
Oxycodone with acetaminophen, 24–26, 36, 41, 42, 59, 61, 66, 75, 77, 80, 137, 170, 171, 178
OxyContin, 6, 36, 61, 74, 75, 76, 92, 93, 94, 103, 105, 128, 129, 151, 164, 166
OxyFast, 6, 177
OxyIR, 76, 151, 164, 166
Oxymorphone, 17, 116
equianalgesic doses, 6, 7, 50
immediate release, 61
long acting, 61
oral, 18
oral, bioavailability, 20
oral, immediate-release properties, 66
oral, switch to oral oxycodone, 45–48
routes of administration, 18
Oxymorphone hydrochloride, 26–27

•••••••••• P

Pain control
and adverse effects, 147–48
rating drop, 58
Pain diary, 60, 62, 130
Pain rhythm, 19
Parenteral administration, 23–24
Parenteral fentanyl, 83
converting from transdermal to IV fentanyl, 99–101, 102
converting from IV to transdermal fentanyl, 101
IV, 98–99
Parenteral methadone, 133
converting from oral, 134
converting to oral methadone, 135
Paroxetine, 111
Patient-controlled analgesia, 134, 135–36, 145–46
adding continuous infusion in opioid-naive patients, 150
advanced illness and, 152
converting from infusion to oral or transdermal therapy, 157, 158–59
converting from multiple opioids, 156–57
converting infusions in opioid-tolerant patients, 154–55
errors with, 150
incident pain, 158
morphine, 154, 158
opioid infusion titration order, 154
opioid-naive patients with advanced illness, 152–53

pain control improvement, adverse effects reduction, 147–48
post-operatively, 146–47
switching from parenteral to oral opioid therapy, 151
switching to oral long-acting opioid therapy, 158
timing, 158
titrating infusion in advanced illness, 153
Patient information, 11
Patient monitoring, 14–15, 58–59, 120, 126
Patient status, change in, 3
Patient-specific variables, 8–9
Penicillin G, 21
Percocet, 2, 6, 24–26, 36, 41, 42–43, 45, 59, 73, 75, 77, 80, 128, 129, 137, 170, 171
Persistent pain, 60, 62
Pharmacodynamic effect, 8, 9
Pharmacokinetics, 4, 9
Phenytoin, 111, 178
Physiochemical properties, 4
Physiochemistry, 4
Plonk, William, 122
Polyanalgesic Consensus Conference 2007, 162
Potency, 4, 42
Potential toxicity monitoring, 1
PQRSTU method, 10–11
Practice problems
acute severe pain in opioid-naive patient, 77, 80
adjusting PCA doses, 163, 165
calculating PCA continuous infusion dose, 163, 165
converting from IV PCA hydromorphone to oral oxycodone, 164, 166
converting from IV PCA to oral morphine, 164, 165
converting from oral to SQ PCA morphine, 164, 166
determining initial PCA dose, 163, 165
opioid dose reduction, 78, 81
oral opioid rescue doses, 77, 80
parenteral opioid dose escalation, 78, 81
same opioid route of administration, different formulation, 35, 36, 37, 38–39
same opioid, different formulation route of administration, 35, 36, 38, 39–40
starting oral methadone in opioid-naive patient, 137, 140
switching from immediate-release to sustained-release oral opioid, 77, 80
switching from IV fentanyl to transdermal fentanyl, 103–4, 106
switching from IV hydromorphone to oral oxycodone, 51–52, 53–54
switching from IV to oral methadone, 138, 142–43
switching from oral acetaminophen/codeine to oral morphine, 52, 55–56
switching from oral long-acting oxycodone to transdermal fentanyl, 103, 105
switching from oral morphine to oral oxymorphone, 52, 54–55
switching from oral morphine to transdermal fentanyl, 103, 105

switching from oral to IV methadone, 138, 142

switching from OTFC lozenges to fentanyl buccal tablets, 77, 80–81

switching from transdermal fentanyl to IV fentanyl, 103, 106

switching from transdermal fentanyl to oral methadone, 137–38, 141–42

switching from transdermal fentanyl to oral morphine, 103, 105

switching oral acetaminophen to oral extended-release morphine, 51, 52–53

switching to oral methadone and interacting drug, 137, 140

volume of co-analgesic oral solution, 176, 180–81

volume of concentrated oral solution, 176, 180

volume of oral solution, 176, 179–80, 181

Pregabalin, 42, 43, 137

Proalgesic effect, 119

Propoxyphene, 60

Psychoactive medications, 109

•••••••••• Q

QTc interval, 131–32

•••••••••• R

Residual drug, 14

Rifabutin, 111, 130

Rifampicin, 111

Rifampin, 111

Ripamonti method, 121, 122, 127, 141

Ritonavir, 111

Route of administration, 17
    buccal or sublingual, 22
    opioid formulations, 18
    oral, 19–21
    parenteral, 23–24
    rectal, 22–23

Roxane Pharmaceuticals, 173

Roxanol, 5, 61, 177

Roxanol Concentrated Oral Solution, 174

Roxicet, 170, 171, 178

Roxicet Oral Solution, 26

Roxicodone, 6, 177

•••••••••• S

Sedation rating, 32

Senna-S tablets, 30

Sertraline, 111, 137, 141

Severe pain, dose escalation, 74

Solubility, 21

Solute, 167

Solution, 167

Solvent, 167

Spironolactone, 111

Spontaneous pain, 63

St. John's Wort, 111

Subcutaneous administration, 23

Subjective Opioid Withdrawal Scale, 76

Sublingual administration, 22, 168

Sublingual opioids, 172

Sufentanil, 162

Suspension, 167, 174

Sustained-release morphine, 99

Sustained-release opioid, 60–62

•••••••••• T

Tegretol, 178

Telithromycin, 111

Temazepam, 30, 31

Therapeutic effectiveness monitoring, 14

Therapeutic response, lack of, 2

Tolerance, 13

Topical products, 12

Total daily dose, 42, 120, 121, 134

Tramadol
    equianalgesic doses, 6, 7
    oral, 18
    routes of administration, 18

Transdermal fentanyl, 72, 83–84, 129, 156, 157, 159
    accidental exposure to, 87
    converting from, 96, 102
    converting to, 87–90, 102
    converting to oral methadone, 137–38, 141–42
    formulations, 85
    important considerations, 86–87
    older adults, cachectic patients, 97–98
    patient monitoring, 95
    pharmacokinetics, 84–86
    switching from multiple opioids to, 92–95
    switching off, 96–97
    switching to IV fentanyl, 103, 106
    switching to oral methadone, 137–38, 141–42
    switching to oral morphine, 103, 105
    switching off, 96–97
    titrating, 95–96, 102

Transmucosal fentanyl citrate lozenges, effervescent tablets, 84, 172

Troleandomycin, 111

Tylenol, 177, 178

Tylenol #3 (with codeine) , 5, 52, 55, 60, 62

•••••••••• U

Unidirectional equivalencies, 9

United States Pharmacopeia, 150, 170

•••••••••• V–Z

VA/DoD methadone guidelines, 117

Valproic acid, 178

Vicodin, 41, 51

Vicodin HP, 52

Volitional pain, 63, 67, 69
    pre-empting, 72

Weissman, David, 73, 154

Zoloft, 137, 141